Primary Health Care

Edited by Ayşe Emel Önal

Published in London, United Kingdom

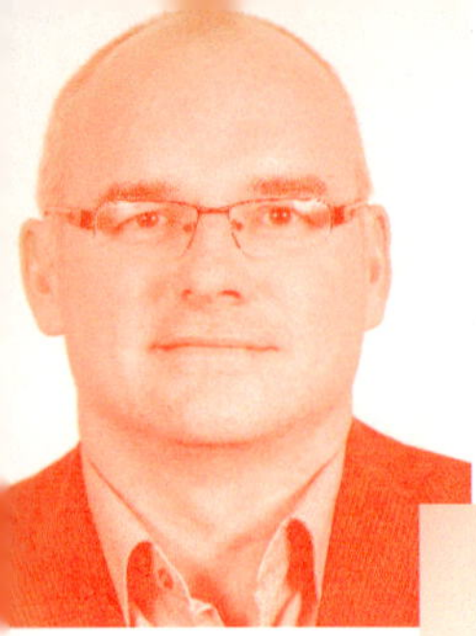
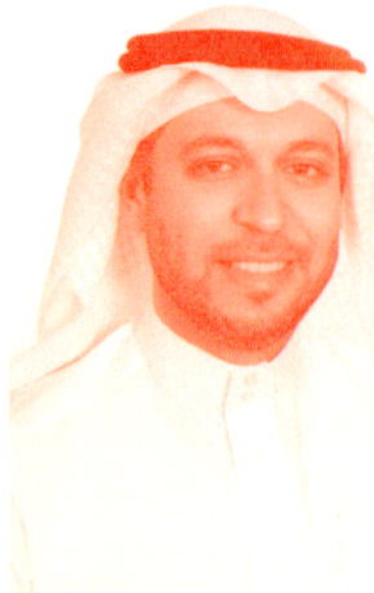
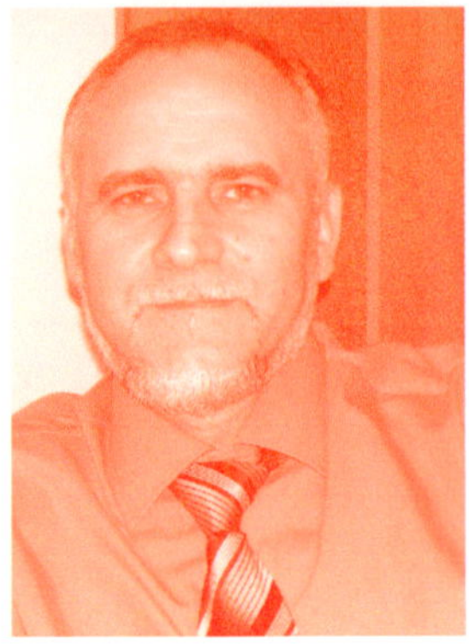
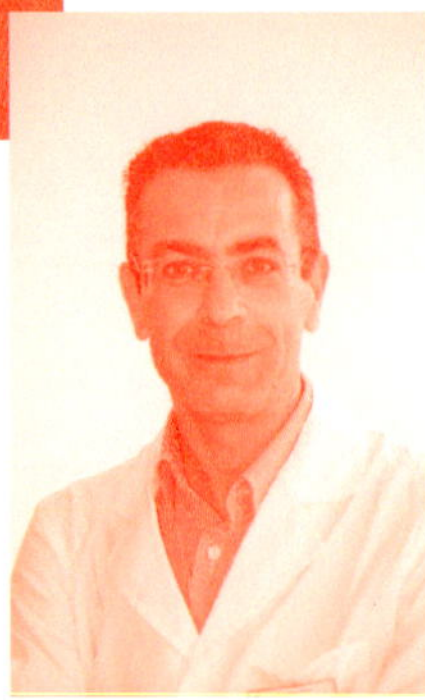
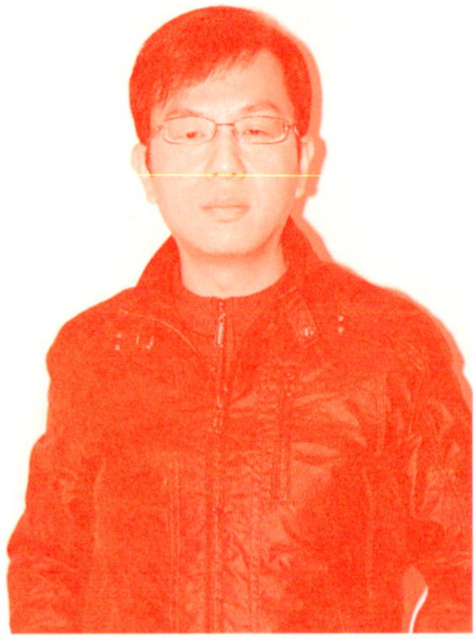
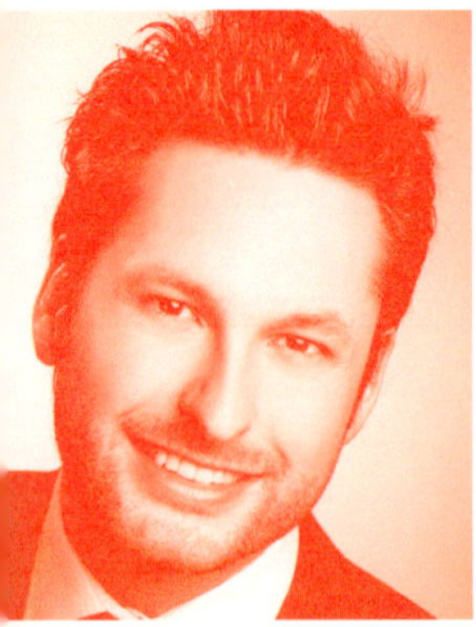
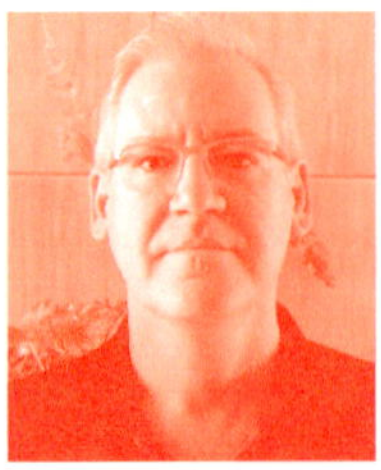

IntechOpen

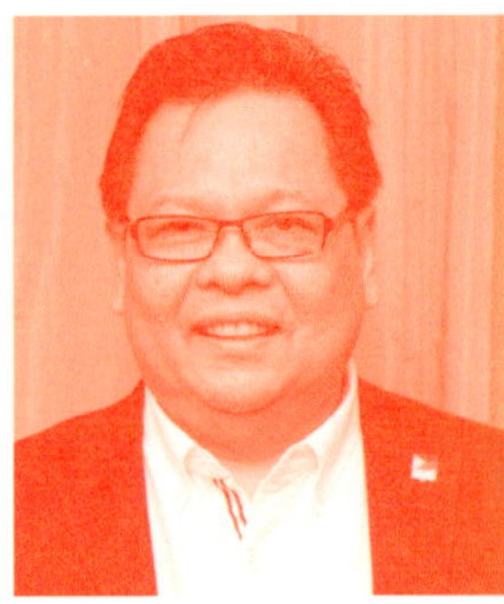
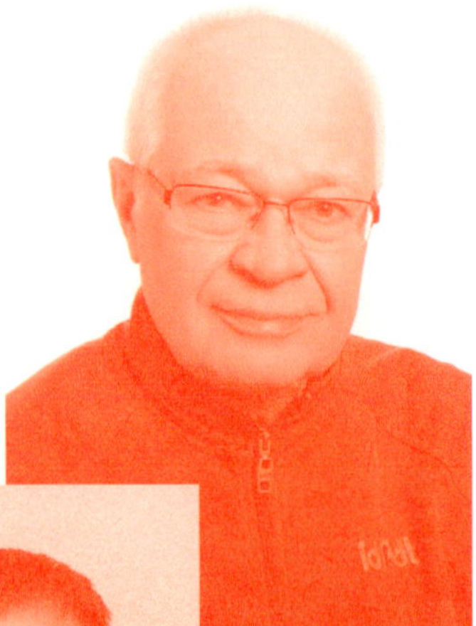
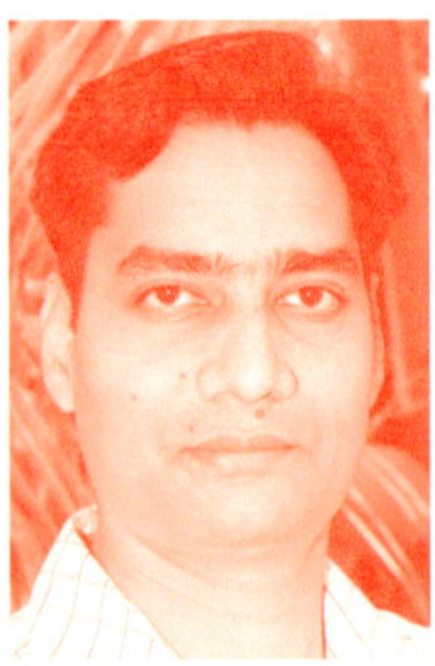
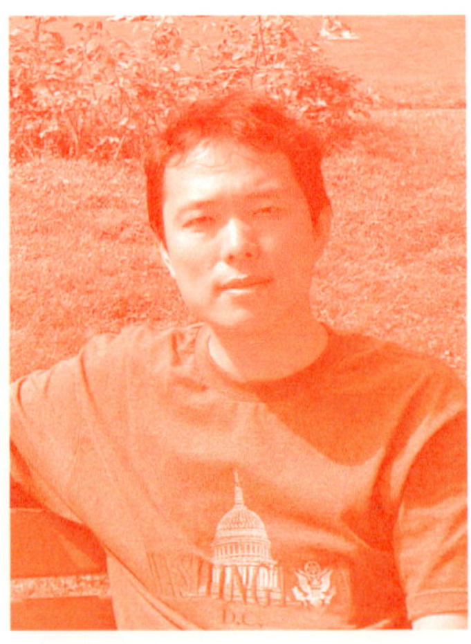
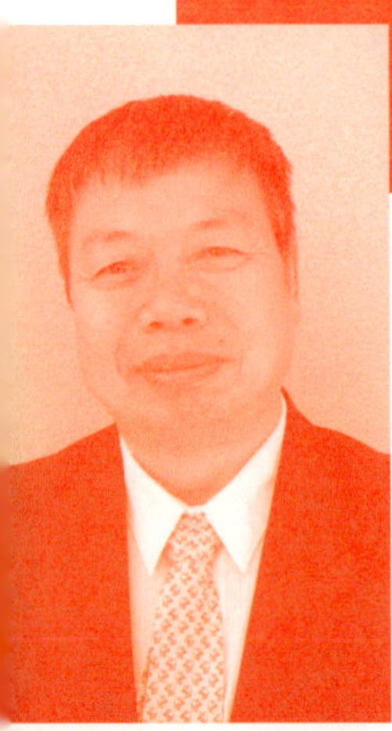
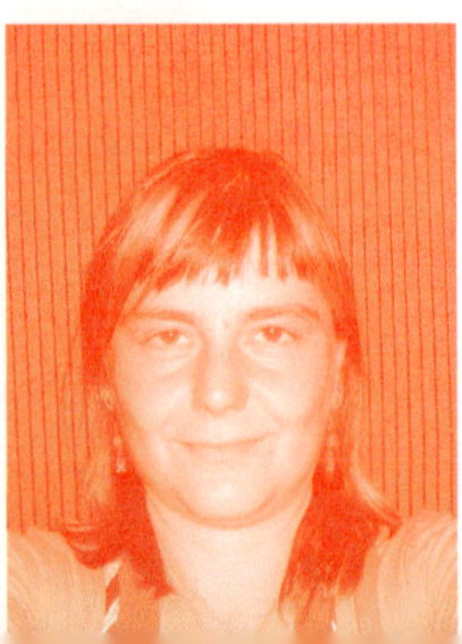

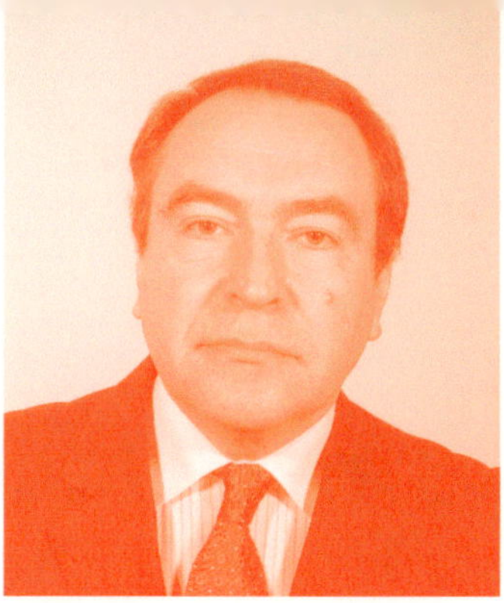

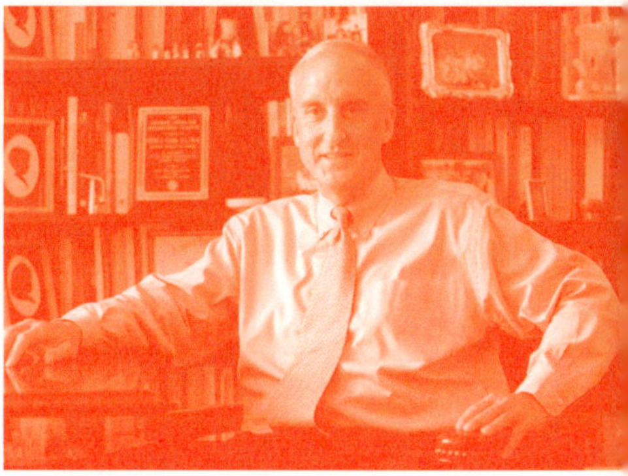

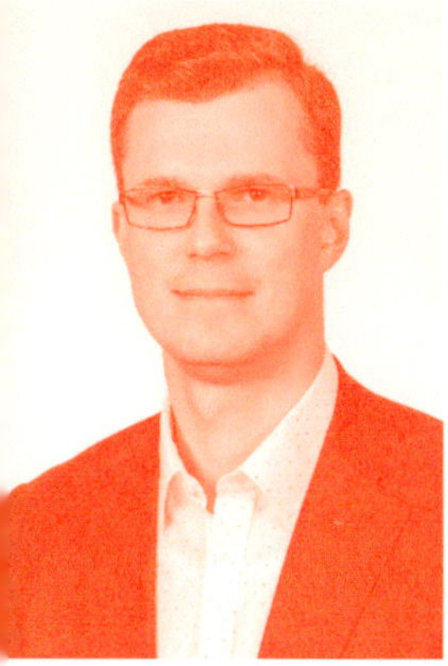

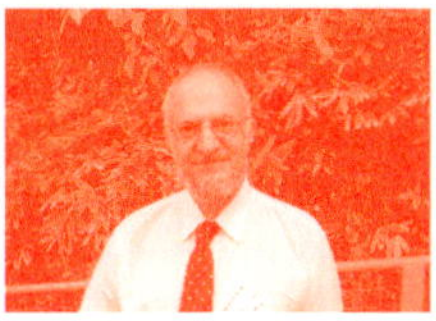

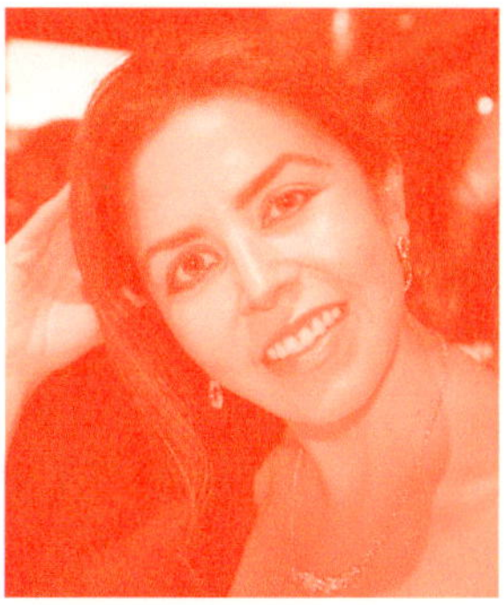

Supporting open minds since 2005

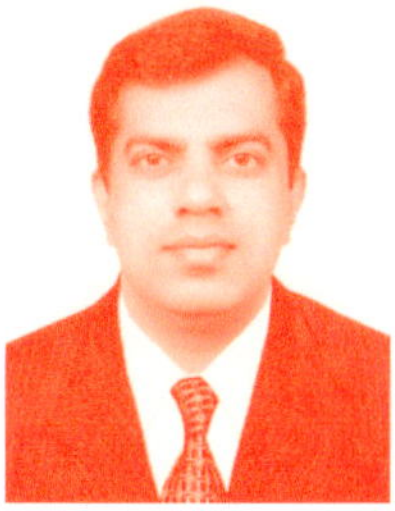

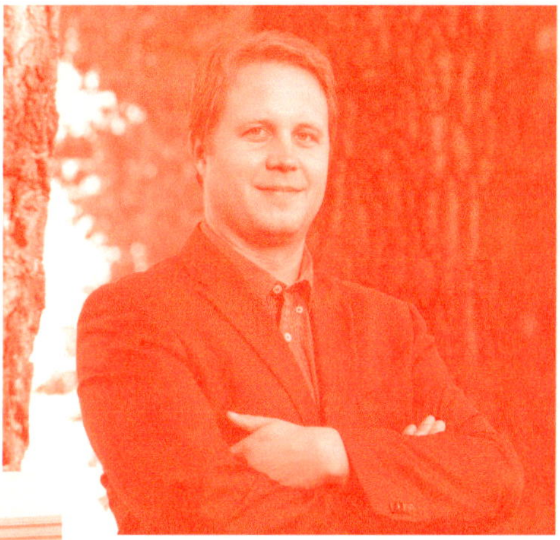

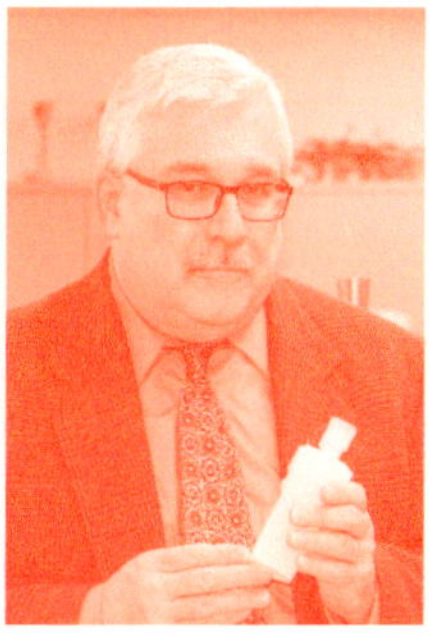

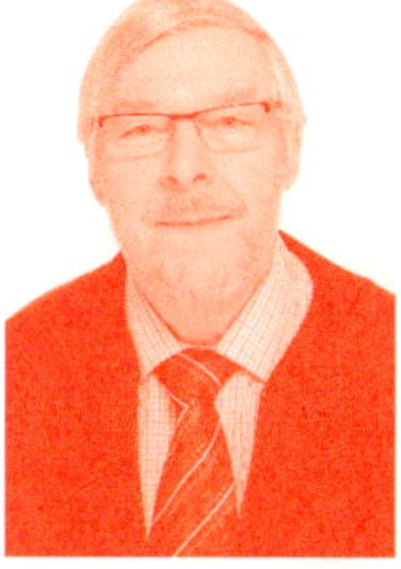

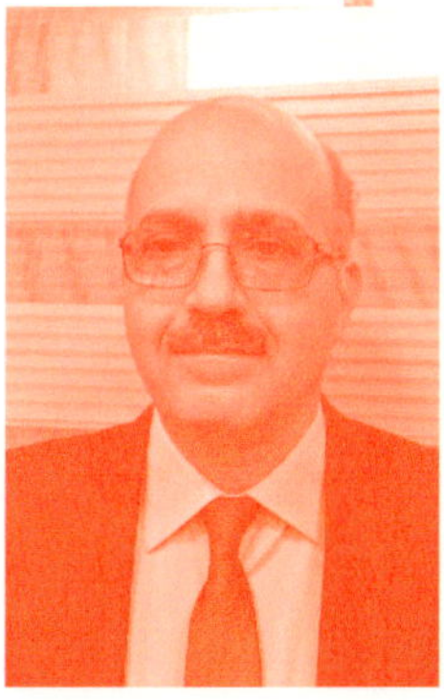

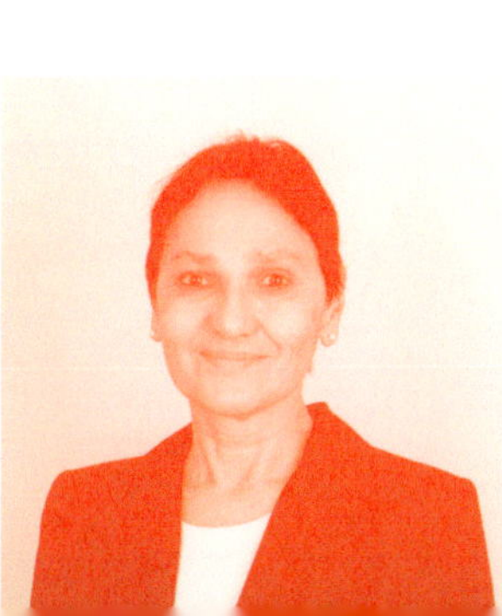

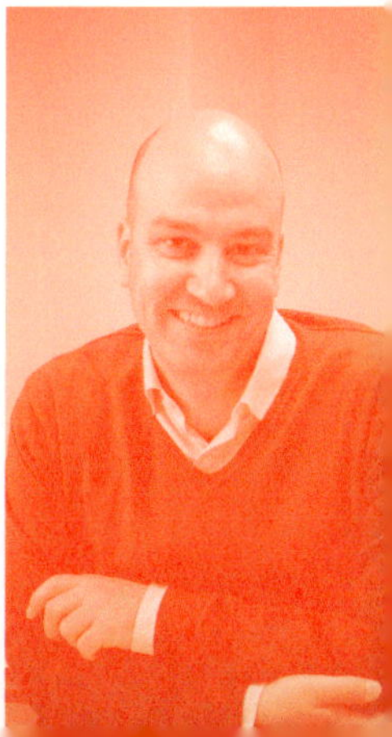

Primary Health Care
http://dx.doi.org/10.5772/intechopen.94677
Edited by Ayşe Emel Önal

Contributors

Florence Tochukwu Sibeudu, Diana Coronel-Martínez, Luis Augusto Moya-Barquín, Aileen Y. Chang, Evelyn Mendoza-Torres, Franklin Torres, Wendy Rosales-Rada, Liliana Encinales, Lil Avendaño, María Fernanda Pérez, Ivana Terán, David Vergara, Estefanie Osorio-Llanes, Paige Fierbaugh, Wendy Villamizar, Jairo Castellar-Lopez, Dimitra Metallinou, Christina Nanou, Antigoni Sarantaki, Eleftheria Lazarou, Anastasia Liagkou, Katerina Lykeridou, Yousef Khader, Mohamad Alyahya, Rami Saadeh, Livhuwani Muthelo, Tebogo Maria Mothiba, Rambelani Nancy Malema, Kebogile Elizabeth Mokwena, Velaphi Anthony Mokwena, Gülden Zehra Omurtag, Neda Taner, John Geyman, Seeta Devi Akyana, Dipali Dumbre, Michael Willie, Sipho Kabane, Neo Nonyana, Dmytro Vakulenko, Liudmyla Vakulenko, Leonid Hryshchuk, Lesya Sas, Maseabata Ramathebane, Sello Molungoa, Lineo Maja, Harishan Tharmarajah, Çiğdem Apaydın Kaya, Susan Janet Matthews, Mark Shephard, Brooke Spaeth, Maleeha Manzoor, Shumaila Sarwar, Madiha Saddique, Khalida Yaqoob, Arshia Muneer, Aisha Fatima, Mohammad Asad Mangat, Ayesha Kabir, Sehar Zulkifal, Laiba Mateen, Zeeshan Javed, Marie Bangsgaard Bang, Tine Bieber Lunn, Tanja Svarre, Margherita Schiavi, Maria Teresa Mascia, Gilda Sandri, Barbara Volta, Erica Keeling, Mxolisi Welcome Ngwenya, Masenyani Oupa Mbombi, Mamare Adelaide Bopape, Tebogo Maria Mothiba

First published in London, United Kingdom, 2022 by IntechOpen
IntechOpen is the global imprint of INTECHOPEN LIMITED, registered in England and Wales, registration number: 11086078, 5 Princes Gate Court, London, SW7 2QJ, United Kingdom
Printed in Croatia

British Library Cataloguing-in-Publication Data
A catalogue record for this book is available from the British Library

Additional hard and PDF copies can be obtained from orders@intechopen.com

Primary Health Care
Edited by Ayşe Emel Önal
p. cm.
Print ISBN 978-1-83969-806-4
Online ISBN 978-1-83969-807-1
eBook (PDF) ISBN 978-1-83969-808-8

For EU product safety concerns:
IN TECH d.o.o., Prolaz Marije Krucifikse Kozulić 3, 51000 Rijeka, Croatia, info@intechopen.com or visit our website at intechopen.com.

Meet the editor

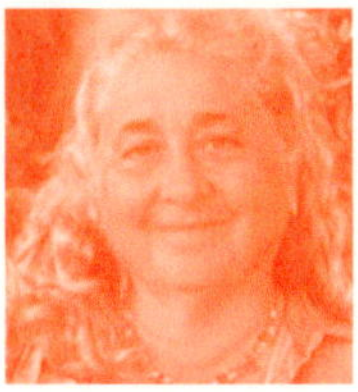

Ayşe Emel Önal is a medical doctor, public health specialist, and professor. She graduated from the Faculty of Medicine, Istanbul University in 1985. After experience in public hospital emergency medicine, health center medicine, maternal and child health, and family planning medicine, Dr. Önal became a public health specialist at the Medical Faculty, Department of Public Health, Istanbul University in 1995. She became an associate professor in 2005 and a full professor in 2010. Since 2013, she has been head of the Department of Environmental Health, Department of Public Health, at the Istanbul University Faculty of Medicine. Since 2014, she has been working as the director of the Istanbul University Community Medicine Practice and Research Center. Since 2016, she has been the head of the Department of Public Health, Istanbul University, where she also provides training in environmental health. She is a member of the Association of Public Health Specialists (HASUDER) and Environmental Health Group. She has been the vice-chairman of the Public Health Competence Executive Board since 2021. She has more than 200 research articles in national and international journals and papers in national and international congresses to her credit. She has more than 30 international publications in the Web of Science. Fluent in French and English, Dr. Önal's main research areas are chronic communicable and non-communicable diseases, epidemiology, gerontology, and environmental health.

Contents

Preface XIII

Section 1
What is Primary Health Care? 1

Chapter 1 3
Health Promotion
by Florence Tochukwu Sibeudu

Chapter 2 23
Primary Care in the USA: The Long Struggle to Build its Foundational Role
by John Geyman

Chapter 3 37
Patient-Centred Point-of-Care Testing: A Life-Changing Technology for Remote Primary Care
by Brooke Spaeth, Susan Matthews and Mark Shephard

Section 2
Child Health in Primary Care 53

Chapter 4 55
The Newborn Baby Check
by Harishan Tharmarajah

Chapter 5 67
COVID-19 Transmission in Children: Implications for Schools
by Evelyn Mendoza-Torres, Franklin Torres, Wendy Rosales-Rada, Liliana Encinales, Lil Avendaño, María Fernanda Pérez, Ivana Terán, David Vergara, Estefanie Osorio-Llanes, Paige Fierbaugh, Wendy Villamizar, Aileen Y. Chang and Jairo Castellar-Lopez

Chapter 6 87
Sexually Transmitted Infections in Pediatrics
by Diana Coronel-Martínez and Luis Augusto Moya-Barquín

Chapter 7 101
Chlamydial Infection
by Dimitra Metallinou, Christina Nanou, Antigoni Sarantaki, Eleftheria Lazarou, Anastasia Liagkou and Katerina Lykeridou

Section 3
Maternal Health in Primary Care 115

Chapter 8 117
The Effects of Multivitamin Use in Pregnancy on Mother and Fetus Health
by Neda Taner and Gülden Zehra Omurtag

Chapter 9 131
Anemia during Pregnancy and Its Prevalence
by Sehar Zulkifal, Shumaila Sarwar, Madiha Saddique, Khalida Yaqoob, Arshia Muneer, Aisha Fatima, Ayesha Kabir, Muhammad Asad Mangat, Laiba Mateen, Zeeshan Javed and Maleeha Manzoor

Section 4
Adult and Elderly Health in Primary Care 147

Chapter 10 149
Managing Polypharmacy and Deprescribing in Elderly
by Çiğdem Apaydın Kaya

Chapter 11 163
Use of Primary Healthcare Facilities for Care and Support of Chronic Diseases: Hypertension
by Maseabata Ramathebane, Maja Lineo and Sello Molungoa

Chapter 12 179
Impact of Cardiovascular Diseases on the Outcome of Patients with COVID-19
by Seeta Devi Akyana and Dipali Dumbre

Chapter 13 193
Aplication Arterial Oscilography to Study the Adaptive Capacity of Subject with COVID-19 in Primary Care
by Dmytro Vakulenko, Liudmyla Vakulenko, Leonid Hryshchuk and Lesya Sas

Section 5
Mental Health Prevention in Primary Care 211

Chapter 14 213
The Need to Strengthen Primary Health Care Services to Improve Mental Health Care Services in South Africa
by Kebogile Elizabeth Mokwena and Velaphi Anthony Mokwena

Section 6
Environmental Health and Infection Control in Primary Care 227

Chapter 15 229
Water, Sanitation, and Hygiene (WASH) and Infection Prevention and Control (IPC) in Primary Healthcare Facilities in Jordan in the Context of COVID-19
by Yousef Khader, Mohamad Alyahya and Rami Saadeh

Section 7
Occupational Health and Safety in Primary Care 257

Chapter 16 259
Strategies to Enhance Compliance to Health and Safety Protocols within the South African Mining Environment
by Livhuwani Muthelo, Tebogo Maria Mothiba and Rambelani Nancy Malema

Chapter 17 277
Early Occupational Therapy Intervention: Patients' Occupational Needs
by Margherita Schiavi, Barbara Volta, Gilda Sandri, Erica Keeling and Maria Teresa Mascia

Section 8
Telehealth and Telemedicine in Primary Care 285

Chapter 18 287
Telephone Consultations by Medical Scheme Patients Consulting General Medical Practitioners, South Africa
by Michael Mncedisi Willie, Neo Nonyana and Sipho Kabane

Chapter 19 299
Utilisation of Digital Health in Early Detection and Treatment of Pre-Eclampsia in Primary Health Care Facilities South Africa: Literature Review
by Mxolisi Welcome Ngwenya, Livhuwani Muthelo, Masenyani Oupa Mbombi, Mamare Adelaide Bopape and Tebogo Maria Mothiba

Chapter 20 317
Evaluating A Mobile App for Data Collection in Occupational Therapy Practice
by Tanja Svarre, Marie Bangsgaard Bang and Tine Bieber Lunn

Preface

To live a long, healthy life, individuals should receive uninterrupted health care starting from the womb until the end of life. Health care is a necessity and a right. Health services, which were defined in 1920 and focused on the necessity of reaching everyone, were defined as Primary Health Care Services in the 1978 Alma-Ata Declaration. The public health approach has come to the fore in primary health care. Today, the development and promotion of health, prevention of illness, early diagnosis and early treatment of diseases, access to multi-faceted rehabilitation services that enable those with chronic illnesses to live active lives in society, and palliative care are possible with a multi-sectoral health service approach. Primary care is important in terms of being a service delivery model and opinion, as well as being the first point of contact for an individual to reach health services. At this point, it is important to be able to start and follow the health service delivery that the individual needs with a holistic approach.

Forty years after Alma-Ata, the "World Conference on Primary Health Care from Alma-Ata to Universal Health Coverage and Sustainable Development Goals" held in Astana, Kazakhstan, in October 2018 has, in a sense, updated the concept of primary health care. It is clear that the environment, peace, security, and socio-economic status are important for health. Environmental factors such as wars, violence, epidemics, natural disasters, and the climate crisis cause premature deaths all over the world. Health should be universal and sustainable. This requires policy-making, knowledge, technology, human resources, and funding.

After 2019, due to the impact of the COVID-19 pandemic, telehealth has been included in primary health services. In cases where distance is a critical factor, as in the definition from the World Health Organization (WHO), health care delivery by health professionals using information and communication technologies has become widespread in the world for preventing diseases and injuries, conducting research, evaluating and improving health, and diagnosing and treating diseases and injuries.

This book presents examples from various countries about the provision of health services at the primary care level. Chapters examine the role of professionals in primary healthcare services and how they can work to improve the health of individuals and communities.

I would like to take this opportunity to thank all the esteemed chapter authors and everyone who contributed to the book.

Ayşe Emel Önal, MD,
Specialist and Professor of Public Health,
Department of Public Health,
Istanbul Medical Faculty,
Istanbul University,
Istanbul, Turkey

Section 1

What is Primary Health Care?

Chapter 1

Health Promotion

Florence Tochukwu Sibeudu

Abstract

Health promotion is one the major interventions employed in healthcare delivery, particularly in primary care. Health promotion enables individuals, families, populations, and communities to adopt and/or adapt lifestyles that promote and improve health. It helps community members to make choices that can improve their health. Every individual, population, and community has factors that influence their health either positively or negatively. Health promotion enables everyone in their context to identify and increase control over these factors to empower them to live a healthy life. This chapter explains actions, approaches, strategies, and steps for effective implementation of health promotion programmes.

Keywords: health, health promotion, health promotion actions, health promotion strategies, health promotion approaches

1. Introduction

According to the Ottawa Charter, health promotion is 'the process that enables people to increase control over their health and improve their overall health'. This can be achieved through education, building skills, and advocating change at the individual, family, and community levels. The responsibility for health promotion extends beyond the health sector and includes wellbeing. Health promotion activities focus on promoting good health and preventing illness, rather than focusing only on people who are at highest risk of developing certain diseases [1–3].

Promoting health is a series of actions; it is not promotion in the usual sense. Promoting health involves more than just telling people how they can take care of themselves. It also involves:

- informing individuals, families, and populations about what they can do to be healthy
- identifying characteristics of communities that influence people's health or wellbeing
- supporting those who are most in need, so they can be helped
- assisting people in improving their control and health
- including all the people in the contexts of their daily lives
- activities that promote health and prevent ill health instead of focusing on specific groups at risk for disease

'Health' is defined by the World Health Organization as 'complete physical and mental well-being, not only the absence of illness or infirmity'. To achieve a state that is complete in terms of physical, mental, and social wellbeing, an individual or group must have the ability to recognize and realize their aspirations, satisfy their needs, and adapt to changing environments.

Therefore, health can be described as:

- a resource for everyday living, not the goal of life
- a positive concept that stresses the importance of personal and social resources along with physical abilities
- being created and lived in daily lives; where one learns, works, and plays
- being capable of taking care of oneself and having control over one's own life.

2. Prerequisite for health

To be healthy, each person, family, and community must have the right conditions and resources. A solid foundation is essential for health improvement and should include:

- peace
- shelter
- education
- food
- income
- a stable ecosystem
- sustainable resources
- social justice and equity

3. Fundamental principles for health promotion

3.1 Advocate

To advocate is to promote good health as a resource for personal, financial, and social development. All factors, including those that are political, economic, social, and cultural, as well as those that affect behavioral and biological behavior, can have a positive or negative impact on health. Through advocacy for health, stakeholders for health promotion make these conditions favorable.

3.2 Enable

Health promotion focuses on equity in health. Health promotion aims to reduce health disparities and provide equal opportunities and support to all people so that they can reach their full potential. This includes a safe foundation and supportive environment that provides information, life skills, and opportunities to make healthy choices. If people are not able take control of the factors that influence their health, they will not be able achieve their fullest potential. This is true for all people.

3.3 Mediate

Without the involvement of all stakeholders, the health sector cannot ensure that there are adequate health conditions and prospects. Importantly, health promotion requires coordination by all stakeholders, including the government, the health sector, other sectors and nongovernmental organizations, industry, local authorities, and media. Individuals, families, communities, and all walks of society are involved. The role of professionals and health personnel, as well as social and professional groups, is to help people reach common goals in the pursuit for health [1–3].

4. Health promotion action

According to the Ottawa Charter (1986), health promotion actions consist of:

1. Building healthy public policy

2. Creating supportive environments

3. Strengthening community actions

4. Developing personal skills

5. Reorienting healthcare services

4.1 Build healthy public policy

Being healthy is much more than being without sickness. Health promotion places health on the agenda of those that make policies in all sectors, directing them to be aware of the burden of diseases on individuals, families, populations, and communities. The consequences of policies on health should be well thought out before these policies are enacted.

Health promotion encompasses legislation, economic measures, taxation, and organizational structure. It is coordinated in a way that results in fitness, profits, and social regulations that foster fairness. Healthy public policies contribute to making sure there are securer and healthier items and offerings, healthier public services, and cleaner, more pleasurable environments.

Health promotion involves identifying limitations to the adoption of healthy public regulations in non-health sectors and approaches to removing them. The goal is to make the healthier choice more attractive to policymakers.

4.2 Create supportive environments

Our societies are complicated and interrelated. The inextricable connections among human beings and their surroundings constitute the premise for a socio-ecological approach to health. A guiding principle for communities worldwide is to take care of each other and the natural environment. Protecting and conserving natural resources as well as built environments is a global responsibility integral for promoting health.

Lifestyle, employment, and leisure have a sizable effect on health, and all of these facets of a person's life should be a source of health. Health promotion should provide living and working conditions that are secure, stimulating, pleasurable, and fun. The world is currently experiencing rapid change in technology, urbanization, and energy use and production and thus systematic evaluation of how a rapidly changing environment affects individual health is critical.

4.3 Strengthen community actions

Health promotion works through concrete and powerful action among all actors in a community in identifying priorities, making decisions, choosing techniques, and implementing strategies to enhance health. At the centre of this process is the empowerment of groups and communities to understand their autonomy and control over their personal pursuits and destinies.

Community improvement calls for the use of existing human and material sources within the community network to improve and broaden flexible structures for strengthening public participation in health matters. This requires complete access to information, health education, and financial investment.

4.4 Develop personal skills

Health promotion helps individual and community development by providing information about health and illness and how to improve life skills. This increases the choices available to people to help them take more control of their personal wellbeing as well as their environments and to make good choices that benefit their health.

It is essential to enable individuals to prepare for all of life's stages and the possibility of chronic illness and injuries. This must be facilitated in all settings of a person's life, including at home, at work, and in community settings. Action is needed through instructional, expert, industrial, and voluntary bodies as well as in the establishments themselves.

4.5 Reorient health services

Health promotion is a shared responsibility among people, networks, corporations, health experts, healthcare providers and institutions, and governments. Everyone should work collectively to develop a healthcare service that contributes to the pursuit of full health. The function of the healthcare sector is not only to provide medical services but also to promote health and wellbeing. Health care should be sensitive to and respectful of cultural wishes to support individuals in the pursuit of a healthier life and open channels among the healthcare sector and broader social, political, economic, and physical institutions.

Reorienting health services additionally calls for more interest in health studies as well as adjustments in health curriculums and training. This will create a mindset and lifestyle of health services that focuses on the individual as a whole person [4–6].

5. Pillars of health promotion

The three pillars of health promotion, as declared at the 9th global conference for health promotion in Shanghai in 2016, are:

1. Good governance

2. Healthy cities

3. Health literacy

5.1 Good governance

Good health policies and equity are highly advantageous to society. Failures in governance are too regularly unfavorable to the pursuit of optimal health both for countrywide and globally. The United Nations Sustainable Development Goals (SDGs) provide universal recommendations for investing in all determinants of health. Governments have an essential duty to deal with the harmful outcomes of unsustainable manufacturing and consumption at local, national, and international levels. This consists of getting rid of economic regulations that create unemployment and dangerous working environments, and allowing advertising, funding, and legislation that enhance health. In addition, business leaders need to be cognizant of health in making company policies that do not value income over employee wellbeing. This is fundamental for disease prevention and health maintenance.

Mechanisms for promoting health include:

- public regulations

- strengthening legislation, regulations, and taxation of dangerous commodities

- implementing economic regulations as an effective device to allow new investments in fitness and health

- creating robust public fitness structures and introducing general fitness insurance as a green way for individuals to attain fitness and economic safety

- ensuring transparency and social duty and allowing the extensive engagement of civil society

- strengthening international governance to manage diseases of international importance

- strengthening and institutionalizing informal and traditional healthcare services for improving health outcomes

A key method for achieving the SDGs is to consider health in all policies. This is possible by having a vision for development without leaving anybody behind, that is, a world that is fair to all, prosperous, peaceful, and exists in a "green" sustainable environment. This situation requires transformed politics and governance through participatory governance, social mobilization, and community participation.

Actions to ensure governance include:

1. Integrating health as a central factor in all regulations and prioritizing regulations that contribute to promoting wellness.

2. Addressing all—social, fiscal, and environmental—determinants of health, implementing city plans and regulations that lessen poverty and inequity, and dealing with person rights and social inclusion.

3. Promoting robust community engagement, integrating health promotion activities in schools, workplaces, and other settings, creating an environment that promotes health literacy, and providing access to health information in communities.

4. Re-positioning health and other social services to the direction of fairness, ensuring unselective access to public services including health services to achieve health for all.

5. Conducting epidemiological studies and monitoring and evaluating evidence on health states and health determinants and disease burden, and using this information to inform policies, guidelines, and programme implementation.

5.2 Healthy cities

More than half of the world's population lives in cities and this number is expected to grow. More now than ever people rely on urban amenities and infrastructure for living a healthy lifestyle.

Health is created within the settings of ordinary lifestyles, within neighborhoods and groups in which people live, work, and play. It is one of the only markers of a city's sustainable improvement and contributes to making cities inclusive, secure, and resilient. As such, there is an urgent need for city leaders and authorities to deal with the adverse effects of rural-to-urban migration, economic stagnation, excessive unemployment and poverty, and environmental deterioration and pollution. People residing in cities are at greater risk of experiencing loneliness, unhappiness, stress, and mental health disorders.

Creating healthy cities calls for collaboration in promoting fitness and health and preventing disease. Cities are on the front line of sustainable improvement.

Urban 'greening' is an example of a transformative approach that promotes health and contributes to the implementation of the SDGs. Examples of greening include planting trees and creating parks, community gardens, living plant walls, and the like. Thus, it is crucial to prioritize regulations that:

- make policies that will be beneficial to the health and wellbeing of people in all sectors

- help cities promote fairness and social inclusion, harnessing the information, capabilities, and priorities of populations through robust network engagement

- re-organize social systems, including heath care, in a way that allows individuals and communities access to needed services

Actions to take to ensure healthy cities include:

1. providing citizens with schooling, housing, employment, and protection

2. implementing measures to remove pollutants from the air, water, and soil

3. investing in younger generations (No Child Left Behind) by offering education, health, and social programmes

4. ensuring the safety of vulnerable populations (migrants, refugees, homeless, etc.), protecting them from violence and harassment and providing them with housing and health care

5. dealing with all forms of discrimination

6. implementing vaccination programs, managing waste and vectors, and providing safe drinking water to prevent infectious disease

7. building cities with infrastructure that promotes walking, biking, and other healthy activities

8. providing access to low-cost healthy meals and safe drinking water, reducing sugar and salt consumption, and decreasing the dangerous use of alcohol through regulations, pricing, education, and taxation

9. banning smoking in indoor, public spaces and limiting or prohibiting tobacco advertising

5.3 Health literacy

Health literacy empowers people and encourages their engagement in collective health promotion. Health literacy is based on inclusive and equitable access to high-quality education.

Health literacy allows people to make more informed decisions about their health and the health of their families and empowers them to make recommendations to their political leaders and authorities. In this era of the Internet, many people regularly obtain their health information online. However, not all online information is accurate or reliable. As such, it may be helpful to consider policies to test unreliable or disputable facts.

It is crucial to:

- understand health literacy as a vital determinant of wellbeing and invest in its improvement

- broaden, enforce, and display intersectoral countrywide and local techniques for strengthening health literacy in all populations and in all instructional settings

- improve residents' management of their personal health and its determinants

- ensure that business environments provide healthful alternatives through business regulations including commodities, standard regulations, consumer rights, and so on

Actions to enhance health literacy include:

- Expanding health promotion actions: One health promotion action can be used as a platform for other health activities thereby broadening the scope of the programme. This is an integrated approach to solve different health problems under a programme.

- Changing health promotion thinking: Connecting health promotion with activities of daily living is integral for health promotion. It entails linking peoples' norms, culture, and responses to health promotion. Making people see health promotion as a way of everyday life is the whole essence.

- Sharing knowledge and information: Exchange of new knowledge and information helps in quality health planning and healthcare delivery across all levels of care. There are better opportunities for healthy living when new knowledge is shared with stakeholders and community members.

- Using new technologies: Use of innovative Information Technology (IT) facilities will help to reform health promotion activities in a way that target populations will be more interested in the programme. Such a transformative approach will increase access to health promotion activities leading to high heath literacy across population groups.

6. Strategies for health promotion

Caring, holism, and ecology are critical factors to consider when developing techniques for health promotion. Therefore, the ones worried must take as a guiding precept that, in every segment of making plans, implementation and assessment of health promotion activities, men and women must emerge as identical partners. The following are techniques for promoting health:

1. Health communication

2. Health education

3. Policy development

4. Systems change

5. Environmental change

6.1 Health communication

Conversations about health consist of verbal and written techniques to persuade and empower people, populations, and groups to make healthy choices. Effective health communication is related to social marketing and includes the following components:

- Use of evidence-based techniques to develop materials and products and to identify channels through which to deliver these products to individuals

- Understanding the traditional wisdom, concepts, language, and priorities for specific cultures and settings

- Consideration of health literacy, Internet access, media exposure, and cultural competency of target populations

- Development of brochures, billboards, newspaper articles, TV broadcasts, radio commercials, public provider announcements, newsletters, pamphlets, videos, digital tools, and other media

Using a variety of communication channels allow the dissemination of health messaging to individuals, communities, and institutions at both the local and national levels. Radio, television, newspapers, flyers, brochures, the Internet, social media, and so on can all be used to communicate health messages. Health communication can be used to alert people to health risks and dangers, reinforce healthy behaviors, influence social norms, increase availability of help and services, and empower people to improve their health.

6.2 Health education

Health education is a social science approach that integrates physical, medical, and other sciences to promote health and prevent illness. It can be delivered in a variety of ways, including through lectures, courses, seminars, workshops, webinars, classes, and so on. Characteristics of health education techniques include:

- Participation of the target population
- Carrying out a community needs assessment to identify community capability, resources, priorities, and wishes
- Planned educational activities that increase participants' information and capabilities
- Using lessons and materials to implement a programme that participants can easily access
- Presentation of facts via multimedia such as videos, websites, software, and so on
- Training staff to ensure they adhere to the programme

6.3 Policy improvement

Policy is a device for promoting and supporting health and preventing disease. Policy decisions are made by organizations and stakeholders. Policy methods consist of legislative advocacy, economic measures, taxation, and regulatory oversight. Examples of health policies include:

- Establishing regulations for smoke-free zones
- Regulating food vendors to provide healthy options to the public
- Taxing unhealthy foods
- Requiring the use of safety equipment in work settings

6.4 Systems change

Systems change refers to an essential shift in the manner in which problematic issues are solved. Within a business enterprise, systems change impacts organizational intent, function, and connections through addressing organizational culture, beliefs, relationships, protocols, and objectives.

Examples of systems change in health promotion include:

- Developing plans for imposing new interventions and strategies
- Adapting or replicating tested and proven health promotion models
- Employing innovative technology

- Creating education, training, or certification programs that align with regulations and policies

6.5 Environmental change

Environmental techniques for promoting health involve fiscal, social, and environmental aspects that influence human health. Examples of environmental health promotion techniques include:

- Increasing the number of parks, greenways, and trails within a community
- Putting up signage that promotes the use of walking and biking paths
- Increasing the supply of fresh, nutritious food in schools, restaurants, and cafeterias [7]

7. Health-promoting approaches

Health promotion methods are primarily based on the idea that health and wellbeing encompass myriad complicated and interrelated elements, including a person's behaviors, beliefs, practices, environment, community, and culture, as well as broader socioeconomic elements like legislation and economics.

There are several different approaches to promoting health. These include medical, behavioral, educational, empowerment, and social approaches.

7.1 Medical approach

This approach focuses on reducing morbidity and mortality. Activity is focused on whole populations or high-risk groups. This type of health promotion seeks to increase clinical interventions to prevent disease and early death.

The clinical method focuses on treatment of diseases to prevent complications and premature death. It targets individuals or groups who are exposed to diseases or those who are already sick. This approach is basically targeting people that are sick to ameliorate their sickness as such it is the center of medical intervention. In the approach, the professional has the responsibility to ensure people adhere to treatment regimens. In most instances, sick people do not have full information of the reasons for their actions, they carry out the health promotion actions because of the directives of the health professionals.

The clinical method to health promotion is unique because:

- It combines scientific evidence through epidemiological studies and medical strategies to manage diseases.
- Prevention and the early detection of sickness are more cost effective than treatment of existing diseases.
- It is a professional-led, or top-down, kind of intervention. This type of health promotion method reinforces the authority of clinical and health experts who are identified as having the professional knowledge about the disease and its management.
- There is enormous evidence on efficacious strategies for disease prevention and management used in health promotion.

The medical approach to health promotion has three levels of intervention:

1. Primary prevention – preventing the onset of illness and disease

2. Secondary prevention – preventing the progression of illness and disease

3. Tertiary prevention – mitigating further illness and suffering in those already ill

The principle of preventive services such as immunization and screening is that they target at-risk groups. Immunization only works if people get their vaccinations. Disease screening is offered to certain groups of people, for example, prostate screening is offered to men who are 55 to 69 years of age. Screening is only effective if the following conditions are met:

- The disease must have an extended preclinical stage so that screening will not miss the symptoms

- Earlier treatment will improve patient outcomes

- The screening test is sensitive, specific, and cost-effective

Preventive strategies should be based on epidemiological proof. The medical approach is predicated on having an infrastructure able to support screening and immunization programmes. This consists of educated personnel, laboratory facilities, information systems, and in the case of immunization, an effective and safe vaccine. It is obvious that the medical approach to health promotion is complicated procedure and may rely on national programmes or guidelines.

7.2 Behavioral approach

Making healthy choices can be complicated and requires self-motivation. A behavioral approach to health aims to inspire individuals to adopt healthy lifestyle behaviors, to use preventive health services, and to take responsibility for their own health. The behavioral approach is popular because it views health as an individual asset and, as such, it can be assumed that people have the ability to make good decisions to improve their health and make healthy lifestyle choices. This approach also assumes that people have only themselves to blame if they do not take steps to look after their health.

It is apparent that the relationship between people's behavior and social and environmental factors is complicated. A person's behavior may be outside of their control due to the conditions in which they live. For example, a person may be unemployed or living in poverty and thus unable to make healthy choices.

The behavioral approach has been undertaken by many health promotion agencies. For example, health campaigns promote quitting smoking, adopting a healthy diet, and regularly participating in physical activities. This method is focused on individuals although mass communication means may be used to reach them. The behavioral approach is typically a professional-led, top-down method, which highlights the divide between the health professional, who knows how to enhance fitness and wellbeing, and the general public who requires education and advice [8, 9].

In some instances, interventions can be directed to clients' needs although these needs will also be identified by the health provider. The behavioral change method is primarily based on trying to change a person's attitudes and behaviors so that they undertake a healthful way of life. For instance, health professionals teach clients how to take care of their teeth, how to prepare their daily food menu, how to lose weight, and so on. This approach underscores the importance of health workers to seize every opportunity to teach healthy lifestyles. However, while it is the duty of health workers to teach, people should also see living a healthy life as their responsibility.

Many healthcare professionals teach their clients about health and wellness via education and individual consultation. Patient education about a health condition or treatment may be used to ensure patient compliance to a certain regimen and thus is focused on the individual and providing them with useful and reliable information.

7.3 Educational approach

The purpose of the educational approach is to provide information and facts, and to develop relevant skills so that individuals can make knowledgeable choices about their health. This approach is different from the behavioral approach. It is not intended to motivate people to move in certain directions, although it does hope to lead them to an outcome. It is based on personal choice regardless of whether the choices made are agreeable to the healthcare promoter.

The goal of the educational method is to offer people facts and encourage them to make their own decisions about their health behavior. Educational interventions require the promoter to understand the concepts the person is studying as well as any factors that assist or preclude the studying.

Psychological theories of learning identify three aspects:

1. Information and understanding (cognition)

2. Attitudes and feelings (affect)

3. Skills (behavior)

The educational method is based on the premise that access to information can help change and modify behavior. When a person is knowledgeable, they are capable of making clear choices acceptable to both health experts and the public.

The educational approach to health promotion involves offering facts to assist people in making informed decisions about their health behavior. This can be accomplished through distribution of materials that contain health information, presentation of health topics, and counseling.

Education offers possibilities for individuals to discuss and discover their attitudes about their personal wellness. Educational programmes may broaden individuals' decision-making capabilities through drama or program designed to discover alternatives. In the educational method, individuals may have the opportunity to role play real-life situations to solidify what they are learning. Educational programmes are typically led through a trainer or facilitator.

7.4 Empowerment approach

Within the context of health promotion, empowerment may be understood as a procedure through which human beings are allowed to control and manage their health and things affecting their health. An empowerment method seeks to allow people as individuals as well as collectively to develop their ability to control their own health status and make their own health decisions. This method focuses on helping people develop decision-making and problem-solving skills and encouraging them to engage in critical thinking and critical action.

In this method, the health expert works with individuals or groups to assist them in identifying what they need to recognize and act on in their body and environment. Then, based on their knowledge and wishes, to make decisions. The function of the health expert is to behave as a facilitator. They assist individuals in identifying their concerns and help them acquire the information and capabilities needed to make adjustments. Empowerment of individuals and communities is vital in health promotion. Individuals or groups have information, capabilities, and competencies to make contributions and decisions. They also have an absolute power to govern their personal health.

7.5 Social change approach

Rather than changing the conduct of individuals, the social change approach focuses on changing societal behavior (physical, economic, and social environments).

The social change approach is concerned with adjusting the physical, social, and fiscal environment to create enabling environment for building health promotion capacity.

Rather than changing the conduct of individuals, the social change approach focuses on changing societal behavior (physical, economic, and social environments). Those that wish to use this method will cause their democratic principles and processes to change the society. The policy makers would place health at the political timetable at all levels in a way that there will be concerted effort to significantly improve the environment where people reside, work, and play to be healthy. This method assumes that if the healthier option is made the less complicated option, people will be more likely to make the healthy choice. Therefore, health promotion is consequently a social and political procedure that regards health as a human right and considers the protection of population health to be a prerequisite for social progress.

8. Health promotion in medical settings

It is essential for all health professionals to integrate health promotion goals and principles in their practice. This section uses the field of nursing as an example of how to incorporate health promotion in medical settings.

8.1 Medical or preventive approach

As previously discussed, the medical approach to health promotion has three levels of intervention:

- Primary prevention – preventing the onset of illness and disease
- Secondary prevention – preventing the progression of illness and disease
- Tertiary prevention – mitigating further illness and suffering in those already ill

Nurses work very closely with sick persons in medical facilities and sometimes even with entire populations or groups who are at risk of sickness. In communities, schools, and industries, nurses have the platform to apply the clinical or preventive method to reduce mortality. It is imperative for nurses to use nursing capabilities in prevention and control of disease.

Nurses who work in this method of health promotion can be involved in immunization programmes, screening for diseases like cancers, or administering medication to individuals in palliative care settings. This method of health promotion also assumes the clinical version of health, which adopts a systematic view of the body whereby the part of the body system can be affected to disorganize the system. This systemic effect can be seen as signs and symptoms of the diseases and the medical approach will just target those signs and symptoms of the diseases. Additionally, sick people are expected to adhere to the instructions of the health expert and conform to treatment regimen for this approach to be effective. This method is in support with a conventional clinical hierarchy that regards the healthcare professional as an expert and the affected person as a clinical subject.

8.2 Behavioral approach

In this approach, nurses are engaged in sensitization and education of people and groups about healthy lifestyles. The behavioral approach makes the essential assumption that the way an individual lives in terms of eating, sleeping, exercising, and so on is critical to being and staying healthy. Nurses who undertake the behavioral method of health promotion offer sick people information about lifestyle and how it affects health, and they encourage individuals to make healthy choices.

8.3 The educational approach

Nurses can also help sick people to broaden their health literacy capabilities and allow them to make significant adjustments to enhance their wellness. The educational method to health promotion assumes that providing people with information about their health will cause more healthy behavior. Nurses who undertake an educational method to health promotion offer individuals and groups information and facts concerning their health, allowing them to make informed decisions. In this method, the information about health is detailed and robust to allow the individual or group to have a clear understanding of the whole situation. This differs from the behavior change method in that the nurse does not try to encourage the person to change their behavior to a pre-determined pattern, but rather supports the individual to make an informed decision based on available information. One crucial result of the educational method is health literacy, which refers to personal, cognitive, and social capabilities that decide the capacity of people to access, comprehend, and use health information to promote and maintain good health.

8.4 The empowerment approach

Nurses are trained to offer nursing services in diverse settings including health facilities, communities, schools, businesses, and so on. The first step in the nursing process in all levels of care is assessment. As such, nurses have information of the socio-cultural background and wishes of individuals and groups, which positions them to empower people in improving their health. For instance, the community health nurse empowers community members to manage their health using what they have in their community. This is possible because nurses will first undertake community assessment and identify their strengths, weaknesses, opportunities, and threats. With this robust data from the community, the nurse will show the community members how to be healthy within their context, and community members are able to live their lives within the community without being sick. Moreover, even at the facility level, by enhancing open conversation with sick persons and their families, nurses are capable of eliciting expressed wishes and available resources that help to broaden personalized care plans. Through therapeutic communication and empathy, nurses can enhance the intellectual wellness of sick people. Nurses are also engaged in industries and schools where they empower management, staff, and students to live healthy lives.

8.5 The social change approach

Nurses recommend for social change that is informed by individual/community assessment and epidemiological reports. Social change includes adjustment of the physical, social, and economic surroundings where people live, work, and play to promote human health. For instance, an occupational health nurse advocates for safe work environments, including provision of personal protective equipment. This method also entails advocacy for the community, which will be taken to the public as well as policy makers.

This method assumes that that if the systems where people live, work, and play are structured for healthy living, people are more likely to make the right choices for healthy lifestyles. Health promotion is a social and political procedure that regards fitness as a human property and considers the protection of population health to be a prerequisite for social progress. Nurses can successfully cause social change for health promotion through advocacy and collaboration. Assessment, which is the first step, provides the platform to obtain complete records that may be informative for social change [8, 9].

9. Developing a health promotion programme for the community

There are eight steps to developing and implementing a health promotion programme:

- Step 1: Manage the plan
- Step 2: Assess the community
- Step 3: Identify goals, population of interest, outcomes, and objectives
- Step 4: Identify strategies, activities, outputs, process objectives, and resources
- Step 5: Develop indicators
- Step 6: Review the programme plan
- Step 7: Implement the plan
- Step 8: Determine results and impact

9.1 Step 1: management of the plan

The objective of this step is to develop a plan to control stakeholder participation, timelines, and resources, and decide strategies for gathering and interpreting data and making decisions. It involves interacting with stakeholders, establishing a timeline, planning allocation of funds and other resources, obtaining records and data for decision-making, and establishing a decision-making procedure through consensus or committee.

9.2 Step 2: conduct a situation analysis

This step examines the current situation of the community and its characteristics, population, trends, and problems that can influence implementation of the programme. It consists of identifying the wants, wishes, strengths, and weaknesses of the community. This step entails the use of records and data obtained through a variety of means, including interviews, surveys, testimonials, guidelines, regulations, polls, research, literature reviews, and so on, to determine the following:

- the present state of the community
- what's making the state of the community better and what's making it worse
- what viable moves can be made to deal with the situation

9.3 Step 3: identify goals, populations of interest, outcomes, and outcome objectives

The purpose of this step is to apply situational evaluation to identify the goals, target population, desired outcomes, and results of the programme. This step consists of:

- Identifying achievable goals: This is price statements outlining what the programme will achieve both at short term and long term.
- Identifying target population: this is a population groups like women of child bearing age, the adolescent, university students and so on that needs the specified health promotion programme.
- Outlining expected outcomes: this refers to short statements specifying the preferred changes that could be due to this program.
- Ensuring that program goals, target populations and expected outcomes of the health promotion programme are aligned with strategic plans of your institution.

These will assist to contextualize the health promotion programme to make sure that it is applicable and sustainable for the community.

9.4 Step 4: identify strategies, activities, outputs, process objectives, and resources

This step involves choosing strategies through brainstorming and situational analysis. At this point, having a clear picture of 'where you want to go' (see Step 3) will help you 'how to get there'. This entails outlining techniques, methods, and activities that will contribute to achieving the goal and objectives of the programme.

- Use of brainstorming techniques. For instance, asking team members to suggest strategies such as health education, health communication, organizational change, and policy improvement for accomplishing goals.
- Use of situation analysis reports to prioritize thoughts from team members.

- Identify unique activities for every approach, including when to start the activity, how long it will run, and when to end each activity.
- Determine outputs (both targets and final outputs) and establish process objectives that you will assess during process evaluation.
- Consider economic, human, and material resources available for the programme.

9.5 Step 5: develop indicators

This step involves developing a list of variables that may be tracked to evaluate the degree to which results and goals are met. To accomplish this, goals should be tested to make sure they are legitimate, reliable, and attainable. Certain goals may need to be subdivided into individual tasks. As such, the indicators that will be used to check the process and outcome of the programme must be clearly described and the validity, reliability, and accessibility of the proposed indicators checked.

For every final result and process goal, there is a need to consider the following:

- the expected end result
- whether or not the expected end result may be divided into separate components
- if the expected end result can be measured
- if there will be suitable time to achieve the end result
- if the required records will be available and accessible
- if the resources needed for checking these results are available

9.6 Step 6: review the programme plan

In this step, the plan for the programme is reviewed and assessed. The reason for this step is to make clear the contribution of every aspect of the plan to the overall programme's goals, to identify any gaps, and to ensure the programme's efficiency and applicability. It is crucial to apply good judgment at this stage.

The plan is reviewed to decide whether:

- techniques successfully contribute to predetermined goals and objectives
- short-term goals contribute to long-term goals
- the most appropriate activities have been selected
- activities are suitable for the audience
- resources are good enough to enforce the activities

9.7 Step 7: implement the plan

This in the step in which the programme is implemented. For a community health programme, it is crucial to make sure community participation is embedded within the programme throughout all stages of implementation. Community participation is the active involvement of human beings from groups and/or communities to ensure acceptance and utilization of the programmme. True community participation entails the involvement of community members in all phases of programme planning and implementation, including community analysis, decision-making, and programme implementation.

9.8 Step 8: Results and impact

This step assesses the programme for its effectiveness, efficiency, fairness, and acceptance. The consequences and effects of the programme are critical benchmarks for assessing programme planners and managers. The programme planners will propose and choose the techniques for assessment to examine the status of the health promotion programme. The results and effects will decide whether the programme is sustainable and can be adapted to other groups [10, 11].

10. Conclusion

Health promotion is a primary technique for ensuring health for all regardless of socioeconomic and geographic status. There is a need to enhance health promotion activities in all areas of healthcare services.

Author details

Florence Tochukwu Sibeudu
Department of Nursing Science, College of Health Sciences, Nnamdi Azikiwe University, Nnewi Campus, Nnewi, Nigeria

*Address all correspondence to: ft.sibeudu@unizik.edu.ng

References

[1] World Health Organization. Health Promotion and Community Participation. 2021. Available from: https://www.who.int/water_sanitation_health/hygiene/emergencies/em2002chap15.pdf

[2] World Health Organization. Health Promotion. 2021. Available from: https://www.who.int/health-topics/health-promotion#tab=tab_1

[3] VicHealth. Health Promotion. 2020. Available from: https://www.vichealth.vic.gov.au/about/health-promotion

[4] WHO. Health Promotion. 2021. Available from: https://www.who.int/teams/health-promotion/enhanced-wellbeing/first-global-conference/actions

[5] Grand River Community Heath Centre. Health Promotion and Community Development. 2021. Available from: https://grandriverchc.ca/in-the-centre/health-promotion-community-development/

[6] World Health Organization. 9th Global Conference on Health Promotion. 2017. Available from: https://www.who.int/publications/i/item/promoting-health-in-the-sdgs

[7] RHIhub. Health Promotion and Disease Prevention in Rural Communities. 2021. Available from: https://www.ruralhealthinfo.org/toolkits/health-promotion/1/introduction

[8] Phillips A. Effective Approaches to Health Promotion in Nursing Practice. 2018. Available from: https://repository.canterbury.ac.uk/download/e5b13fb82eb016e6c2bae128f962f54291a459571e774b8ec99c0b0d6d27f297/298377/Effective%20approaches%20to%20 health%20promotion%20in%20 nursing%20-%20Nursing%20Standard%20Oct%202018.pdf

[9] Nurse Key. Models and Approaches to Health Promotion. 2017. Available from: https://nursekey.com/models-and-approaches-to-health-promotion/

[10] Public Health Ontario. At a Glance: The Six Steps for Planning a Health Promotion Program. 2015. Available from: https://www.publichealthontario.ca/-/media/documents/S/2015/six-steps-planning-hp-programs.pdf

[11] The Health Communication Unit. Health Introduction to Health Promotion Planning. 2001. Available from: http://www.mentalhealthpromotion.net/resources/introduction-to-health-promotion-program-planning.pdf

Chapter 2

Primary Care in the USA: The Long Struggle to Build its Foundational Role

John Geyman

Abstract

Family practice was recognized as the 20th specialty in American medicine in 1969. With the hope that primary care would become the foundation of an improved health care system, vigorous efforts were launched in medical education, research and practice to achieve that goal. This chapter traces the history of that effort, together with negative system changes that have obstructed that goal. Although primary care physicians have been shown to improve access to care, contain costs, decrease inequities, and improve patient outcomes, they are still too few in number to meet national needs for primary care. The COVID-19 pandemic revealed the extent of inadequacy and vulnerability of the system. The U. S. still lacks a system of universal access as has been in place for many years in most other advanced countries around the world. Corporate stakeholders in a largely privatized financing and delivery system continue to challenge the future of primary care. Lessons from the failure of reform initiatives over the last 50 years are discussed, as are current reform alternatives, only one of which would at last bring universal access to health care in this country.

Keywords: primary care, family practice; access, costs, quality and outcomes of care; corporatization, medical-industrial complex, health care reform, Medicare for All

1. Introduction

The need for primary care to serve as the foundation of U. S. health care has been recognized for years. Many efforts have been taken to make that happen through medical education and practice. However, despite considerable progress toward that goal, the U. S. still lacks such a foundation, as international studies of 11 advanced countries clearly show.

This chapter has three goals: (1) to bring historical perspective to the evolution and progress of primary care in this country, despite system obstacles; (2) to describe current attempts to rebuild primary care; and (3) to briefly consider the road ahead.

2. Historical perspective

2.1 How primary care developed

Family practice, which became its own board-certified specialty in 1969, evolved from general practice, which just 20 years earlier represented 50 percent of all U. S.

physicians [1]. But specialization in the aftermath of World War II changed the ratio of generalist physicians to specialists from 80 percent of all physicians in 1930 to just 20 percent in 1969 when family practice was recognized as a specialty.

Medical care was fragmented by the 1960s among many non-generalist specialties to the point that three national groups issued three major reports—the Millis Report, the Willard Report and the Folsom Report. All strongly stated the urgent need for the primary or family physician as the backbone of personalized comprehensive medical care.

Those reports, together with a shift of federal and state funding priorities, led to new family medicine teaching programs in U. S. medical schools and hospitals. By 1990, impressive progress had been made, as shown by these markers:

- Clinical departments of family practice in more than one-half of departmentalized U. S. hospitals.
- Active clinical departments of family practice in most medical schools.
- 384 family practice residency programs with about 7,300 residents in training.
- More than 40,000 board-certified family physicians.
- Active research in many academic departments of family practice, together with some collaborative research networks involving community settings.
- Family practice in high demand, with leading role in managed care [2].

Fast forward, however, to 30 years later in 2020, and we still have an acute shortage of primary care physicians in an upside-down pyramid dominated by other specialties, with fragmented care the rule. A 2010 conference sponsored by the Josiah Macy, Jr. Foundation that brought together leading experts in health policy came to this conclusion:

> *The lack of a strong primary care infrastructure across the nation has had significant consequences for access, quality, continuity, and cost of care in this country. It also has had consequences for our health profession educational enterprise and the healthcare workforce, resulting in numbers and geographic distributions of primary care providers that are insufficient to meet current and projected needs ... We are facing an economic situation in which the current rate of rise of medical cost is unsustainable, and this situation is exacerbated by an aging population with higher care needs and expectations. These events have created a climate in which it is necessary and appropriate to question the models of care and health professions education on which we have relied [3].*

As the shortage of primary care persists with stagnation of the primary care physician workforce, part of this growing need has been filled by the rapid growth of nurse practitioners and physician assistants, typically working in teams with primary care physicians but sometimes more independently [4].

3. Negative system changes as obstacles to primary care

Other advanced countries around the world ensure universal access to health care with a stronger role of primary care. The U. S. has evolved a profit-driven medical-industrial complex with deregulated markets and little oversight and accountability by government. Much of U. S. health care has been corporatized, with a shift to for-profit health care, increased privatization, and growth of investor-owned corporate health care. These changes have resulted in:

- prices to what the traffic will bear;
- uncontained costs;
- decreased choice and access to care;
- variable, often poor quality of care;
- erosion of a safety net; and
- rampant profiteering, even fraud.

These changes have worked against the further development of family practice. Private equity firms have driven purchases of many physician-owned medical practices, driving many to become hospital-affiliated employees [5]. Almost two-thirds of U. S. physicians are now employed by others, especially by large hospital systems, where they are under pressure to maximize revenues for their employers. This is a far cry from a generation ago when family physicians ran their own practices, rounded in the hospital, and worked in the community [6]. Not surprisingly, small group practice has almost disappeared, while practice satisfaction has declined for many physicians together with increasing burnout rates [7].

Other generational changes have been taking place over the past 30 years which change the landscape for traditional primary care. One of these is the increasing numbers of millennials who do not want a family doctor, but instead value the convenience of dropping in to an urgent-care facility with an acute need without any continuity or comprehensiveness of ongoing care. National polls have found that up to one-third of millennials take this approach [8]. That change is further enabled by the increasing wait times for those who want to visit a family physician, which has gone up to almost a month because of their shortage [9].

Primary care physicians in practice are besieged by electronic health records, which have become billing instruments, and having to spend an average of $99,000 a year per physician for their billing activities that take away many hours from patient care [10]. They have to spend additional time in dealing with the different and changing policies of more than 1,000 private insurers over such everyday issues as restricted networks, drug formularies, pre-authorizations, and other requirements related to reimbursement.

The mantra of our unfettered marketplace holds that competition will bring efficiency and contain costs. That claim, however, has been proven false for years. As one example, the non-profit U. S. Center for Studying Health System Change conducted a nine-year study of 12 major health care markets in its Community Tracking Study involving 60 communities, 60,000 households and 12,000 physicians. It found four major barriers to efficiency: (1) providers' market power, (2) absence of potentially efficient provider systems, (3) employers' inability to push the system toward efficiency and quality; and (4) insufficient health plan competition [11].

The U. S. compares poorly among 11 countries periodically measured by the Commonwealth Fund, as illustrated by cost barriers for high-need older adults (**Figure 1**). Despite spending more for health care than any other country in the world (about $1.3 trillion a year), the U. S. lags behind other countries in terms of mortality amenable to health care [12].

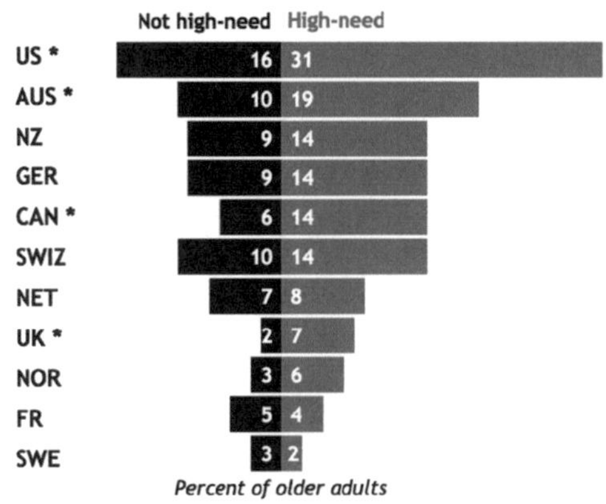

Source: 2017 The Commonwealth Fund International Health Policy Survey of Older Adults

Figure 1.
High-need older adults experience greater cost barriers to receiving care.

3.1 Positive system impacts by primary care physicians despite obstacles

Despite their relatively small numbers system-wide, primary care has been found to be markedly beneficial by many studies around the country, as these illustrate.

- A study at Dartmouth Medical School in New Hampshire found that costs of care in regions with the most primary care physicians were 23 percent lower than in regions with the fewest number thereof. Medicare patients with most access to primary care patients also had fewer physician visits (including to other specialists), spent less time in the hospital, and were less likely to die in the hospital [13].

- A study conducted from 2005 to 2015 found that every increase of 10 primary care physicians per 100,000 population was associated with reductions of mortality of 0.9% to 1.4% from cardiovascular, cancer, and respiratory diseases [14].

- Another study found that the more primary care is used, the less use of emergency room visits and hospitalizations [15].

- Other studies have documented that increased density of primary care physicians is associated with reduced overall mortality [16–18].

- The business community, which pays the freight for our widespread system of private employer-sponsored health insurance (ESI), has found that it spends one-third less money for health care in places where primary care is available, with 19 percent lower mortality within its workforce [19].

3.2 Negative system impacts due to shortage of primary care physicians

The critical shortage of primary care physicians has led to these adverse system problems, which include increased costs and fragmentation of care of lower quality:

- Polypharmacy is a common problem among patients without primary care physicians who seek multiple physicians, who do not communicate with each other, for chronic health problems [20].

- A 2009 study found that about one-half of patient visits to specialists were already follow-up visits that could more appropriately have been handled by their primary care physicians [21].

- Although emergency physicians account for just 5 percent of the physician workforce, they handle one-quarter of all acute care encounters and more than one-half of those visits for the uninsured [22].

The COVID-19 pandemic has further exposed the fragility and inadequacy of primary care, as shown by these markers:

- With so many in-person physician visits being canceled across the country, the future financial viability of primary care practices was being called into question [23].

- Primary care physicians in smaller, independent practices faced such a large drop in patient volume that they thought that they may be forced to close their practices [24]; nine months into the pandemic, 16,000 had done so due to the stress of the pandemic [25].

- Only about 5 percent of all U. S. health care spending goes to primary care compared to an average of 14 percent in other wealthy nations [26].

- The lack of a national physician workforce plan by specialty was again made crystal clear, with serious shortages in primary care, psychiatry, and public health.

With our continued lack of a national physician workforce plan, despite all the warnings along the way, the U. S. still confronts a shortage of between 21,000 and 55,200 primary care physicians by 2032, according to the Association of American Medical Colleges [27]. Money has everything to do with that challenging prognosis as U. S. medical graduates continue to seek out more highly reimbursed specialties, such as orthopedic surgery, anesthesiology, radiology, and dermatology.

4. Current approaches to rebuild primary care

It has long been apparent that system reform will be required in the U. S. before primary care can grow and thrive at its foundation. Our non-system has been taken over by corporate stakeholders dancing to the tune of Wall Street investors, not the needs of patients, families and taxpayers. Before we can move back to a traditional service ethic in health care based on the public interest, major reforms will be needed. As the distinguished medical historian, Rosemary Stevens, observed 20 years ago:

> *The most important impediment to a clear-cut role for family practice has been the lack of a formal administrative structure for primary care practice on a nationwide basis in the United States [28].*

4.1 Lessons learned from past reform initiatives

Before having any success in bringing about change, we need to better understand the forces that blocked previous attempts. It has been more than a century since Teddy Roosevelt, running as a presidential candidate on the progressive ticket in 1912, proposed universal coverage through national health insurance. These are the major lessons that we can take from every attempt to reform health care since then, including passage of the Affordable Care Act (ACA) in 2010:

1. "Turning to the stakeholders, who themselves crafted the system's problems, for recommended solutions does not work.

2. The more complex a bill becomes, in an effort to respond to competing political interests, the more its legislative and public support erodes.

3. Strong presidential leadership from the start and throughout the legislative process is critical to enactment of health care reform.

4. Corporate power in our enormous medical-industrial complex, accounting for one-sixth of the nation's gross national product, trumps the democratic process.

5. The "mainstream" media are not mainstream at all, and have conflicts of interest based on their close ties to corporate stakeholders in the status quo.

6. We can count on opponents to use fear mongering to distort the health care debate.

7. Centrist middle of the road reform proposals for health care are bound to fail.

8. Framing the basic issues in the health care reform debate has been inadequate; the alternatives have been controlled by the special interests resisting reform so they will win.

9. History repeats itself, and we do not learn from our mistakes" [29].

A comprehensive report was published by the Institute of Medicine in 1996, *Primary Care: America's Health in a New Era*, calling for an urgent priority to prioritize primary care. But its recommendations were largely unheeded by legislators and policy makers as underinvestment in primary care continued. A recent 2021 report from the National Academies of Sciences, Engineering and Medicine again strengthened the case for primary care as the foundation of the U. S. health care system. Its 448-page report, *Implementing High-Quality Primary Care: Rebuilding the Foundation of Health Care,* calls for policies that:

- "Pay for primary care teams to care for people, not doctors to deliver services;

- Ensure that high-quality primary care is available to every individual and family in every community;

- Train primary care teams where people live and work;

- Design information technology that serves the patient, the family and the interprofessional care team; and

- Ensure that high-quality primary care is implemented in the United States" [30].

That report went further to recommend, with a sense of urgency, that major government programs such as Medicare and Medicaid shift money to primary care and away from the non-primary care specialties, which are so highly reimbursed in our present system. The report concluded that:

> *High-quality primary care is the foundation of a robust health care system, and perhaps more importantly, it is the essential element for improving the health of the U. S. population. Yet, in large part because of chronic underinvestment, primary care in the United States is slowly dying [31].*

4.2 Coalition of primary care organizations

A coalition of 7 primary care organizations, representing 400,000 members and diplomates, has come together to emphasize the urgent need for primary care to serve as the foundation of the U. S. health care system. These include the national organizations in family practice, general internal medicine, and general pediatrics. Together, they call for a new paradigm for primary care to be established based on coordination and continuity of comprehensive person-based care for the majority of health care conditions, with the capacity to decrease disparities and inequities. They also bring a unified voice calling for payment and regulatory reform to stabilize and strengthen practice [32].

4.3 Current approaches to health care reform

Three major reform alternatives will be considered in a deeply polarized Congress with corporate lobbyists descending on Washington D. C. to try to ward off reform one more time. Here are briefly encapsuled summaries of the alternatives.

4.3.1 Building on the ACA

The ACA has been helpful as an incremental step to needed reform by bringing health insurance to some 20 million people since its passage in 2010, mostly through expansion of Medicaid in 31 states. It has also provided coverage to 8 million Americans who lost coverage during the pandemic [33].

On the other hand, these points show how far short from needed reform that this alternative is:

"It will still be just another Band-Aid on a broken system without universal coverage.

- It has failed to contain costs, and will continue to do so since a profiteering, inefficient private insurance industry is left in place.

- Insurance and health care will remain unaffordable and inaccessible for a large part of our population.

- Continuing inequities, with many Americans still delaying or foregoing essential care.

- Health insurance still pricey and volatile as employer-based coverage is further stressed.
- Regulation of network size has been inadequate as has been gaming by insurers.
- Many insurers abandon markets that are not sufficiently profitable, often with little advance notice.
- A continued Medicaid coverage gap exists in the 12 states that refused to expand Medicaid" [34].

4.3.2 A public option

This was included in the ACA in 2010 whereby private non-profit CO-OPs were established to sell insurance in an effort to compete with private insurers under the same rules and on a level playing field. The hope was that they could compete, reduce costs, and increase the value of health insurance. They failed to do so, however, and only 5 of the initial 23 CO-OPs survive to this day, serving just 1 percent of the 11 million people who initially obtained this coverage through the ACA's exchanges [35].

Unfortunately, the public option of one kind or another is still being talked about in some circles, despite this lesson that we should have learned—incremental steps leaving the private health insurance industry in place, which has been subsidized by government funds for many years, will never achieve universal coverage.

4.3.3 Single-payer Medicare for all

This is the only way forward that can get bring system reform to our present non-system, with its inadequate access, unaffordable prices and costs, unacceptable quality, and widespread disparities. A fix can be on the way if we can muster the political will to enact an updated Medicare for All bill now in the House of Representatives in Congress, H. R. 1976. As stated by Rep. Pramila Jayapal (D-WA), one of its two lead sponsors, when the bill was introduced:

> *While this devastating pandemic is shining a bright light on our broken, for profit health care system, we were already leaving nearly half of adults under the age of 65 uninsured or underinsured before COVID-19 hit. And we were cruelly doing so while paying more per capita for health care than any other country in the world [36].*

Among its many benefits, H. R. 1976, when enacted, will bring:

- A new system of national health insurance with comprehensive benefits based on medical need, not ability to pay, and with full choice of hospitals,
- physicians, and other health professionals anywhere in the country.
- Coverage for all medically necessary care, including outpatient and inpatient services; laboratory and diagnostic services; dental, hearing and vision care; prescription drugs; reproductive health, including abortion; maternity and newborn care; mental health services; and long-term care and supports.

- Administrative simplification with efficiencies and large-scale cost controls, including negotiated fee schedules for physicians and other health professionals, global annual budgeting of hospitals and other facilities, and bulk purchasing of drugs and medical devices.

- Cost savings that will enable universal coverage through a single-payer, not-for-profit public financing system.

- Elimination of cost-sharing at the point of care, such as co-pays and deductibles, as well as the current need for pre-authorization through private insurers.

- Establishes an Office of Health Equity to monitor and eliminate health disparities and promote primary care.

- Sharing of risk for the costs of illness and accidents across our entire population of 330 million Americans [37].

It is little known that our multi-payer private health insurance industry has been propped up by various subsidies from the federal government for many years,

	ACA	Public option	Medicare for all
Access	Restricted	Restricted	Unrestricted
Choice	Restricted	Restricted	Unrestricted
Cost containment	Never	Never	Yes
Quality of care	Unacceptable	Unacceptable	Improved
Bureaucracy	Large, wasteful	Large, wasteful	Much reduced
Universal coverage	Never	Never	Yes
Accountability	No	No	Yes
Sustainability	No	No	Yes

Table 1.
Comparison of three reform alternatives based on evidence.

	ACA	Public option	Medicare for all
Health care a human right?	No	No	Yes
Commodity for sale?	Yes	Yes	No
Profits to service ethic?	No	No	Yes
Medical need vs. ability to pay?	No	No	Yes
Full choice of physician & hospital?	No	No	Yes
Accessible, reliable, efficient?	No	No	Yes
Not for profit, reduced waste?	No	No	Yes
Population-based shared risk?	No	No	Yes
Science-based?	No	No	Yes
Common good, public interest?	No	No	Yes

Table 2.
Comparison of three reform alternatives based on values.

averaging about $685 billion a year today [38]. Well known economist Gerald Friedman, who has studied the costs of Medicare for All for more than ten years, estimates that we would have saved more than $1 trillion in 2019 had it been in place at that time [39].

The U. S. has tried market-based alternatives for many years, and they have all failed the public interest. Privatization and commodification of health care leads to higher prices and costs, decreased access and worse outcomes of care, as well as more bureaucracy and waste. **Table 1** compares our three reform alternatives in terms of experience and evidence, and **Table 2** compares them in terms of values [40].

5. Whither the future of primary Care in the U. S.?

5.1 Corporate alliances against reform

The COVID-19 pandemic exposed the inadequacy of our system to deal with its disastrous consequences. As the urgency for health care reform has grown in its aftermath, including support for universal coverage through a public financing system under Medicare for All, reactionary opposition from corporate stakeholders and their allies has increased apace, as these examples illustrate:

- Major insurers, hospitals, and some unions joined together under the banner of the Alliance to Fight for Health Care [41].

- The private health insurance industry has spread propaganda and disinformation about how unaffordable, disruptive, and unwanted such a government-based program would be [42].

5.2 Some continuing threats to primary care

5.2.1 Telehealth and corporatization

The growth of telehealth during the COVID-19 pandemic filled a pressing need for safe virtual medical visits. Because of its prevalence, it soon became reimbursed by insurers, typically at the same price as in-person consultations. Despite its utility in some circumstances, as we move beyond the pandemic, it poses a risk of worse care, price gouging, and more inequities since many patients in need may not have access to high-speed internet [43, 44]. Some employers and insurers, such as Amazon and United Healthcare, are promoting virtual first care plans as if they are as effective as in-person physician visits, despite the accumulating evidence that major conditions can be missed. Wall Street and venture capital have also discovered the profit potential of expanded telehealth [45]. with one recent example being the acquisition by Walmart of MeMD, a big telehealth provider [46].

5.2.2 Continued underinvestment in primary care

Primary care visits in the U. S. account for 35 percent of health care visits but make up about 5 percent of health care expenditures, compared to an average of 14 percent of all health care spending in OECD countries [47]. A promising development now is the expected introduction of legislation by Senator Bernie Sanders authorizing 14,000 new Medicare-supported residency programs over seven years. That bill, if enacted, would also importantly establish new criteria for the distribution of residency slots, with one half allocated for primary care [48].

Another way that the government could, and should address the shortage of primary care physicians is to establish ways that can cover their debt, now averaging $200,000 for medical school graduates, if they enter primary care. Reimbursement policies should also be changed to more highly value time-intensive care involved in primary care with fewer currently overly reimbursed procedures driving high costs of care by other more procedurally oriented specialties [49].

6. Conclusion

As is obvious from the foregoing, the U. S. still lacks a primary care base for its health care system, despite a long struggle over many decades. Health care services are still treated as a commodity for sale on in a largely unfettered marketplace. Although the ideologic claim that the competitive free market will contain costs has been proven conclusively false, the political battle continues over the role of government vs. an open market. It has become obvious to much of the public and many health policy experts that the time has come to put in place a system of universal coverage based on a service ethic for the common good. As Winston Churchill observed many years ago:

> *You can always count on Americans to do the right thing— after they've tried everything else.*

That time has finally come, so let us hope for the future!

Author details

John Geyman
Emeritus of Family Medicine, University of Washington School of Medicine, Seattle, WA, USA

*Address all correspondence to: jgeyman@uw.edu

References

[1] 1931-1967 distribution of physicians in the U.S. by major professional activity and specialty. GP, 1969; 40: 193.

[2] Geyman, JP. Family medicine as an academic discipline: progress, challenges and opportunities. J Fam Pract 1990: 31 (3): 297-303.

[3] *Co-Chairs' Summary of the Conference. Who will provide primary care and how will they be trained?* New York. Josiah Macy, Jr. Foundation, 2010.

[4] Auerbach, DI, Buerhaus, PI, Staiger, DO. Implications of the rapid growth of the nurse practitioner workforce in the U. S. *Health Affairs* 2020; 39 (2): February.

[5] Zhu, JM, Polsky, D. Private equity and physician medical practices—Navigating a changing ecosystem, *N Engl J Med* 2021; March 18.

[6] Hancock, C, Garrison-Jakel J, Jordan, V et al). Why family physicians should not "just" be family physicians: Rethinking physician roles in community health centers and beyond. *FPM* 2020; January/February.

[7] Abbott, B. Burnout strikes mid-career physicians hard. *Wall Street Journal* 2020; January 16: A 3.

[8] Boodman, SG. lSpurred by convenience, millennials often spurn the 'family doctor' model. *Kaiser* Health News 2018; October 9.

[9] Franki, R. Wait times for family physician visits up almost 10 days since 2014. Family Practice News 2017; April 6.

[10] Tseng, P, Kaplan, RS, Richman, JD et al. Administrative costs associated with physician billing and insurance-related activities at an academic health system. JAMA 2018; February 20.

[11] Nichols, LM et al. Are market forces strong enough to deliver efficient health care systems? Confidence is waning. Health Affairs 2004; 23 (2): 8-21.

[12] Blumenthal, D, Collins, SR, Radley, DC. 2017 Commonwealth Fund International Health Policy Survey of Older Adults in 11 countries. New York. *The Commonwealth Fund* 2017; December 1.

[13] Bynum, JPW, Fisher, ES. *Is primary care worth saving? Access to primary care and health system performance.* Ibid # 3.

[14] Basu, S, Berkowitz, SA, Phillips, RL et al. Association of primary care physician supply with population mortality in the United States, 2005-2015. *JAMA Intern Med* online 2019; February 18.

[15] Kravit, SJ, Shore, AD, Miller, R, Green, GB, Kolodner, K et al. Health care utilization and the proportion of primary care physicians. Am J Med 2008; 121 (2): 142-148.

[16] Starfield, B. Shi, L, Macinko, J. Contribution of primary care to health systems and health. Milbank Q 2005; 83 (3): 457-502.

[17] Franks, P, Fiscella, K. Primary care physicians and specialists as personal physicians: health care expenditures and mortality experience. J Fam Pract 1998; 47: 103-104.

[18] Baicker, K, Chandra, A. Medicare spending, the physician workforce, and beneficiaries' quality of care. *Health Affairs* (Millwood) 2004; 23: 184-189.

[19] Ibid# 3, p. 19.

[20] Landro, L. Medication overload. *Wall Street Journal* 2016: October 1: D 1.

[21] Valderas, JM, Starfield, B, Forrest, CB, Sibbald, B, Roland, M. Ambulatory

care provided by office-based specialists in the United States. Annals Fam Med 2009; 7 (2): 104-111.

[22] Pitts, SR, Carrier, ER, Rich, EC, Kellermann, AL. Where Americans get acute care: Increasingly, it's not at their doctor's office. Health Affairs 2010; 29 (9): 1620-1628.

[23] Basu, S, Phillips, RS, Phillips, R et al. Primary care finances in the United States amid the COVID-19 pandemic. *Health Affairs* online 2020; June 25.

[24] Slavitt, A, Mostashari F, COVID-19 is battering independent physician practices, STAT 2020; May 28.

[25] Ungar, L. Thousands of doctors' offices buckle under financial stress of COVID. *Kaiser* Health News 2020; November 30.

[26] Levy, NN. A primary care physician for every American, science panel urges. *Kaiser Health News* 2021; May 4.

[27] Knight, V. American medical students less likely to choose to become primary care doctors. *Kaiser Health News* 2019; July, 3.

[28] Stevens, RA. *The Americanization of family medicine: Contradictions, challenges and change, 1969-2000*. In Keystone III. The Role of Family Practice in a Changing Health Care Environment: A Dialogue. Conference Proceedings. The Robert Graham Center. American Academy of Family Physicians. Washington, D.C., 2001:19, 22.

[29] Geyman, JP. *Hijacked: The Road to Single Payer in the Aftermath of Stolen Health Care Reform*. Friday Harbor, WA. *Copernicus Healthcare* 2010, 227-231.

[30] News staff. NASEM report heralds primary care evolution, urges action. *AAFP News*, American Academy of Family Physicians. Kansas City, MO, 2012; May 4.

[31] Ibid # 26.

[32] New Primary Care Paradigm. Primary care speaks as one. (https://www.newprimarycareparadigm.org/) [Accessed 2021-05-28]

[33] Goldstein, A. Pandemic job losses drive more people to sign up for ACA plans. The Washington Post 2020; December 19.

[34] Geyman, JP. *America's Mighty Medical-Industrial Complex: Negative Impacts and Positive Solutions*. Friday Harbor, WA. *Copernicus Healthcare*, 2021, 264.

[35] Galewitz, P. *Kaiser Health News*. Only three of 26 Obamacare-era non-profit co-ops will soon remain. Fortune 2020; September 6.

[36] Jayapal, P. As quoted by Wilkins, B. 'Everyone in, nobody out': Jayapal, Dingell introduce Medicare for All Act with 112 co-sponsors. Common Dreams 2021 March 17.

[37] Rogers, S. Introducing the new (and improved) Medicare for All Act of 2021. Press release. Physicians for a National Health Program. Chicago, IL, 2021; March 17.

[38] Ockerman, E. It costs $685 billion a year to subsidize U. S. health insurance. *Bloomberg News* 2018; May 23.

[39] Friedman, E. *The Case for Medicare for All*. Medford, MA, *Polity Press*, 2020, 62-63.

[40] Ibid # 34, 272-273.

[41] Grant, C. PhRMA heads for a deals spree. Wall Street Journal 2020; December 31.

[42] Potter, W. I used to be a propagandist for insurance companies. Learn the four truths the insurance industry doesn't want Americans to see. *Tarbell* 2019; April 30.

[43] Rosenthal, E. Telemedicine is a tool, not a replacement for your doctor's touch. *New York Times* 2021; April 29.

[44] Kendrick, K. As telemedicine replaces the physical exam, what are doctors missing? *NPR* 2020; August 31.

[45] Gormley, B. Telemedicine startups seek to build on 2020 momentum. *Wall Street Journal* 2021; January 5: B 3.

[46] Walmart Health to acquire telehealth provider MeMD, *Business Wire* 2021; May 6.

[47] News staff. NASEM report heralds primary care evolution, urges action. *AAFP News* 2021; May 4.

[48] Cohen, A. Sanders says U. S. physician shortage is a 'solvable problem.' *Roll Call* 2021; May 20.

[49] Lazris, A, Roth, A, Brownlee, S. No more lip service; it's time we fixed primary care (Part Two). *Health Affairs Blog* 2019; November 18.

Chapter 3

Patient-Centred Point-of-Care Testing: A Life-Changing Technology for Remote Primary Care

Brooke Spaeth, Susan Matthews and Mark Shephard

Abstract

Point-of-care (POC) testing has proven to be a life-changing and transformational technology for patients with acute, chronic, and infectious diseases who live in regional and remote Australia. This technology facilitates patient-centred test results, of equivalent laboratory quality, that are rapidly available to inform clinical and public health decisions with immediate impact on case management. Traditionally, POC testing in high-middle income countries has been most widely used in tertiary or acute care settings to provide rapid diagnostic results for emergency departments, intensive care units, operating theatres and outpatient clinics. However, in low-middle income countries, POC tests are commonly used during antenatal and perinatal care for infectious disease detection, such as Human immunodeficiency virus (HIV) or syphilis, where laboratory services are too expensive, inaccessible, or non-existent. Similarly, the application of POC testing in primary care settings in Australia offers improved healthcare benefits to geographically isolated regional and remote communities, where access to laboratory-based pathology testing is poor and the burden of disease is high. Evidence-based data from research in established primary care POC testing networks for acute chronic, and infectious disease is used to describe the clinical, cultural, and economic effectiveness of POC technologies. Innovative solutions to address current barriers to the uptake of POC testing in primary care settings, which include clinical and cultural governance, high staff turnover, operator training and competency, device connectivity, quality testing, sustainable funding strategies, and the need for regulatory requirements are also discussed. POC testing can provide practical and resourceful opportunities to revolutionise the delivery of pathology services in rural and remote primary care sectors, where the clinical and community need for this technology is greatest. However, several barriers to the scale-up and sustainability of POC testing networks in these settings still exist, and the full potential of POC testing cannot be realised until these limitations are addressed and resolved.

Keywords: Primary health care, point-of-care testing, patient-centred care, remote, Australia

1. Introduction

Primary health care describes the first contact an individual with a health concern has with the health system that is not related to a hospital visit. This may include health promotion, prevention, early intervention, treatment of acute conditions, and management of chronic conditions or infectious disease [1].

In 2015–2016, the proportion of the Australian health budget spent on primary health care (approximately 35%, representing approximately $AUS 59 billion) was similar to that of country's hospital services (39%, representing approximately $AUS 66 billion), reflecting the vast and diverse geographical and cultural requirements for health care services in the country [2]. In rural and remote Australia, healthcare services in primary care differ to that in urban or metropolitan areas. Primary healthcare facilities are generally small, with less infrastructure to provide a broad range of health services to a wide geographically distributed population [3]. In addition to a lack of resources, the health of those living in rural and remote Australian locations is also poorer, with the life expectancy for both males and females decreasing with increasing remoteness [3]. The workforce of Australian rural and remote primary health care relies more on general practitioners (GPs) to provide health care services, either on-site, or more recently via telehealth consultations [4, 5]. The remote primary healthcare sector is also largely supported by nurses and Aboriginal Health Practitioners [6]. Due to the high proportion of Aboriginal and Torres Strait Islander people living in remote Australia, health services in these regions are provided by either: (i) Aboriginal Community Controlled Health Services (ACCHOS), which are funded by the Australian Government and administered by a Board comprising Aboriginal and Torres Strait Islander representatives from the respective community or (ii) State or Territory funded health services [7]. With the burden of acute, chronic, and infectious diseases amongst Aboriginal and Torres Strait Islander people higher than that of the non-Indigenous population and the highest Indigenous disease rates correlating with degree of geographic remoteness [3], the overarching Indigenous governance of ACCHOs assists in the delivery of culturally safe health services to address health inequity in Australia [7].

Point-of-care (POC) testing refers to pathology testing performed in a clinical setting at the time of patient consultation, generating a rapid test result that enables timely clinical decision making for patient care [8]. POC testing has proven to be a transformative and life-changing technology for health services and patients in remote Australian communities. From the patient perspective, POC testing provides a convenient and accessible 'one-stop' health service. In this context, POC testing empowers the patient to be accountable for their own health, eliminating the need for multiple follow-up visits to the health services to access diagnostic test results and commence treatment or other interventions. It is also assumed that POC testing reduces patient anxiety associated with waiting for pathology results as test results can be obtained quickly and discussion with the treating clinician can commence immediately. From a clinical perspective, POC test results allow the health practitioner to make immediate and informed decisions for patient management, including the rapid initiation of treatment and/or alternative health intervention strategies. From a cultural perspective, POC testing has enabled Aboriginal and Torres Strait Islander people without life-threatening conditions to be safety monitored and/or treated in their own community [9]. Thus, POC testing not only averts costly medical evacuations, but also allows First Nation people to remain on 'Country' with community and cultural support during the recovery period. Additionally, POC testing assists remote communities by building local health workforce capacity and facilitating an extended scope of practice for Aboriginal Health Practitioners, who can be trained to conduct POC testing. In qualitative surveys, Aboriginal Health Practitioners reported being trained and competent in POC testing as "empowering them to care for patients in their local communities" [10].

DOI: http://dx.doi.org/10.5772/intechopen.100375

2. Examples of primary care POC testing networks in Australia

The Flinders University International Centre for Point-of-Care Testing (ICPOCT) is a specialist POC test provider, with over 20 years of experience in the establishment, management, and evaluation of best-practice POC testing to improve access to routine pathology services. At present, the ICPOCT independently manages five POC testing networks and is a collaborating partner with the Kirby Institute at the University of New South Wales (UNSW) on a further two POC testing networks. **Table 1** summarises the ICPOCT and collaborative partnership POC testing programs indicating the POC test device used, the POC test/s performed, the time taken to generate the POC test result, and the number of participating health clinics. The complexity of the POC methodologies and device types used across these POC testing programs ranges from simple, lateral flow rapid antibody tests with qualitative results (e.g. used to detect *Treponema pallidum* (Syphilis) infection) to complex, gold-standard, nucleic acid amplification tests (NAATs) which utilise safe, closed cartridge test systems for the qualitative detection of infectious disease RNA (e.g. used to diagnose SARS-CoV-2 (COVID-19) infection) or DNA (e.g. used to detect *Chlamydia trachomatis* (Chlamydia), *Neisseria gonorrhoeae* (Gonorrhoea) and *Trichomonas vaginalis* (Trichomonas) infections) or the quantitative detection of infectious disease RNA viral load (e.g. used for diagnosis and monitoring of Hepatitis C (HCV) infection).

POC testing program name	POC device used	POC test/s performed	Time for POC test result/s (mins)	No. of clinics
QAAMS	Siemens DCA	HbA1c^	7 min	238
	Vantage	Urine ACR#	6 min	
NT i-STAT	Abbott i-STAT	Electrolytes (sodium and potassium), glucose, Hb~, urea, creatinine, Cardiac troponin I Blood gases – pH, pO2, pCO2, base excess; lactate INR*	2 min 10 min 2 min 5 min	86
COVID-19**	Cepheid GeneXpert	SARS-CoV-2+	45 min	83
TTANGO (Test, Treat and Go)**	Cepheid GeneXpert	Chlamydia, Gonorrhoea and Trichomonas	60–90 min	55
ESR	Abbott Syphilis TP	Syphilis	15 min	84
Syphilis WA	Abbott Syphilis TP	Syphilis	15 min	41
NT WBC DIFF	Radiometer (HemoCue) WBC DIFF	Total WBC count plus five-part differential	5 min	20

*^Haemoglobin A1c, #albumin:creatinine ratio, ~Haemoglobin, *International Normalised Ratio, +Severe Acute Respiratory Syndrome Coronavirus 2, **Partnership POC testing program with the Kirby Institute, University of New South Wales.*

Table 1.
Summary of primary care POC testing networks managed by the ICPOCT (Flinders University) alone, or in collaborative partnership with the Kirby Institute (UNSW).

The POC testing programs described in **Table 1** are primarily focussed in rural and remote Australian primary care settings, with the general location of health services participating in the seven networks represented in the series of maps in **Figure 1(A–F)**. Indicative of the clinical need for diagnostic test provision by POC testing, it is notable that over 50% of the health services participating in the Aboriginal and Torres Strait Islander COVID-19 POC testing program are located more than 10 hours' drive from a laboratory testing facility and thus complement laboratory services [11]. In addition, primary health care services particularly in the most remote parts of Australia (notably the Northern Territory and north-west and central Western Australia) actively participate concurrently in up to six POC testing networks so that they can facilitate a broad range of on-site diagnostic tests for patient centred-care (**Figure 2**).

The Quality Assurance in Aboriginal Medical Services (QAAMS) POC testing program for diagnosis and management of diabetes and renal disease, the Aboriginal and Torres Strait Islander COVID-19 (COVID-19) POC testing program, the Test, Treat ANd GO (TTANGO) POC testing program for sexually transmitted disease

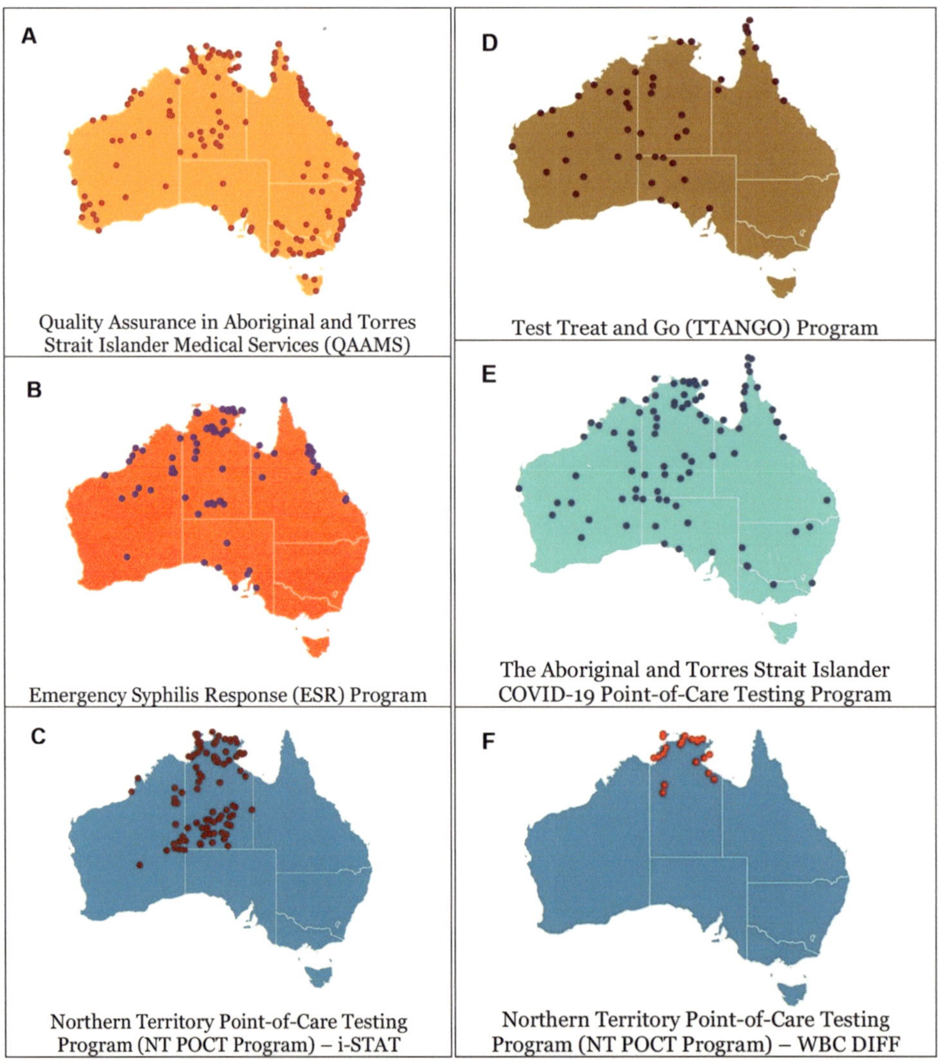

Figure 1.
(A–C). *Point-of-care testing network maps under the jurisdiction of the ICPOCT.* **(D–F)**. *Point-of-care testing network maps under the jurisdiction of the ICPOCT.*

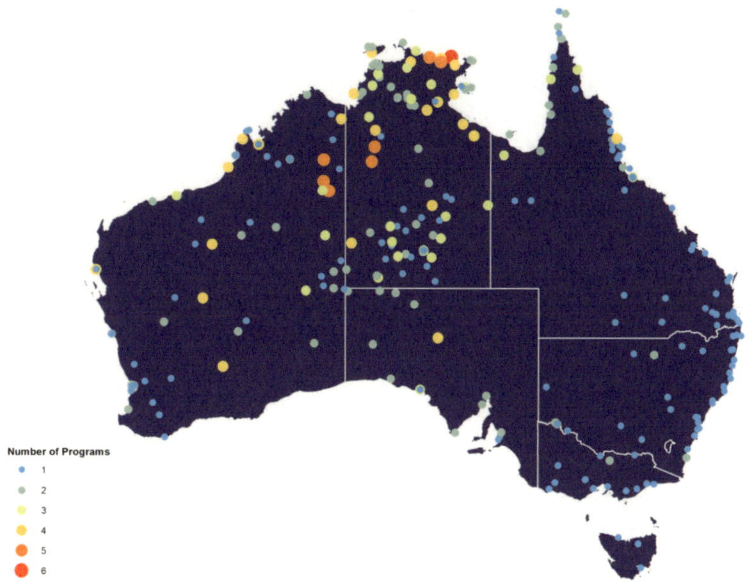

Figure 2.
Merged ICPOCT point-of-care network maps.

diagnosis and monitoring and the Enhanced Syphilis Response (ESR) POC testing program are all funded by the Australian Government and thus include site selection criteria for national testing coverage, complementary to regional and urban laboratories. The COVID-19 and ESR POC testing programs were both established as 'emergency response' initiatives under the directive of the Australian Government [12]. The Northern Territory (NT) i-STAT POC testing program for acute disease management (blood gas, urea/electrolytes and cardiac troponin I), and Prothrombin (PT)/International Normalised Ratio (INR) monitoring and the White Blood Cell (WBC) Differential (DIFF) POC testing program for sepsis diagnosis are both funded by the NT Government Department of Health and include site selection criteria and enrolled health services specific to the remote Central and Top End regions of the NT. Similar to the NT funded POC program, the Western Australian (WA) Syphilis POC testing program is a state-based network funded by the WA Government Department of Health, facilitating syphilis POC testing in broad range of decentralised setting including: remote, regional, and urban community services, hospital maternity wards, peer harm reduction outreach services, homeless health care services and prisons.

The QAAMS Program has been operational for 22 years [13], and is economically sustainable at the health service level due to the availability of specific public health (Medicare Benefits Schedule (MBS)) rebates for: (i) glycated haemoglobin A1c (HbA1c) POC testing for diabetes diagnosis or management and (ii) urine albumin to creatinine ratio (UACR) POC testing for monitoring of renal disease, when the quality management is compliant under the auspices of the QAAMS program. At present, the QAAMS program supports the only POC testing performed outside of an accredited laboratory facility within Australia to have approved MBS item numbers. Dependant on regulatory system development to facilitate accreditation processes, an equivalent MBS rebate may soon expand to HbA1c POC testing performed independently within GP clinics in Australia.

Like the QAAMS program, the NT i-STAT POC testing also has significant longevity, with 13 years of continuous operation and government funding [14]. The sustainability of the NT i-STAT POC testing program is largely associated with the demonstrated economic benefits of POC testing in acute clinical management in remote primary health care, due to averted medical evacuations [15]. The NT government has also recently expanded the NT POC testing network to facilitate twenty total white blood cell (WBC) count POC devices (HemoCue, Radiometer) with 5-part WBC differential for sepsis management in the Top End NT sites.

The COVID-19 and TTANGO POC testing programs, and more broadly a National Health and Medical Research Council (NHMRC) Centre for Research Excellence for Infectious Disease POC Testing in the Asia-Pacific, are representative of a long-term, collaborative partnership between the ICPOCT and the Kirby Institute (UNSW). The COVID-19 and TTANGO POC networks use gold-standard NAATs within a safe, closed cartridge testing system to detect the respective infectious disease RNA or DNA, using the Cepheid GeneXpert POC device [11]. Some POC devices, including the GeneXpert (Cepheid), offer broad clinical application with extensive test menus as well as the rapid development of newer *in vitro* diagnostic tests utilising the same test cartridge design and device infrastructure. Utilising this capability, a new collaborative POC testing network (with the Kirby Institute) for capillary (fingerstick) hepatitis C viral load using the GeneXpert will be established in late 2021 to early 2022. Funded by the Australian Government, the National Hepatitis C (HCV) POC testing program, will focus on the application of a Class IV *in vitro* diagnostic POC test in a broader range of primary care settings. Justice health services, safe drug injection rooms, community needle and syringe programs and homeless health services will be eligible as high prevalence, decentralised test sites for enrolment into the National HCV POC testing program. The overall aim of the National HCV POC testing program is to support Australia's contribution to the World Health Organization's global goal to eliminate hepatitis as a public health threat by 2030 [16]. In addition, future infectious disease research to investigate the potential advantages of using multiplexed POC test cartridges, such as respiratory panel, including Influenza A, Influenza B (Flu A/B), COVID-19 and Respiratory Syncytial Virus (RSV) in primary care settings using the GeneXpert in Australia may also be warranted.

3. Clinical outcomes

In the Australian primary care POC testing programs described above, the evidence-based clinical outcomes that benefit patient care following the introduction of POC testing as summarised in **Table 2**.

POC network	Clinical focus	POC test	Outcome measure
QAAMS	Chronic	HbA1c^	Improvement in glycaemic control
NT i-STAT	Acute	Cardiac Troponin I	Early risk stratification for acute coronary syndrome
		Potassium	Stabilisation of patients with severe vomiting or diarrhoea
	Chronic	INR*	Improved time in therapeutic range
NT WBC DIFF	Acute	White blood cell count	Assisted with patient triage
TTANGO	Infectious	Chlamydia and Gonorrhoea	Reduction in time to treat
COVID-19	Infectious	SARS-CoV-2+	Early detection/reduced time to treat

*^Haemoglobin A1c, *International Normalised Ratio, +Severe Acute Respiratory Syndrome Coronavirus 2.*

Table 2.
Summary of key clinical outcome measures from Australian primary care POC testing networks.

Briefly, some of these benefits include: (i) improved glycaemic control in patients with type 2 diabetes [17], (ii) improved time in therapeutic range for warfarin-treated patients [18], (iii) early risk stratification for acute coronary syndrome [19], (iv) assisted triaging and determination of need for medical evacuation in septic patients with four different medical presentations and [20] (v) reduced time to treat sexually transmitted disease [21, 22]. These positive clinical outcomes associated with the introduction of POC testing in remote primary health care services highlight some of the life-changing impact that this type of technology can offer in decentralised patient care settings.

4. Patient-centred outcomes

POC testing enables the patient to be at the centre of healthcare processes. Diagnostic POC test results are rapidly available within the initial on-site consultation, inform prompt patient management decisions and even may fast-track additional clinical investigations, as required. For the patient, this eliminates the need to attend separate phlebotomy collection services and return for a follow-up visit to discuss laboratory test results, thus making POC testing patient-centric and linkage to care convenient. Other cited patient benefits for POC testing include: (i) increased adherence to diabetes medication [23], (ii) reduced pain and/or anxiety associated with capillary, rather than venous blood collection, particularly for elderly or paediatric patients, and (iii) an increased likelihood of patients consenting to diagnostic testing [24]. Furthermore, the wait for the return of diagnostic test results is a reported cause of anxiety [25, 26], so in this context, POC testing may also reduce overall patient anxiety or stress related to waiting for laboratory test results [27].

In acute care settings, POC testing changes lives, with rapid results informing prompt diagnosis and rapid initiation of patient stabilisation and/or treatment. An example is the use of i-STAT cardiac troponin I POC testing within the NT POCT Program for the immediate diagnosis of non-ST elevation myocardial infarction (non-STEMI) in remote patients [19]. In this scenario, if cardiac troponin I POC testing was not available, non-STEMI events may not be quickly diagnosed and treated [19]. Without POC testing, remote patients who often miss scheduled dialysis due to cultural and community obligations may also become acutely ill. In these cases, the i-STAT POC device can be used to detect critical levels of hyperkalaemia, so that immediate treatment with calcium gluconate to lower cardiac risk can be initiated [19]. In dehydrated patients, with acute vomiting or diarrhoea, i-STAT POC testing facilitates frequent monitoring of the patient's electrolyte levels during stabilisation with IV or oral fluid administration [19]. In these remote primary care settings, POC testing facilitates information to avert the time, inconvenience and cost of unnecessary transfer to a tertiary medical facility. Averting unnecessary medical evacuations can be particularly significant for Aboriginal and Torres Strait Islander people who live in remote communities, where the dislocation from community and Country can cause significant mental distress [28, 29]. Though brief, these examples illustrate how POC testing can be a life-changing technology at the individual patient level, particularly for those who would not otherwise be able to access timely pathology results.

5. Public health outcomes

Beyond the individual patient level, POC testing programs have the capability to facilitate broader public health benefits. For example, one of the site selection criteria for the COVID-19 POC Program was that primary health care services were located a minimum of 2 hours' drive from an existing COVID-19 testing laboratory facility and serviced predominately Aboriginal and Torres Strait Islander communities of greater than 500 people. Indicative of the clinical need of the COVID-19 POC testing program for remote, priority communities, by the completion of site enrolment, approximately half of the participating health services were located more than 10 hours' drive from a laboratory testing facility and included several health services located on remote islands requiring dedicated flights to reach mainland COVID-19 testing services [11]. To provide wider COVID-19 testing access, a hub and spoke model was established, whereby nasopharyngeal swab samples were collected from patients in neighbouring spoke communities, placed into virus inactivating molecular transport media and transported to the hub testing sites. The hub and spoke POC testing model expanded total testing capability to approximately one hundred and fifty at-risk communities (from eighty-eight hub testing sites). With over 32,000 patient COVID-19 POC tests performed nationally to date, the Aboriginal and Torres Strait Islander COVID-19 POC testing program has significantly reduced the time required for isolation/quarantining for vulnerable individuals who test negative as the turn-around time for COVID-19 results is reduced from an average three-day turn-around time for laboratory testing to less than one hour per test for POC testing. Applying similar assumptions of community size, remoteness and access to laboratory test facilities as those reflected in the site selection criteria for the COVID-19 POC testing program, mathematical modelling used to inform the Australian Government, indicated that by reducing the time for COVID-19 case identification and isolation from ten days, the COVID-19 transmission rate changed from that associated with an uncontrolled outbreak to a either a significant surge or controlled condition, for reductions of five or three days, respectively [30]. The ability to reduce isolation and quarantining duration for negative COVID-19 cases is particularly relevant to remote communities within Australia, where self-isolation may be difficult due to a lack of suitable housing and/or over-crowding, or impacted by other social and cultural determinants [31]. Most recently, the Aboriginal and Torres Strait Islander COVID-19 POC testing program rapidly scaled-up the number of GeneXpert devices, competent staff and test cartridges available to deliver COVID-19 results required for case identification, contact tracing and public health response in emergency outbreak local government areas of New South Wales (NSW), as opposed to waiting several days for laboratory results [32]. In addition, in outbreak response areas and other under-resourced remote communities, the COVID-19 POC testing program has enabled mobile employees to be rapidly screened using molecular-based COVID-19 testing. In these circumstances, POC testing has assisted with crisis workforce capacity, whilst also providing a level of protection to the local communities by minimising COVID-19 infection transmission risk.

For the TTANGO Program, a significantly improved "time to treat" sexually transmitted Chlamydia and Gonorrhoea infections in comparison to regular test processes was demonstrated by the application of rapid POC molecular-based test results in remote Australian communities [22]. For sexually transmitted diseases, prompt diagnosis and public health notification, patient education and treatment hasten STI contact tracing aiming to decrease the onward and/or vertical transmission of STIs in the community.

For chronic diseases, such as type 2 diabetes and the associated renal complications, the availability of POC testing provides extended scope for consented screening tests of at-risk populations. In these patients, POC testing facilitates linkage to early education of the disease and lifestyle interventions that can afford the patient improved long-term monitoring and improvement of their long-term health outcomes, without a loss to follow-up [33]. Early identification and treatment of chronic disease, such as type 2 diabetes, that slows the progression of disease complications, may in turn may lead to reduced burden on tertiary care facilities.

6. Economic outcomes

Data which demonstrates the cost effectiveness of POC testing, comparative to laboratory testing, is essential for ensuring the initial feasibility and sustainability of POC testing models worldwide. Previously, our research demonstrated savings of over $21 million per annum for the NT Government through averted unnecessary medical retrievals as a result of acute i-STAT POC test results in the remote communities within the NT POCT program [15]. Similarly, economic savings have been reported in rural New Zealand hospitals, where an annual cost reduction of more than $NZ 450,000 was realised from POC testing through a decreased number of hospital transfers and an increase in the hospital discharge rates [34]. In the United Kingdom, a primary care study also reported that POC testing was cost effective, in comparison to laboratory testing, when used to perform routine health checks as the results were available at the first consultation [33]. A review of POC testing health economics in remote primary health care settings also provided general support for POC testing benefits to health services outweighing the associated costs [35]. In Australia, the Medical Services Advisory Committee (MSAC), is an independent, non-statutory committee established by the Minister for Health, that is responsible for the appraisal of new medical services proposed for public funding, including POC testing. MSAC provides advice to the Australian Government on whether a new medical service should be publicly funded, based on an assessment of its comparative safety, clinical effectiveness, cost-effectiveness, and total cost, using the best available evidence. Amendments and reviews of existing Medical Benefits Schedule (MBS) services, including POC tests, are also considered by MSAC. In this regard, evidence-based Australian economic cost-effectiveness data that supports the application of POC testing in primary care is paramount to ensure the economic sustainability of POC testing through public funding models.

7. Key elements of POC testing networks

Best-practice POC testing models are underpinned by a common set of core elements as illustrated in **Figure 3**. These include: (a) a defined clinical or public health need for POC testing, (b) appropriate site selection, targeting priority populations with high disease prevalence or risk, (c) clinical and cultural governance of the POC testing procedures and patient test results, (d) engagement with the community to ensure patients are educated in understanding the health benefits of POC testing and can be easily linked to appropriate models of healthcare, (e) robust training and competency assessment processes for health professionals conducting POC testing to minimise patient harm, (f) continuous surveillance of analytical quality using internal quality control and external quality assurance programs, with prompt and appropriate actioning to maintain satisfactory analytical quality standards, (g) provision of an intensive level of technical and scientific troubleshooting support to maximise device operation and result quality, (h) connectivity and real-time reporting systems to ensure rapid patient result transmission, complete patient result audit trails and allow appropriate public health notification of required patient infectious diseases (noting that POC connectivity systems can be complex to integrate and sustain in primary care settings and are not always cost-effective) and (i) supply and logistical management of equipment, reagents and consumables, often to remote locations with sub-tropical or tropical climates. Once established, ongoing evaluation of the clinical effectiveness and utility, cultural effectiveness, benefits to patient and community, cost-effectiveness, risk management assessments and limitations of each POC testing program is integral to ensure

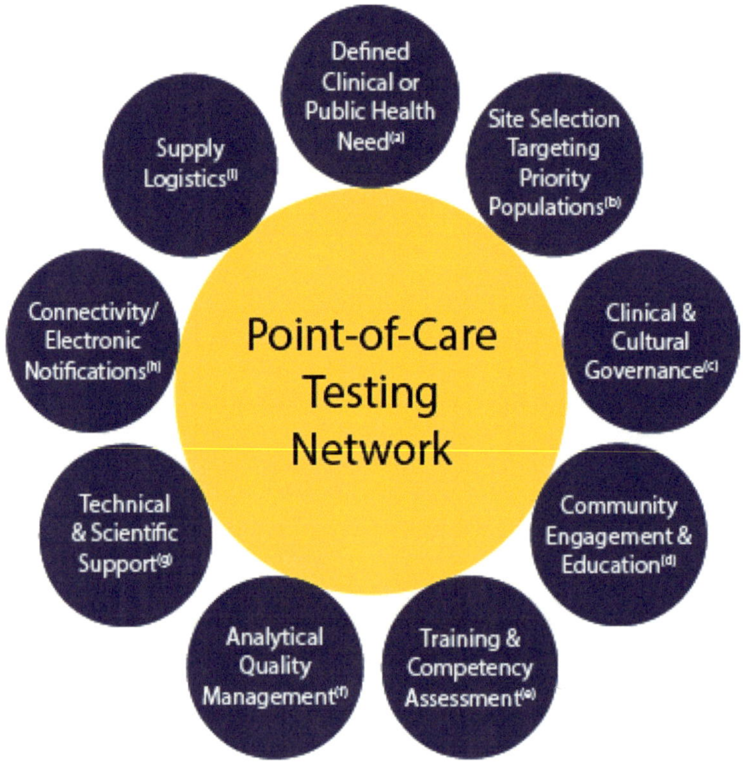

Figure 3.
Key elements of a best-practice point-of-care testing network.

continual quality process improvement. The sustainability of best-practice POC testing is reliant on the continual development of national and international of POC testing implementation and management policies and robust guidelines that arise from translational research of best-practice POC testing networks [36].

Whilst the POC testing models described have been implemented with financial support from Australian Commonwealth and/or State Governments, several challenges currently exist when considering the sustainability and viability of POC testing in remote locations. These are summarised in **Table 3**. At a local community level, there can be saturation of health services with POC testing network requirements regarding staff capacity. This is particularly evident when individual health services enrol in multiple POC testing programs and experience rapid staff turnover. For ACCHOS, Commonwealth support for targeted POC testing remote staff, to be managed through the national leadership body for Aboriginal Community Controlled Health Organisations (NACCHO) may assist in alleviating future workforce shortages. More broadly, feasibility studies and predictive modelling can be applied to remote primary care scenarios prior to implementation to ensure POC testing networks are scaled to maximise reach and outcome benefits. At a national level, the existing regulatory framework for POC testing performed outside a clinical laboratory setting is somewhat rudimentary, with newer POC technologies superseding the 2015 National Pathology Accreditation Advisory Council (NPAAC) Guidelines for POC testing. Broader clinical acceptance and public health funding of POC test results performed in decentralised Australian primary care settings is reliant of the development and evaluation of a formal regulatory system for best-practice POC testing performed outside that of an accredited laboratory framework. In addition, further integration of patient POC test results from primary

Challenge	Comment
Governance	A multidisciplinary management committee, with representatives from clinical, scientific, nursing, Indigenous, industry, collaborative research partners and Government stakeholder groups, provides maximum support for the POC testing model
Staff Turnover	There is a requirement for flexible options for training delivery to ensure operator competency standards are maintained in the face of high staff turnover
Devices and Consumables	There needs to be commitment from industry for continuity of cold-chain supply of cartridges and QC material to remote health services
Connectivity	A cost-efficient solution for the electronic capture and transfer of pathology results to a patient management system is critical for network sustainability
Government funding/ support	Government support for POC testing and a reimbursement (rebate) mechanism for cartridge costs is essential for long-term viability of a POC testing network
Accreditation	Accreditation frameworks for POC testing networks need to be flexible and adaptable to the many different clinical settings in which POC testing is undertaken
Saturation of POC testing uptake	When a service is engaged in multiple POC testing networks, the imposition of training needs and different quality management testing materials and regimes can impede the uptake and acceptability of POC testing, even in settings where significant clinical needs exist
Scalability of POC testing networks	Prior to implementation of POC testing, the capacity for scalability of the POC testing model needs to consider not just analytical quality and clinical benefits of POC testing but also factors such as acceptability and cost effectiveness

Table 3.
Summary of key challenges for POC testing in the primary care setting.

care settings into patient management systems and/or electronic medical records is required to overcome the current lack of accessibility of historical POC test results which may be useful for patient management (e.g. past history of sexually transmitted diseases). It is only when the current challenges POC testing are overcome that the full benefits of POC testing in decentralised primary care settings can be widely recognised, accepted, and sustained [37].

In summary, POC testing in Australia can be considered a life-changing technology as it can: a) provide equity of access to pathology services in remote and under-resourced locations, b) support prompt medical evacuation and public health decisions c) be cost-effective, in comparison to laboratory testing or overall health service savings, if the network scale-up is optimised prior to implementation, and d) has capacity to deliver individualised patient-centred care. If the current challenges and barriers to POC testing sustainability can be further addressed, a wider range of clinical, public health and economic benefits could be realised through new and/or additional POC testing initiatives for high priority, at-risk populations, especially in rural and remote Australian communities.

Author details

Brooke Spaeth, Susan Matthews* and Mark Shephard
Flinders University International Centre for Point-of-Care Testing, Flinders Medical Health and Research Institute, College of Medicine and Public Health, Flinders University, Adelaide, South Australia, Australia

*Address all correspondence to: susan.matthews@flinders.edu.au

References

[1] Australian Government, *Primary Health Care - Frequently asked questions*, Department of Health, Editor. 2018, Public Health Network: Canberra, ACT. p. 2

[2] Australian Institute of Health and Welfare, *Australia's Health 2018: in brief*. 2018, AIHW: Canberra

[3] Australian Institute of Health and Welfare, *Rural & remote health*. 2019, AIHW: Canberra.

[4] Wakerman, J., et al., *Primary health care delivery models in rural and remote Australia – a systematic review*. BMC Health Services Research, 2008. **8**(1): p. 276

[5] Fisk, M., Livingstone, A. and Pit, S.W. *Telehealth in the Context of COVID-19: Changing Perspectives in Australia, the United Kingdom, and the United States*. Journal of Medical Internet Research, 2020. **22**(6): p. e19264

[6] Australian Government, *National Strategic Framework for Rural and Remote Health*. 2016, Department of Health,: Canberra

[7] Ong, K.S., et al., *Differences in primary health care delivery to Australia's Indigenous population: a template for use in economic evaluations*. BMC Health Services Research, 2012. **12**(1): p. 307.

[8] Shephard, M., Causer, L. and Guy, R. *Point-of-care testing in rural, remote and Indigenous settings*, in *A Practical Guide to Global Point-of-Care Testing*, M. Shephard, Editor. 2016, CSIRO: Melbourne, Australia. p. 343-354

[9] Shephard, M. and Gill, J. *The National QAAMS Program - A Practical Example of PoCT Working in the Community*. Clinical Biochemist Review, 2010. **31**: p. 105-109

[10] Shephard, M., et al., *Review of the cultural safety of a national Indigenous point-of-care testing program for diabetes management*. Australian Journal of Primary Health, 2016. **22**(4): p. 368

[11] Hengel, B., et al., *A decentralised point-of-care testing model to address inequities in the COVID-19 response*. The Lancet Infectious Diseases, 2020. 21(7): p. e183-190.

[12] Equity Economics, *Blueprint for the Future: Evaluation of NACCHO's Role under the Enhanced Syphilis Response*. A Report prepared for the National Aboriginal Community Controlled Health Organisation (NACCHO). 2021

[13] Regnier, T., et al., *Results From 16 Years of Quality Surveillance of Urine Albumin to Creatinine Ratio Testing for a National Indigenous Point-of-Care Testing Program*. Archives of Pathology & Laboratory Medicine, 2020. **144**(10): p. 1199-1203

[14] Matthews, S.J., et al., *Sustained Quality and Service Delivery in an Expanding Point-of-Care Testing Network in Remote Australian Primary Health Care*. Archives of Pathology & Laboratory Medicine, 2020. **144**(11): p. 1381-1391

[15] Spaeth, B., et al., *Economic evaluation of point-of-care testing in the remote primary health care setting of Australia's Northern Territory*. ClinicoEconomics and Outcomes Research, 2018. **10**: p. 269-277

[16] Australian Government, *Fifth National Hepatitis C Strategy 2018-2022*, Department of Health, Editor. 2018, Australian Government Department of Health: Canberra

[17] Shephard, M., *Cultural and Clinical Effectiveness of the 'QAAMS' Point-of-Care Testing Model for Diabetes*

Management in Australian Aboriginal Medical Services. Clinical Biochemist Reviews, 2006. **27**: p. 161-170

[18] Spaeth, B. and Shephard, M., *Clinical and Operational Benefits of International Normalized Ratio Point-of-Care Testing in Remote Indigenous Communities in Australia's Northern Territory.* Point of Care, 2016. **15**(1): p. 30-34

[19] Spaeth, B., Shephard, M. and Omond, R., *Clinical Application of Point-of-Care Testing in the Remote Primary Health Care Setting.* Quality in Primary Care, 2017. **25**(3): p. 164-175.

[20] Spaeth, B., et al., *Impact of point-of-care testing for white blood cell count on triage of patients with infection in the remote Northern Territory of Australia.* Pathology, 2019. **51**(5): p. 512-517

[21] Guy, R.J., et al., *A randomised trial of point-of-care tests for chlamydia and gonorrhoea infections in remote Aboriginal communities: Test, Treat ANd GO- the "TTANGO" trial protocol.* BMC Infectious Diseases, 2013. **13**(1): p. 485

[22] Guy, R.J., et al., *Molecular point-of-care testing for chlamydia and gonorrhoea in Indigenous Australians attending remote primary health services (TTANGO): a cluster-randomised, controlled, crossover trial.* The Lancet Infectious Diseases, 2018. **18**(10): p. 1117-1126

[23] Gialamas, A., et al., *Does point-of-care testing lead to the same or better adherence to medication? A randomised controlled trial: the PoCT in General Practice Trial.* Medical Journal of Australia, 2009. **191**(9): p. 487-491.

[24] Tang, R., et al., *Capillary blood for point-of-care testing.* Critical Reviews in Clinical Laboratory Sciences, 2017. **54**(5): p. 294-308

[25] Leekha, S., et al., *Patient Preferences for and Satisfaction with Methods of Communicating Test Results in a Primary Care Practice.* The Joint Commission Journal on Quality and Patient Safety, 2009. **35**(10): p. 497-501

[26] Meulbroek, M., et al., *BCN Checkpoint: same-day confirmation of reactive HIV rapid test with Point Of Care HIV-RNA accelerates linkage to care and reduces anxiety.* HIV Medicine, 2018. **19**: p. 63-65

[27] Shephard, M., et al., *Results of an Aboriginal community-based renal disease management program incorporating point of care testing for urine albumin:creatinine ratio.* Rural and Remote Health, 2006. **6**(4): p. 591.

[28] Conway, J., et al., *Indigenous patient experiences of returning to country: a qualitative evaluation on the Country Health SA Dialysis bus.* BMC Health Services Research, 2018. **18**:1010

[29] Worrall-Carter, L., et al., *Exploring Aboriginal patients' experiences of cardiac care at a major metropolitan hospital in Melbourne.* Australian Health Review, 2016. **40**(6): p. 696

[30] Australian Government, *Impact of COVID-19 in remote and regional settings: Theoretical modelling of how the health system can respond*, Department of Health, Editor. 2020, Commonwealth of Australia: Canberra

[31] Bailie, R.S. and Wayte, K.J., *Housing and health in Indigenous communities: Key issues for housing and health improvement in remote Aboriginal and Torres Strait Islander communities.* Australian Journal of Rural Health, 2006. **14**(5): p. 178-183.

[32] Australian Government, *Aboriginal and Torres Strait Islander Advisory Group on COVID-19*, Department of Health, Editor. 2020, Commonwealth Government of Australia: Canberra

[33] El-Osta, A., et al., *Does use of point-of-care testing improve*

cost-effectiveness of the NHS Health Check programme in the primary care setting? A cost-minimisation analysis. BMJ Open, 2017. **7**(8): p. e015494

[34] Blattner, K., et al., *Changes in clinical practice and patient disposition following the introduction of point-of-care testing in a rural hospital.* Health Policy, 2010. **96**(1): p. 7-12

[35] Wong, H.Y., et al., *Review of Health Economics of Point-of-Care Testing Worldwide and Its Efficacy of Implementation in the Primary Health Care Setting in Remote Australia.* Risk Management and Healthcare Policy, 2020. **13**: p. 379-386

[36] Shephard, M., *Principles of establishing and managing a point-of-care testing service*, in *A practical guide to global point-of-care testing*, M. Shephard, Editor. 2016, CSIRO Publishing: VIC. p. 16-28

[37] Shephard, M., et al., *The Benefits and Challenges of Point-of-Care Testing in Rural and Remote Primary Care Settings in Australia.* Archives of Pathology & Laboratory Medicine, 2020. **144**(11): p. 1372-1380

Section 2

Child Health in Primary Care

Chapter 4

The Newborn Baby Check

Harishan Tharmarajah

Abstract

The newborn baby check is often the first encounter a General Practitioner (GP) has with an infant and their family. It is an excellent opportunity to review the journey the family has taken antenatally, at the time of delivery and the weeks that have followed. It is also a time to detect and identify conditions that can be managed in their early stages. If untreated, some conditions can result in major morbidity. In this chapter we will look at what makes up a newborn baby check and important considerations to think about when undertaking this assessment. The examination is also performed in a systematic way to maximise the chance of detecting any abnormalities.

Keywords: newborn baby check, physical examination, screening, developmental hip dysplasia, cradle cap

1. Introduction

The newborn baby check is often the first encounter a General Practitioner (GP) has with an infant and their family. It is an excellent opportunity to review the journey the family has taken antenatally, at the time of delivery and the weeks that have followed. It is also a time to detect and identify conditions that can be managed in their early stages. If untreated, some conditions can result in major morbidity.

At the time of birth and discharge from hospital, the newborn will often have an examination performed [1]. Following this period, the family is introduced to their local maternal child health nurse who monitors the infant and discusses important topics such as feeding, growth, family supports and maternal and paternal mental health. Provided no concerns have been raised, the family will only need to present for the first time to the doctor at around 6–8 weeks. For this reason, the newborn examination we refer to in this chapter is one taken around this time.

Although the routine examination performed prior to a child being discharged from hospital is thorough, conditions can evolve or go unnoticed. It is important that we do not solely rely on the discharge check but it can serve as a good reference if the nurse or doctor raised a concern at the time.

2. History

Before the examination is performed, a brief history should be taken to help understand the infant in front of you.

The history should include the following:

- The antenatal history including maternal conditions that may impact the child

- Birth history
  - Mode of delivery
  - Time spent in hospital
    - Were any interventions required? i.e., oxygen, antibiotics etc.
  - Elaborate on feeding i.e., when it was established and if there have been difficulties
  - Weight, length and head circumference measured to date and how it is trending
- Any parental concerns
- Any concerns raised by the maternal child health nurse

3. Examination

From here, we can move onto the examination. A summary of the steps involved in the examination can be found at the end of the chapter. The examination should be systematically performed and an ideal method is to examine the front of the infant from head to toe and then turn them over and examine them from top to toe again. This chapter has been designed with that in mind and the examination should follow this structure were possible.

3.1 Exposure and positioning

The correct exposure for the examination is important because signs can be easily missed if they are not obvious to us. The best level of exposure is with the infant fully undressed and their nappy on. The nappy can be removed and replaced at the time of the genital and hip examination which gives the examiner confidence that they will not encounter any unfortunate surprises.

Positioning the newborn for the examination should rely on the principle of ensuring both the examiner and infant are comfortable. It would be appropriate to have the infant resting supine on a firm standard examination bed. Have the infant laying straight in front with their legs towards you and head away. If the infant is larger where it may compromise your ability to visualise distal parts of their body, laying them as you would an older patient perpendicular to you and examining them from their right is also fine. Being able to appreciate subtle asymmetry is the key so if you cannot achieve this, position the patient so you can.

3.2 General inspection

Look at the infant from a distance and comment on any dysmorphic features, deformities, rashes, skin lesions or skin colour changes [2–4]. Remember to repeat this process when examining the infants back.

Make a note of whether the child is comfortable or distressed. This can influence how we interpret signs throughout the examination.

3.2.1 Dysmorphic features

Being familiar with congenital conditions such as Down's syndrome (trisomy 21) can help the examiner look out for signs that are seen more often in these patients by association [5]. In trisomy 21 this may include epicanthic folds, hypotonia, a sandal gap, Simian creases, upslanting palpebral fissures and a protruding tongue [5].

3.2.2 Skin

Gross skin changes seen include pallor, cyanosis or icterus (jaundice).

Identify any obvious skin rashes at this step. Categorise skin rashes into normal and abnormal with normal rashes including those that are transient or birth marks and abnormal skin rashes being those that can indicate a congenital abnormality [6].

Initially comment on the type of rash identified i.e., pustules, vesicles, bullae, whether the skin is dry, erythematous or scaly [6]. From here it would be worth reviewing possible differentials for these findings as there may be several causes.

In the authors experience, commonly encountered skin lesions include heat rashes, haemangiomas, resolving milia, cradle cap, Mongolian spots and occasionally pityrosporum folliculitis [6].

3.3 Head

The head examination is next. At the level of the head, a few areas should be focussed on:

- Head shape
- Scalp
- Fontanelles
- Suture lines

3.3.1 Scalp

The main condition seen within the scalp at this age is seborrheic dermatitis or cradle cap [6, 7]. It presents from 2 weeks of age in some infants [6, 7]. It can present as redness through the scalp along with redness behind the ears and skin folds [6, 7]. More severe cases will have thick yellow plaques on the scalp [6, 7]. Although the cause is not clear, it is thought to be due to a combination of a type of yeast called *Malassezia* and abnormal sebum production [6, 7].

3.3.2 Fontanelles

At birth, the infant will have 6 fontanelles with the anterior fontanelle being the largest [8]. The anterior fontanelle is located between the two frontal and two parietal bones of the skull. The anterior fontanelle size varies greatly between infants with an average size of 2.1 cm reported in one study [8]. The initial size of the anterior fontanelle is not a strong indicator of when it will eventually close [8]. The average time for closure is 13.8 months [8]. Craniosynostosis is associated with early fontanelle closure, but given that approximately 1% of infants have closed fontanelles by the age of 3 months, a small fontanelle is not necessarily an indicator of an abnormality but careful reviews of head circumference can assist with knowing if a timely referral is required [8].

3.3.3 Shape, symmetry and suture lines

The shape and symmetry of the skull will give clues about plagiocephaly and craniocynostosis [9]. During the examination, carefully check if the skull appears asymmetrical or misshaped, feel the fontanelles and the suture lines. A hard raised suture line may indicate premature closure and careful review of the infant's head circumference will help determine if this finding is significant [9].

3.3.4 Head circumference

Remember to review the head circumference and trends from previous measurements to ensure there is no significant change within the period since birth.

3.4 Face

The face consists of structures including the eyes, nose, mouth and ears [10].

3.4.1 Eyes

Red reflex examination can help detect early stages of disease [11]. Using an ophthalmoscope, shine the light directly into both eyes through the pupil. If the retina appears white, it can indicate retinoblastoma and the absence of this red reflex with lens opacity may indicate congenital cataracts [11–13]. A prompt referral to an ophthalmologist is appropriate in these cases or if you are not sure a red reflex is properly elicited. To complete the eye exam, remember to comment on the external eye, eye movements and visual fixation. At this age, monitor concerns raised about visual fixation as strabismus might need to be considered and may only be obvious in the following months [14].

3.4.2 Nose

Remember that infants are obligate nose breathers and nasal congestion is common. Observe the nasal passage visually and describe whether they are patent and symmetrical.

3.4.3 Mouth

Using a gloved finger, place it in the infant's mouth and observe their suck reflex and check if it's coordinated. Also remember to feel the palate [10].

You may be asked to comment on whether the infant has a lip tie or tongue tie especially if the infant has had difficulties with feeding. A tongue tie (ankyloglossia) refers to a short lingual frenulum [15]. You can observe this by seeing if the tongue fails to stick out or converts to a heart shape when protruding out. The tongue tie can impact on a tongues range of movement and ability to function [15]. A lip tie refers to a short labial frenulum and this results in a lip that looks like it's stuck to the gum [15]. This may affect the infant's ability to latch properly when feeding [15].

3.4.4 Ears

Comment on the position and structure of the ear. Preauricular sinuses, skin tags or cysts should be followed up as they can be associated with congenital syndromes. It is hoped that these conditions have already been identified by this stage.

To complete the head exam, remember to comment on the neck. Torticollis is a condition that can affect an infant's range of neck movement [16]. Observing if the head looks tilted or if there's a preference to one side and restriction to full neck movement on examination can suggest torticollis [16]. Other opportunistic signs to look for are neck masses which can be associated with the thyroid or cervical chain lymph nodes [10].

3.5 Upper limbs

The upper limb exam is not too complicated. The aim is to check the general range of movement of the shoulder joints, elbows, hands and fingers. Assess the brachial pulses in both arms by placing a finger over the antecubital fossa. Count the number of fingers and look for webbing and check the palm for any deep creases.

3.6 Anterior chest

Comment on the shape and symmetry of the chest. Respiratory effort and rate should be looked at but in a well-baby this is usually normal. Using your thumb, check capillary refill time by placing it over the sternum and holding it there for 5 seconds. After letting go, the blood should return to the area within 4 seconds [17].

Auscultation of the heart will help identify any murmurs and additional heart sounds. In a child that is failing to thrive, looking for underlying heart disease is important [18].

Comment on the shape and position of the nipples. Evidence of breast buds and galactorrhoea may be present due to the maternal oestrogen effect and will resolve around the 2-month mark [19]. Seeking an endocrinologist opinion would be advisable if breast buds or galactorrhoea persists.

3.7 Abdomen

Comment on the shape and symmetry of the abdomen. Organomegaly can be detected by palpating the abdomen and feeling the liver, spleen and kidneys. It may be difficult to assess the abdomen if the infant is unsettled. Follow this by auscultating the abdomen for bowel sounds.

3.7.1 Umbilicus

Umbilical hernias are common and present in about 20% of newborns [20]. They can increase in size over the first few months of life [20]. Multiple references report that an umbilical hernia can be monitored if asymptomatic at this age [20]. Australian guidelines recommend that referral for such hernias wait until a child is 2 to 3 years of age and it is expected that up to 90% of hernias will close on its own by 5 years of age [20]. This is helpful to know when faced with a common presentation of a soft reducible umbilical hernia at this check.

3.7.2 Inguinal hernias

Inguinal hernias are common and present in up to 5% of newborns with a higher percentage seen in those born prematurely [20]. If present in an infant, a timely referral within 2–4 weeks is recommended [20]. This referral interval may vary for a neonate or an older child.

3.8. Genitourinary

3.8.1 Male genitalia

The penis should be observed and commented on for size, chordee and hypospadias [20, 21]. Chordee is when the penis is curved during an erection. Hypospadias is common and occurs in 1 in 125 males born [21]. It is a defect resulting in an opening of the urethra along the penile shaft, scrotum or perineum [21].

The scrotum should be felt for the presence of testes [21]. If they are empty, the examiner should locate the position of the testes. Maldescended testes may be "undescended" or "ectopic" [21]. The term undescended refers to a testis that presents within the normal line of descent and an ectopic testis is one outside this line. A retractile testis may be brought down by milking it down. A technique for examination would be to use one hand to lift up the suprapubic fat and then use two fingers of the other hand to palpate the areas of interest in the inguinal region with a circular motion [21].

Whilst examining the scrotum, look for the presence of a hydrocoele. This can be normal up until the age of 1 year for most infants [21]. If suspected, use an examination torch pressed against the side of the testis (transillumination) to confirm the presence of fluid surrounding the testis [22].

Signs of ambiguous genitalia may include a micropenis or bilateral undescended testes [23].

3.8.2 Female genitalia

The aim is to observe whether the genitalia is developing normally. Abnormal findings that may indicate ambiguous genitalia include clitoromegaly and fused labia [23].

3.9 Anus

After the genital examination, briefly look between the buttocks to observe the anus and particularly the skin around it. It's not uncommon to see a significant rash hidden within this area. There is no reason for performing a per rectal examination and this should not be done.

3.10 Lower limbs

3.10.1 Hips

The hip examination is a critical step during this examination as a delayed diagnosis of hip dysplasia can result in significant morbidity to the infant involved.

When taking the initial history, remember to go through potential risk factors for developmental hip dysplasia (DDH). Risk factors for DDH include being female, being a breech birth and having a family history of DDH [24]. Postnatally, some risk factors include tight swaddling of lower limbs in extension and adduction [24].

In those babies up to the age of 8 weeks, the Ortolani and Barlow test are the preferred tests to detect DDH [24]. Leg length discrepancy, asymmetric gluteal creases and restricted hip abduction are also helpful signs to work up a DDH.

The Ortolani and Barlow test are performed as follows. The Ortolani test checks to see if a dislocated hip can be relocated or reduced back into the hip joint [24]. By holding the flexed and adducted hip, abduct the hip while putting gentle upward pressure with your fingers on the greater trochanter [24]. If the test is positive, a "clunk" should be heard as the hip is reduced back into the joint [24]. The Barlow test aims to dislocate a hip that is sitting within the joint [24]. The test is performed with the hip adducted while gently putting pressure down in the direction of the examination bed [24]. During this step, the examiner may feel the hip move out of the acetabulum. This is a Barlow-positive test.

In situations where a hip is dislocated and irreducible, it will be interpreted as an Ortolani negative and Barlow negative test. In this scenario, checking if the hip can abduct completely will pick up this uncommon presentation [24].

3.10.2 Legs and feet

With both hands on the infant's knees, straighten their legs to see if the knees, medial malleoli and feet line up. Leg length discrepancy can be a sign of unilateral hip dysplasia.

As we did for the upper limbs, check the range of movement of the lower limbs by moving the joints at the level of the hips, knees and ankles. Check the feet to see if there is evidence of talipes [25]. Again, count the number of digits on the infant's feet as you did for the hands earlier.

3.11 Back

Now that the front of the examination is complete, you can turn the baby over onto their tummy and continue with the remainder of the examination with the infant in a prone position.

Observe the back of the head to look for skull moulding or rashes. If you are able to, observe the degree of neck control and position of the head. This may not be possible with all infants due to immaturity.

Look at the back to see if there are any skin rashes. Skin lesions are discussed earlier in the chapter but one in particular that is seen on the back are Mongolian spots.

Look at the positions of the scapula and buttocks to see if they are roughly symmetrical and in line with each other and then run your hand along the infant's spine to see if it's straight [10]. At the base of the spine, you may find clues for spina bifida including sacral dimples or tufts of hair [10].

3.12 Newborn reflexes

To finish off the examination, a screen for reflexes can be performed. This includes the stepping reflex, palmar grasps, moro reflex and rooting reflexes. Most of these reflexes should still be present. The stepping reflex tends to disappear around 2 months of age so this might not be illicited if the infant is close to 8 weeks when the exam is done.

3.13 Measurements and finishing the exam

Finish off by checking the infant's weight, head circumference and length. Remember to document the findings of the examination and arrange appropriate follow up for any abnormalities that need attention. Thank the patient's family and allow the family to dress the infant.

Newborn baby check
Introduce yourself and ask parents identifying questions i.e. name, age, date of birth
Wash hands
Exposure – undress the child leaving them in a nappy which will be removed at the time of the genital and hip exam.
Position – place the child on an examination bed which is relatively firm and start with them in the supine position
General inspection
• Is the child comfortable or not? • Look for skin rashes • Dysmorphic features
Head
• Scalp – palpate fontanelles, palpate sutures, head shape and symmetry, look for cradle cap. Opportunistically measure head circumference • Eyes – red reflex • Ears – low set, pre-auricular skin tags, deformity • Nose – patency of nostrils and symmetry • Mouth – Suck reflex, cleft lip, tongue tie and lip tie
Shoulders and arms
• Check the shoulders are well aligned with appropriate range of movement • Check arm movements including general tone. Comment on palmar creases, number of fingers (more = polydactylyl or less = syndactyly)
Anterior chest
• Capillary refill time • Observe breathing • Auscultate heart and comment on heart sounds
Abdomen
• Comment on size including distension and observed masses • Palpate for masses and organomegaly • Auscultate for bowel sounds • Comment on the umbilicus for hernia
Femoral region
• Check pulse • Check for inguinal hernias
Genital examination
• Male – palpate testes and comment on if they have descended, review penis and comment on presence of hypospadias or chordee. Check for signs of ambiguous genitalia including a micropenis or absent testes. • Females – check for fusion of labia and clitoromegaly to suggest ambiguous genitalia

Newborn baby check
Hips and legs
• Check for asymmetric creases • Look for limited abduction of both hips • Perform Barlow and Ortolani test • Check leg length – both true and apparent • Check range of movement of lower limbs • Comment on feet for talipes or deformities • Count the number of toes (more or less)
Change baby's position so they are now on their tummy (prone position)
• Assess head control
Posterior chest
• Auscultate lung fields • Feel the spine – comment on how straight it is • Look for signs of spina bifida distally including tufts of hair and sacral dimples • Look for any more skin rashes
Reflexes
• Grasp • Rooting reflex • Moro (startle reflex) • Walking reflex

Table 1.
Summary of the newborn baby check.

4. Conclusion

This completes the overall baby check. A summary of the key steps to the examination can be found in **Table 1**.

Conflict of interest

The author declares no conflict of interest.

Notes/Thanks/Other declarations

Thank you to my wife Dr. Majuri Tharmarajah for your support and encouragement during this chapter writing process.

Key Points

- The newborn check performed at roughly 6–8 weeks is often the first encounter the GP has with the infant and their family

- Having a systematic approach to the newborn check will reduce the chance of missing important signs

Author details

Harishan Tharmarajah
Monash University, Victoria, Australia

*Address all correspondence to: harishan.tharmarajah@monash.edu

References

[1] Ghabra K et al. Streamlining the process of Newborn and Infant Physical Examination (NIPE). Arch Dis Child Educ Pract Ed. 2019;104:270-271. DOI: 10.1136/archdischild-2018-314914

[2] Drapkin Z et al. Is my baby normal? A review of seemingly worrisome but normal newborn signs, symptoms and behaviours. American Journal of Emergency Medicine. 2019;37:1153-1159. DOI: https://doi.org/10.1016/j.ajem.2019.03.028

[3] Fasher M. The 6 week check. Australian Family Physician. 2012;41(5):288-290.

[4] Piejko W. The postpartum visit. Australian Family Physician. 2006;35(9):674-678.

[5] Devlin L, Morris PJ, Accuracy of the clinical diagnosis of Down syndrome. Ulster Med J. 2004;73(1):4-12.

[6] Su J. Common rashes in neonates. Australian Family Physician. 2012;41(5):280-286

[7] Clark GW, Pop SM, Jaboori KA. Diagnosis and treatment of seborrheic dermatitis. Am Fam Physician. 2015;91(3)185-190.

[8] Kiesler J, Ricer R. The Abnormal Fontanel. Americal Family Physician. 2003;67(12):2547-2552.

[9] CDC. Facts about Craniosynostosis [Internet]. 2020. Available from: https://www.cdc.gov/ncbddd/birthdefects/craniosynostosis.html [Accessed: 2021-07-15]

[10] Quach A. Common neonatal presentations to the primary care physician. Australian Journal of General Practice. 2018;47(4):193-198.

[11] Leong SS et al. The Red Reflex Exam: Highlighting the Importance of Physical Exam Maneuvers. 2020;34:383-384. DOI: https://doi.org/10.1016/j.pedhc.2020.04.003

[12] Viquez MV, Wu L. Sensitivity and specificity of the red reflex in Costa Rican newborns. Arch Soc Esp Oftalmol. 2020;95(1):4-8.

[13] Prajantawanich K et al. Clinical outcomes and prognosis of Thai retinoblastoma patients. Paediatrics international. 2021;63:671-677. DOI: 10.1111/ped.14498

[14] Ahmed N, Fashner J. Eye Conditions in Infants and Childre: Amblyopia and Strabismus. FP Essent. 2019;484:18-22.

[15] Ray S, Golden WC, Walsh J. Anatomic Distribution of the Morphologic Variation of the Upper Lip Frenulum Among Healthy Newborns. JAMA Otolaryngology-Head & Neck Surgery. 2019;145(10):931-938. DOI: 10.1001/jamaoto/2019/2302

[16] Mikov A. Torticollis in an infant. Am Fam Physician. 2007;76(8):1197-1198.

[17] Fleming S et al. Capillary refill time in sick children: a clinical guide for general practice. Br J Gen Pract. 2016;66(652):587-588. DOI: 10.3399.bjpg16X687925

[18] Menon G, Poskitt EM. Why does congenital heart disease cause failure to thrive? Arch Dis Child. 1985;60(12):1134-1139. DOI: 10.1136/adc.60.12.1134

[19] Madlon-K DJ. 'Witch's Milk' Galactorrhea in the Newborn. Am J Dis Child. 1986;140(3):252-253.

[20] Teague W, Sebastian KK. Paeditric surgery for the busy GP – Getting the referral right. Australian Family Physician. 2015;44(12):890-894.

[21] Stokowski LA. Hypospadias in the neonate. Adv Neonatal Care. 2004;4(4):206-215. DOI: 10.1016/j.adnc.2004.05.003

[22] Koski ME et al. Infant communicating hydroceles – do they need immediate repair or might some clinically resolve? J Pediatr Surg. 2010;45(3):590-593. DOI: 10.1016/j.jpedsurg.2009.06.026.

[23] Mayo Clinic. Ambiguous Genitalia – Symptoms and Causes [Internet]. 2018. Available from: https://www.mayoclinic.org/diseases-conditions/ambiguous-genitalia/symptoms-causes/syc-20369273 [Accessed: 2021-07-15]

[24] Williams N. Improving early detection of developmental dysplasia of the hip through general practitioner assessment and surveillance. Australian Journal of General Practice. 2018;47(9):615-619.

[25] Gray K, Gibbons P. Clubfoot – Advances in diagnosis and management. Australian Family Physician. 2012;41(5):299-301.

Chapter 5

COVID-19 Transmission in Children: Implications for Schools

Evelyn Mendoza-Torres, Franklin Torres, Wendy Rosales-Rada, Liliana Encinales, Lil Avendaño, María Fernanda Pérez, Ivana Terán, David Vergara, Estefanie Osorio-Llanes, Paige Fierbaugh, Wendy Villamizar, Aileen Y. Chang and Jairo Castellar-Lopez

Abstract

The COVID-19 pandemic poses multiple issues of importance to child health including threats to physical health and disruption of in-school learning. This chapter reviews what is currently known about COVID-19 epidemiology, presentation, pathophysiology, case definitions, therapies, and in-school transmission in children. COVID-19 has some unique characteristics in children including the rare yet severe Multisystem Inflammatory Syndrome in Children (MIS-C) that may be related to acquired immune responses. There are limited studies to date to define therapeutic guidelines in children, however consensus recommendations from multiple organizations are summarized including the use of immunomodulatory therapies (intravenous immunoglobulin, steroids, anakinra and tocilizumab), antiplatelet (aspirin) and anti-coagulant (low molecular weight heparin) therapies. Finally, considerations for safe return to the classroom are discussed including strategies for optimized student to teacher ratios, hand washing, social distancing, sibling pairing and staged re-opening strategies.

Keywords: COVID-19, children, SARS-CoV-2, MIS-C, Kawasaki

1. Introduction

Coronavirus disease (COVID-19) is caused by a virus in the beta-coronavirus family, SARS-CoV-2. The specific characteristics of COVID-19 infection in children are of particular interest. Little is unknown about the epidemiology of SARS-CoV-2 transmission in children. The transmissibility of COVID-19 in general is greater than other coronaviruses [1]. COVID-19 is typically asymptomatic or presents with mild symptoms [1, 2]. Coronavirus causes up to 14% of respiratory infections in children however influenza virus infections remain the most common pediatric infections. Those most likely to be infected with SARS-CoV-2 are children under three years of age [1] and more specifically, children under one year of age. Furthermore, according to a metanalysis, 50% of children under the age of five infected with COVID-19 were infants under one year of age, male and were exposed to the infection via community transmission [3]. This highlights the importance of testing and disease monitoring in families with infants and young children.

COVID-19 disease is less common in children than adults [1, 2]. The lower incidence of COVID infection in children may be explained by the lower expression of Angiotensin Converting Enzyme 2 (ACE2) and TMORSS2 (protease) in alveolar epithelial cells in children in comparison to adults and decreased viral transmission [2–4]. The higher rates of infection seen in infants may be due to their immature immune system, which not only increases their risk of infection, but also makes vaccination less effective [1, 3]. Maternal immunization may provide maternal-fetal protection [1, 3, 4]. In addition, maternal immunization may protect young children as transmission from COVID-positive mothers to children has been documented [1, 4]. Therefore, targeted maternal vaccination may be an important tool to protect vulnerable infants and children.

2. SARS-CoV-2 overview

Since the discovery of SARS in 2002, including the recent detection of SARS-CoV-2, seven strains of human coronavirus have been identified, defined by the WHO as "A broad family of viruses that cause various conditions, from the common cold to more serious illnesses, such as the Middle East respiratory syndrome coronavirus and the one that causes severe acute respiratory syndrome." Among them, SARS-CoV-2, the virus responsible for the 2019 coronavirus disease, originated in Wuhan (Hubei, China) in December 2019, was declared a pandemic by the WHO in March 2020 and is defined as an "enveloped positive-sense single-stranded RNA virus 80-220 nm in diameter. The envelope has corona-shaped peaks 20 nm in length that resemble the corona of the sun under electron microscopy" [5].

The coronaviral genome encodes four major structural proteins, the spike protein (S), the nucleocapsid protein (N), the membrane protein (M), and the envelope protein (E), all of which are necessary to produce a structurally complete viral particle. Unlike the other major structural proteins, N is the only protein that functions primarily to bind to the CoV RNA genome, forming the nucleocapsid. Although N is largely involved in processes related to the viral genome, it is also involved in other aspects of the CoV replication cycle and the host's cellular response to viral infection [6]. Furthermore, protein S plays a crucial role in the entry of the virus into host cells and the structural capabilities of this newly discovered SARS-CoV-2 enhance its intended actions. Because these prominent peaks are the first point of contact with host receptors, therapeutic strategies can be applied to prevent their binding to target receptors and prevent viral entry into host cells [7].

The WHO reported that the most common symptoms of COVID-19 are fever, dry cough and tiredness. Other less frequent symptoms include nasal congestion, headache, conjunctivitis, sore throat, diarrhea, loss of taste or smell, skin rashes or changes in the color of the fingers or toes [8]. These symptoms are usually mild and begin gradually. Approximately 80% of people recover without the need for hospital care, while approximately 1 in 5 people who contract COVID-19 end up with severe symptoms and experience breathing difficulties. Elderly people with underlying diseases, such as high blood pressure, heart disease, lung problems, diabetes or cancer are more likely to suffer from an aggravated clinical stage [8].

The primary route of transmission to humans was zoonotic, via interaction with animals. A hypothesis that was later confirmed and defined by the WHO was that the virus was spread through droplets that are expelled from the nose or mouth of an infected person by coughing, sneezing, or talking, and even by touching infected objects and surfaces, such as tables, doorknobs, and railings, so that healthy people can become infected if they touch those objects or surfaces and then touch their eyes, nose, or mouth [9].

Kotfis & Skonieczna-Żydecka identified viral cells in gastrointestinal biopsy samples, including those that belonged to patients who had left the hospitals, which may partially explain gastrointestinal symptoms, potential recurrence, and transmission of SARS by persistent shedding in stool as well. Specifically, the virus is protein molecule covered by a protective lipid layer that is absorbed into ocular, nasal, oral and gastrointestinal mucosal epithelial cells and replicates there [10].

2.1 ACE2: The door to SARS-CoV2

The renin angiotensin aldosterone system (RAAS) is the primary regulator of plasma volume, maintaining cardiovascular and fluid homeostasis. This system plays a protective and adaptive role against risk phenomena, such as hypotension, sodium or water deprivation, and in turn, its dysregulation has implications in the development of hypertension and other cardiovascular diseases [11].

Activation of the classic RAAS pathway begins in the juxtaglomerular apparatus with the release of preformed renin from its prorenin precursor, secondary to baroreflex, beta-adrenergic or molecular stimuli in the macula densa. Renin takes the hepatic precursor angiotensinogen and converts it into angiotensin I (Ang I) [11]. This decapeptide has no specific known physiological action and ends up being converted into octapeptide angiotensin II (Ang II) by angiotensin converting enzyme (ACE), which is located primarily in cells of the pulmonary endothelium, as well as other tissues [11].

Ang II acts on AT1 receptors and exerts powerful vasoconstrictive, profibrotic and proinflammatory effects [6]. The action of Ang II on the AT2 receptor generates the opposite vasodilator and antiproliferative effect [11].

ACE is an essential component of the renin angiotensin aldosterone system, functioning as a transmembrane protein with two N- and C-terminal active catalytic domains. The C-terminal domain generates the soluble carboxypeptidase that removes the carboxy-terminal dipeptide of Ang I, generating Ang II, while hydrolysis of the vasodilator peptides, called bradykinins, occurs by the enzymatic action of both domains. ACE2 is a monocarboxypeptidase homologous to ACE but has only one transmembrane helix, an intracellular segment, and N- and C-terminal domains with a single enzymatic active site, endowing ACE with distinct characteristics [11].

ACE2 is also homologous to ACE, which plays a role in the cleavage of angiotensin I into angiotensin-(1–9) and the vasoconstrictor peptide angiotensin II in the vasodilator angiotensin-(1–7). Consequently, ACE2 acts as the entry point into cells for various coronaviruses [12]. By cleaving angiotensin II and increasing vasodilator angiotensin-(1–7), it can act as an important regulator of cardiac function and plays a protective role in acute lung injury.

Possible antitumor effects of ACE2 and future therapeutic prospects for cancers have been reported for ACE2. Unfortunately, ACE2 has a high affinity for severe acute respiratory syndrome coronavirus 2 (SARS-CoV-2) [7], which may explain its manifestations at the respiratory level.

2.2 SARS-CoV-2 and ACE2

Viral infections bind their viral structures with receptors on the host cell surface. Although it has been shown that there are several coronaviruses that cause human diseases, only three of them bind ACE2: SARS-CoV, SARS-CoV-2 and HCoV-NL63, with SARS-CoV being responsible for a health emergency known as severe acute respiratory syndrome (SARS) in 2003 in China. Curiously, glycoprotein S is characterized as the critical determinant for viral entry into host cells, consisting of two functional subunits, S1 and S2. The S1 subunit recognizes and binds to the host receptor through the receptor-binding domain (RBD), while S2 is responsible for fusion with the host cell membrane. MERS-CoV uses dipeptidyl peptidase-4 (DPP4) as an entry receptor, while SARS-CoV and SARS-CoV-2 use ACE2, which is abundantly expressed in pulmonary alveolar epithelial cells and enterocytes, suggesting glycoprotein S as a potential drug target to stop SARS-CoV-2 entry [13].

However, SARS-CoV infection downregulates surface expression of the binding protein (ACE2), a fundamental component for the entry of the host cell. Low ACE2 expression is associated with a greater severity of the infection in epithelial cells of the human respiratory tract [14].

3. Presentation of COVID-19 in children

The presentation of COVID-19 in children differs somewhat from the presentation seen in adults. COVID-19 in children most commonly present with fever and cough [15] and gastrointestinal symptoms such as diarrhea and vomiting. Gastrointestinal symptoms are reported in a considerable portion of cases [1, 3, 15] which is less characteristic of adult cases. While some patients develop respiratory distress syndrome, the severe form of COVID-19 is less common in children as compared to adults [15] and the mortality rate of COVID-19 in children is <0.1%. COVID-19 infection in children may present with anemia, thrombocytopenia, hypoalbuminemia, and altered INR [12]. Other laboratory abnormalities may include leukopenia, lymphopenia, increased transaminases and inflammatory markers such as procalcitonin and C-reactive protein [1, 16]. While patchy lesions in pulmonary lobules of children are identified on chest computed tomographic scans with moderate infection, the ground-glass opacities which are a typical feature in adults are rare in pediatric patients [15]. The mechanisms underlying the unique presentation of COVID-19 in children are unknown and further study is required to understand why the presentation differs in children.

IgA antibodies have been found both in Kawasaki disease and in COVID-19 cases with vasculitis. This suggests that MIS-C could be triggered by a COVID-19 infection and that similar to Kawasaki disease, IgA antibodies are produced. These antibodies have receptors in endothelial, mucosal, and cardiac cells [1]. This hypothesis that the vasculitis is mediated by IgA antibodies may explain the similarities between the two pathologies and the potential post-infectious origin [1].

Another common pathology associated with COVID-19 in children is "COVID toes", or chilblains. This primarily affects the toes but can also be seen in the heels and fingers, presenting as red-purple, tender, or itchy bumps [17]. The cause appears to be the result of vascular damage through the impact of the SARS-CoV-2 virus on endothelial cells as well as T-cells CD4, CD8, and B-cells [1].

3.1 Multisystem inflammatory syndrome in children (MIS-C)

While most cases of COVID-19 in children range from asymptomatic to mild/moderate disease, severe disease has been documented in children. Some countries have documented cases of COVID-19 in children under the age of five [1, 18] with an acute inflammatory syndrome called Multisystem Inflammatory Syndrome in Children (MIS-C) [1, 3] that is similar to Kawasaki disease [1, 3, 19] that is a medium-vessel vasculitis [1, 18] and typically presents 2 weeks after initial infection. The most commonly affected vessels in MIS-C are the coronary arteries [20].

Most infants (more than 80%) infected with SARS-CoV-2 develop mild COVID-19 with a natural history similar to other self-limited respiratory viruses, without complications [21]. But in the case of children who develop MIS-C, severe systemic inflammation occurs with elevated pro-inflammatory cytokines and acute phase reactants, affecting multiple organ systems including the gastrointestinal, respiratory, cardiovascular, renal, hepatic, hematological and nervous systems among others [22, 23]. The most comprised organ systems include the gastrointestinal, dermatologic and cardiovascular organ systems.

MIS-C typically presents with fever lasting more than 4 days [1, 12, 16] as the universal characteristic. Gastrointestinal symptoms [1, 3, 12] may also present as the first symptoms [24]. These include abdominal pain, vomiting [1, 3, 12], and diarrhea [24]. Neurological symptoms such as headache, sensory disturbances, and meningeal signs [1, 24] can also be present. Hemodynamic instability can be present as well as cardiovascular complications including heart failure, myocarditis and pericarditis. Laboratory values may demonstrate elevations in troponin, proBNP, ferritin, C-reactive protein, and D-dimer with neutrophilia and lymphopenia [1, 12, 16]. Patients may also develop shock [1, 16] with single or multi-organ dysfunction requiring intensive care, mechanical ventilation [1, 12] and/or extracorporeal membrane oxygenation (ECMO) [3, 12]. Cytokine storm and ferritin counts >1400 μg/L may present in older patients [1]. In summary, MIS-C presents as a hyperinflammatory syndrome with gastrointestinal, neurologic and cardiac manifestations.

3.2 Epidemiology of MIS-C

In April 2020, the United Kingdom reported a series of cases with clinical presentation similar to Kawasaki disease (KD), toxic shock syndrome (TSS) and hyper-inflammatory state that had an epidemiological link with SARS-CoV-2 [25]; since that event, clinically similar cases have been reported in other parts of the world, including France, Switzerland, the United States, Canada, Norway, among others [18, 26–28]. After the notification of these cases, an expert consensus among critical care, infectiology, rheumatology and hematology pediatric subspecialists named this new clinical condition "Multisystemic inflammatory syndrome in children".

The worldwide incidence of SARS-CoV-2 in children under 18 years of age is 322 cases per 100,000 inhabitants and the incidence of MIS-C is 2 per 100,000 inhabitants [29]. The first cases were reported in the United Kingdom, as well as in other places in Europe (France, Germany, Greece, Italy, Luxembourg, Portugal, Spain, Switzerland, Sweden), later in Canada and the United States [30]. Most cases of MIS-C occur in previously healthy children older than 8 years and adolescents. Children of African-American and Latino ancestry are the most affected, in contrast to classic KD, which typically affects children under 5 years of age and has a higher incidence in East Asia and in children of Asian descent [31].

The first report of MIS-C was a series of 8 cases receiving medical assistance in southeast England [25]. Subsequently, 3 series of cases were reported in England ($n = 58$), France and Switzerland ($n = 35$) and New York ($n = 33$). In most cases, the children were previously healthy, that is, without underlying comorbidities (88% in the United Kingdom, 89% in France, and 79% in the New York series) [12, 18]. In those with comorbidities, obesity and asthma were the most frequent. The average age was 10 years with an age range of 1 to 17 years [32].

To date, the prognostic factors of severe disease in children are not known, however, a French prospective study that took data from 397 children admitted for COVID-19 in 60 hospitals identified three factors that were independently associated with severe evolution of the disease in the univariate analysis: age ≥ 10 years (OR: 3.4; $p = 0.034$), hypoxemia (OR: 8.9; $p = 0.0004$) and C-reactive protein ≥80 mg / L (OR: 6; $p = 0.012$) [33]. Meanwhile, research presented at the 2021

ENDO Virtual Congress revealed that children with type 1 diabetes whose glycated hemoglobin (A1c) is greater than 9% have a higher risk of severe forms of COVID-19 [34]. At the moment many efforts are being carried out in order to better characterize the pediatric population at risk, with the aim of identifying susceptible populations early and preventing life-threatening events in infants.

3.3 The epidemiology of MIS-C in the Americas

As of January 14, 2021, a total of 17 countries in the Region of the Americas have officially notified PAHO / WHO or have published information through an official website a total of 2,737 cumulative confirmed cases of MIS-C that coincide chronologically with COVID-19, including 78 deaths [18]. Of the total reported cases, 66% were between 0 and 9 years old at the time of illness and only 10% were in the age group between 15 and 19 years. Regarding the outcome of these cases, the highest proportion of deaths is observed in the age group of 15 to 19 years. Regarding the distribution by sex, 56% of the cases are male [35].

The countries with the highest number of confirmed cases are the United States with 1,659 cases, Brazil with 631 cases, Chile with 151 cases, the Dominican Republic with 102 cases, and Argentina with 65 cases [36]. So far in Colombia, 3 cases of MIS-C have been identified in the district of Cartagena. These cases were detected through media monitoring. The incidence rate of COVID-19 in people under 18 years of age per 100,000 inhabitants in Colombia by department, shows us that the departments and districts above the 75th percentile are: Amazonas, Barranquilla, Atlántico, Bogotá, Cartagena, Chocó, Cesar and Nariño; Between the 50 to 75 percentiles are the departments of Valle del Cauca, Cundinamarca, Santa Marta, Sucre, Tolima, Bolívar, Magdalena, Antioquia. At the 25th percentile are Risaralda, Arauca, Cauca, Santander, Córdoba, Quindío, Caldas and Norte de Santander and below the 25th percentile are Boyacá, Guajira, Meta and Huila [37].

3.4 Pathophysiology of MIS-C

MIS-C is a clinically severe event that mimics other pathologies that present with hyper-inflammatory status in the pediatric population, in mention: KD, SST, Hemophagocytic Lymphohistocytosis (HHL), Macrophage Activation Syndrome (SAM), among others [38]. It is characterized by persistent fever (≥38°C) for more than 24 hours, with involvement of vital organs and consequent cardiological, renal, gastrointestinal, respiratory and / or hematological affection. Patients may present with maculopapular rash, arthritis, and aseptic bilateral conjunctivitis, similar to KD [39].

Symptoms begin 2 to 6 weeks after the resolution of COVID-19 symptoms (in those symptomatic), so it is suggested that it is not due to an effect of the acute event, but to an event mediated by the mechanisms of acquired immunity (cellular and / or humoral) [40]. In the initial stage, fever is usually documented, accompanied by constitutional symptoms, intense headache, general malaise, irritability, GI manifestations such as abdominal pain, vomiting or diarrhea, palmar and / or plantar erythema, mucosal edema, among others less frequent [41].

A range of cardiac dysfunctions are commonly seen with MIS-C, including but not limited to, myocarditis, pericarditis, aneurysms or dilatation of the coronary arteries, valvular insufficiency [1, 16], heart failure [16, 24] and electrocardiographic abnormalities. Other common findings include elevation of troponin, proBNP, C-reactive protein, ferritin, IL-6, D-dimer and need for intensive care [12, 16]. The presence of pericarditis, coronary aneurysms and myocarditis suggest that patients with COVID-19 could have an incomplete form of the Kawasaki disease.

Immunomodulators used in treatment have yielded positive results restoring normal left ventricular function [1] in echocardiographic reports after six weeks of treatment.

Subsequently, the patient presents a hyper-inflammatory state, characterized by an increase in pro-inflammatory cytokines such as: Interleukin 1 (IL-1), Tumor Necrosis Factor alpha (TNF-α), Interleukin 11 (IL-11), Interleukin 12 (IL-12), and especially, Interleukin 6 (IL-6) [42]. Proinflammatory cytokines exert a pleiotropic and redundant effect, which favors the elevation of acute phase reactants and products of the coagulation system, processes termed "immunothrombosis and thromboinflammation" [43]. Lactate Dehydrogenase (LDH), Procalcitonin (PCT), Globular Sedimentation Rate (ESR), C-Reactive Protein (CRP), Serum Ferritin, Serum Amyloid A, Fibrinogen, and D-dimer among other biomarkers may elevated. This state can produce functional alterations at the endothelial level, generating an imbalance between the homeostatic mechanisms of vasoactive control, leading to a state of severe hypotension and the consequent cardiogenic shock. These conditions may lead to multiple organ failure and death in some cases [44].

Immunologically, the mechanisms underlying the hyperinflammation state are not known; however, there are some findings that suggest certain molecular and cellular mechanisms. Regarding immunogenetics (Major Histocompatibility Complex, MHC, and HLA molecules), Nguyen and Cols, by immunoinformatic analysis, examined how HLA variation could affect the cellular immune response against coronavirus peptides that infect humans [45]. The researchers found that the HLA-B * 46: 01 allele has few SARS-CoV-2 peptide binding sites, while the HLA-B * 15: 03 allele showed greater ability to recognize and display highly conserved peptides in SARS-CoV-2, which suggests that host genetic factors may play a role in cellular immune response and clinical presentation in response to SARS-CoV-2 infection [46].

The superantigen hypothesis has also been proposed to understand and clarify the immunological events that support MIS-C [47]. This hypothesis suggests that the SARS-CoV-2 virus produces super antigens that activate the immune system. A superantigen refers to peptides (sometimes motifs and / or proteins) that bind to T lymphocytes of an individual, expressing a particular group or family of genes on the β chain of the variable region (Vβ) of the T-cell receptor (TCR) [48]. The binding of the superantigen with the Vβ domains of the TCR leads to their polyclonal activation, leading to the production of large amounts of cytokines and a clinical syndrome similar to septic shock, similar to what occurs in MIS-C. Superantigens are presented to T-cells through binding to non-polymorphic regions of HLA-II molecules located on antigen presenting cells (APC) and interact with conserved regions of the Vβ domains of the TCR. For example, several staphylococcal enterotoxins are SAg [49].

By structure-based computational modeling Rivas and Cols discovered that the SARS-CoV-2 Spike (S) protein possesses a high affinity motif located close to the S1 / S2 cleavage site with a highly conserved sequence to superantigens [50]. The region containing this motif exhibits a high binding affinity to the complementarity determining regions (CDRs) present in the variable domains of the α and β chain of the TCR. This region is highly similar to the primary sequence and three-dimensional structure of a superantigen fragment corresponding to staphylococcal enterotoxin B (SEB), which interacts with the TCR and CD28 of T cells [51].

Next-generation immuno-sequencing of the TCR repertoire of COVID-19 patients indicated that the severity of the infection may be associated with some genes that encode the Vβ region of the TCR [52]. Using structure-based computational modeling, Cheng and cols. Demonstrated that the SARS-CoV-2 protein S exhibits a high-affinity TCR-binding motif, being able to form a complex with

HLA-II molecules. The researchers argue that this interaction between the virus and human T cells could be enhanced by a rare mutation (D839Y / N / E) from a European strain of SARS-CoV-2 [52]. The studies also found that the SARS-CoV-2 protein S possesses a neurotoxin-like sequence motif in the receptor-binding domain, which exhibits a high tendency to bind to TCR. These findings are consistent with the clinical presentation of patients with MIS-C, who exhibit hyperinflammation and neurological symptoms suggestive of neurotoxicity [53, 54].

3.5 Cases definition

Most children with Covid-19 infection are asymptomatic or present mild symptoms, however, children who may develop a significant systemic inflammatory response have been identified, which may require hospitalization, ICU admission and even management for different medical specialties [55]. This syndrome, although it is a rare complication, can be fatal in children and adolescents. Due to the risk to the health of this population, it is necessary to characterize this disease and its risk factors, as well as to initiate immediate epidemiological surveillance. WHO has developed a preliminary case definition and case report form for MIS-C in children and adolescents. The preliminary case definition reflects the clinical and laboratory features observed in children reported to date and are used to identify suspected or confirmed cases (**Figure 1**) [56]. The National Institute of Health of Colombia, in its technical document of January 21, 2021, defines the operational concepts of cases as follows (**Table 1**; **Figures 2** and **3**) [57].

3.6 MIS-C treatment

Currently, studies comparing clinical efficacy of various treatment options are lacking. According to the United States Center for Disease Control, Colombian Association of Infectious Disease and American College of Rheumatology treatments have consisted primarily of supportive care and directed care against the underlying inflammatory process. Supportive care may include that may include fluid resuscitation, inotropic support; respiratory support and in rare cases, ECMO [58, 59].

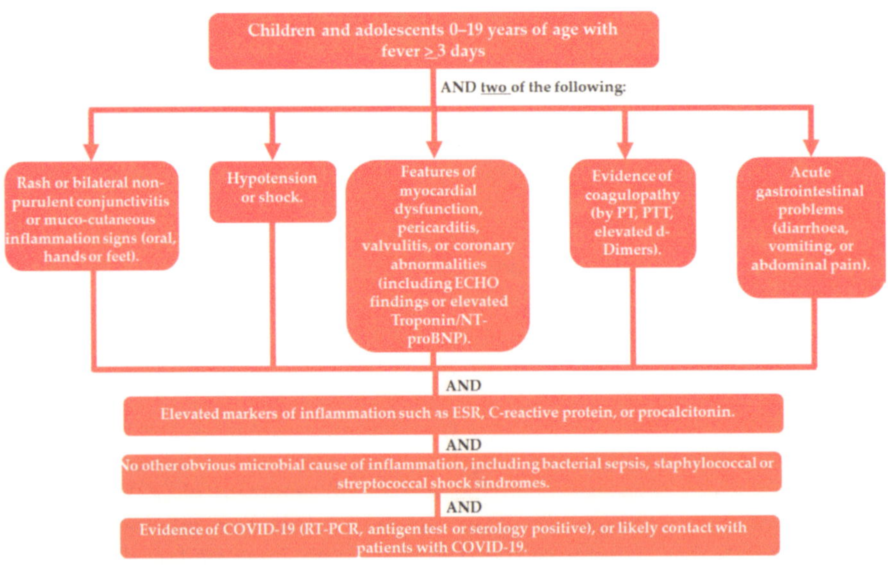

Figure 1.
Preliminary case definition according to the World Health Organization.

Case	Case characteristics
Probable MIS-C Covid-19 Case	• Under 18 years of age with fever for >24 hours, current or recent infection for SARS-CoV-2 evidenced by RT-PCR or IgM / IgG antibody serology or close contact with a COVID-19 confirmed case in the prior 4 weeks. • Also presenting with any of the following symptoms: abdominal pain, vomiting, diarrhea, skin rash, non-purulent bilateral conjunctivitis, erythema on the soles or palms or mucosal edema, headache or altered state of consciousness. • Without alternative diagnosis or other possible causes that explain this clinical picture.
Confirmed MIS-C Covid-19 case	• Probable case with clinical findings in at least 2 organ systems (Gastrointestinal symptoms: abdominal pain, vomiting, diarrhea or Mucocutaneous; skin rash, non-purulent bilateral conjunctivitis, erythema on soles or palms or mucosal edema or Neurological symptoms such as headache or conscious state alteration or Cardiological symptoms: myocardial dysfunction, pericarditis, abnormalities in the coronary arteries or Hematological: evidence of renal or respiratory coagulopathy). • At least one of these altered laboratory findings: Neutrophilia, thrombocytopenia or lymphopenia or elevation of ESR, Fibrinogen, C-reactive protein, Ferritin, lactate, D-Dimer, interleukin-6 orThrombocytopenia.
Dismissed MIS-C Covid-19 case	None of the conditions listed in the probable or confirmed case definitions are met

Table 1.
Case definition according to National Institute of health of Colombia.

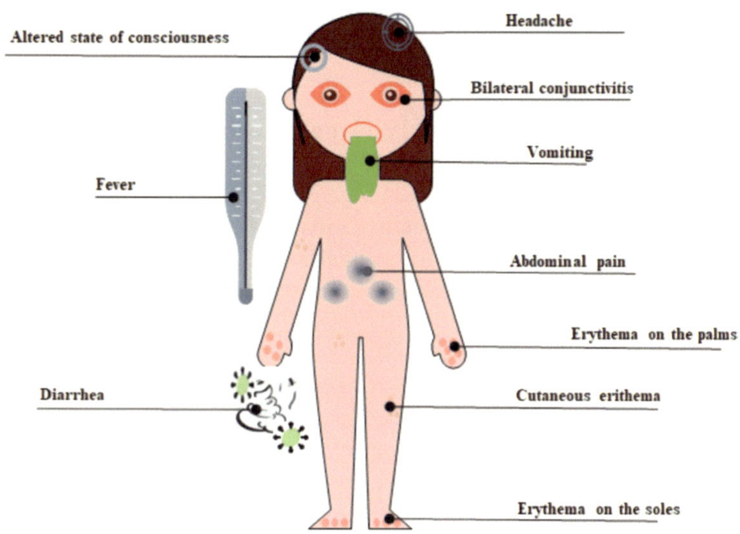

Figure 2.
Probable MIS-C COVID-19 case.

Anti-inflammatory measures may include the use of intravenous IgG (IVIG) and steroids. Aspirin may be used due to concerns for coronary artery involvement and antibiotics are sometimes used to treat potential sepsis while awaiting bacterial cultures. Thrombotic prophylaxis is often used to treat the hypercoagulable state typically associated with MIS-C.

The Colombian Association of Infectious Diseases (CAID) [60] and the American College of Rheumatology (ACR) (cite website shown above) have provided consensus statements for the management of MIS-C related to the immunomodulatory, antiplatelet and anticoagulation that are summarized below:

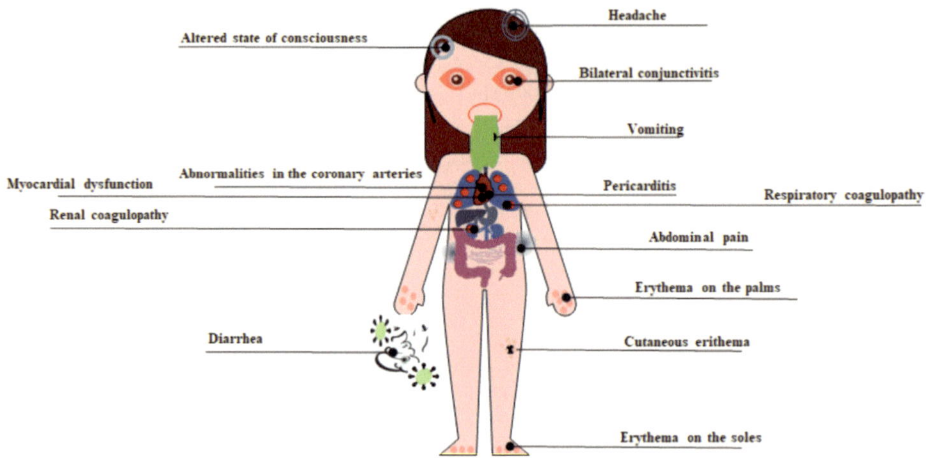

Figure 3.
Confirmed MIS-C COVID-19 case.

Immunomodulatory management of MISC:

- A stepwise progression of immunomodulatory therapies should be used to treat MIS-C with IVIG and/or glucocorticoids considered as first tier treatments (ACR)
  The use of human polyclonal IVIG at a dose of 2 g / kg is suggested for all patients who meet MIS-C diagnostic criteria (CAID) with stable cardiac function and fluid status (ACR).

- In patients that do not respond to IVIG the following approaches may be considered:

  - Low to moderate doses of glucocorticoids may also be considered (ACR) noting that in endemic countries antiparasitic management with albendazole or ivermectin is needed to avoid hyperinfestation syndromes of strongyloides (CAID).

  - The use of a second dose of IVIG at a dose of 2 g / kg in case of no response within 36 hours of the first dose, with or without steroid at a low dose (prednisolone orally at a maximum of 1 mg / kg / day or its intravenous equivalent if there is intolerance to the oral route, according to response) may be applied (CAID).

  - High dose intravenous pulse glucocorticoids may be considered in shock (ACR) such as the administration of pulses of methylprednisolone at 30 mg / kg / day for 3 days (CAID).

  - Children with severe respiratory symptoms due to COVID-19 should be considered for immunomodulatory therapy if any of the following are present: ARDS, shock/cardiac dysfunction, substantially elevated LDH, d-dimer, IL-6, IL-2R, CRP, and/or ferritin levels, and depressed lymphocyte count, albumin levels, and/or platelet count (ACR). Risks and benefits suggest that anakinra (intravenously or subcutaneously) be used as first-line immunomodulatory treatment of children with COVID-19 and hyperinflammation (ACR).

  - Tocilizumab may be effective in reducing mortality and intensive care admission in patients with severe COVID-19 pneumonia and signs of the hyperinflammation while causing higher risk for bacterial and fungal infections (ACR). When tocilizumab is used to treat children with COVID-19, weight-based dosing should be employed (body weight < 30 kg, 12 mg/kg IV; body weight ≥ 30 kg, 8 mg/kg IV, maximum 800 mg) (ACR). Currently there is no evidence to support the benefits of tocilizumab in the pediatric population, even in special populations such as cancer patients and patients with primary or secondary immunodeficiencies. Current evidence is based on adult patients with a therapeutic dose of 8 mg / kg of body weight (requiring a second dose 8–24 hours after the first), however, the results have also demonstrated adverse events such as gastrointestinal perforation and greater susceptibility to secondary infections when used concomitantly with dexamethasone 6 mg IV every 24 hours or equivalent corticosteroid dose [58].

- Taper of immunomodulatory medications is recommended in 2–3 weeks after recovery (ACR and CAID).

Antiplatelet and Anticoagulation management of MISC:

The use of aspirin at anti-inflammatory doses (3–5 mg / kg / day maximum 81 mg/day) is recommended in MIS-C (CAID and ACR) in the event of thrombocytosis (≥450,000 / μL) or dilatation of the coronary arteries until resolution and if there is no thrombocytopenia (≤80,000/μl), gastrointestinal bleeding, abnormal liver function tests (up to 5 times normal values of transaminases), uncontrolled asthma, oral intolerance, or influenza A or B virus infection (CAID). In cases of thrombocytosis (platelet count ≥450,000/μl), aspirin should be continued until the platelet count normalizes (ACR). Furthermore, patients with MIS-C and documented thrombosis or an ejection fraction <35% should receive therapeutic anticoagulation with enoxaparin until at least 2 weeks after discharge from the hospital (ACR).

4. Back to school

School re-opening is critical to support academic progress, mental health and access to essential services. Considerations of transmission and case severity in children may guide childcare and school policies. Many countries have reported that children under the age of ten have the lowest population based COVID infection rates [2]. Furthermore, while serious infections in children under the age of two are known to occur [2], studies have shown low infection in schools and low probability of transmission between children and teachers suggesting that safe school re-opening may be possible [60].

Despite uncertainties regarding the safety of returning to the classroom, some data collected suggests a partial or total return to face-to-face classes by taking measures to reduce community transmission may be possible. Schools in multiple countries have already reopened their classrooms with little published evidence that schools implementing COVID-19 control policies contribute significantly to COVID-19 transmission [61].

Some studies of COVID-19 transmission demonstrate that school-acquired infections are limited in comparison to community-acquired infections [62]. For example, a case–control study from Mississippi, USA carried out in children over 18 years of age described a total of 154 with SARS-CoV-2 infections and 243 without infection. In this group having attended social gatherings outside the home and receiving visitors was associated with a greater risk of infection, while attending school in person was not associated with a greater risk [62].

Despite this promising data, there have been school-related outbreaks. For example, in Israel 2 weeks after the reopening of the schools in mid-May 2020 there was a large outbreak in a high school when 2 students attended school with mild symptoms. Students (n = 1,161) and the school staff (n = 151) were tested and infection was confirmed in students (n = 153) and staff (n = 25). However, some factors reported that may have contributed to this massive outbreak were full classrooms with insufficient physical distancing, the lack of mask use in some people and the continuous air conditioning that allowed recycle indoor air in closed classrooms. Therefore, perhaps implementation of these preventative measures may mitigate school transmission [61, 62].

Some measures implemented in schools and nurseries to mitigate the contagion are:

- Use of universal mask
- Adequate physical distancing
- Models of alternation classes (face-to-face-virtual)
- Avoid overcrowding
- Increase air ventilation in classrooms
- Increased coverage of rapid screening tests to quickly isolate asymptomatic infected
- Online education options for those who are at higher risk of serious illness or death if they contract COVID-19
- Limit groupings in classrooms to a maximum of 10 people
- Thorough cleaning of classrooms before and after activities
- Contingency plan in case someone is exposed to the virus
- Staged re-opening by year groups (eg, primary and secondary) or by geographic region to allow close monitoring and changes to the re-opening strategy as needed [63].

It is important to mention that athletic activities may increase the spread of SARS-CoV-2. For example, January 26 the CDC reported an outbreak associated with a wrestling tournament in a high school that occurred in December 2020 including 10 schools and 130 student-athletes, coaches and referees, of the students 38 (30%) contracted laboratory-confirmed SARS-CoV-2 infection [63]. Contact tracing identified 446 contacts of the positive cases that were considered to have had a high risk of transmission. One death of reported in one of the contacts of the students. However, limitations of the evaluation include that fewer than half of the participants were evaluated therefore some cases may have been unrecognized [64].

Simulation models have been used to determine how fast the virus spreads, how easily it is contained, effectiveness of containment strategies, social and economic impacts of closure, and the role of schools in transmission [63]. For example, some simulated transmission control strategies include placing siblings or children who cohabit together in classrooms, assigning one group of children attends face-to-face one week while another group interacts online and then switching roles the following week, or school closure for 14 days if a symptomatic child attends school with those who are asymptomatic returning and symptomatic students staying at home. Another simulation evaluated the effect of child-educator ratios per classroom including 7: 3, 8: 2 and 15: 2. The most favorable transmission profile was shown with 7 students for every 3 educators and group assignment of siblings or students who cohabit together [65]. Whereas the worst transmission profile was shown with 15 students for 2 educators and the random assignment of students [64].

Virtual learning has been used to substitute for in-classroom experiences for many children globally. 143 countries had transitioned to online learning by August 2020, generating stress for both students and their families [66]. Virtual instruction has placed increased demands on family members in terms of time and other resources [67]. Fantini et al. suggests that we must take a deep look into the policies that have led to the necessary closure of the schools and the impacts they have [2]. The isolation school closures cause have great impacts on children, impacting not only their social life, but also their identity and personality development. Without proper social interaction, children may develop anger, guilt, and even depression in addition to anxiety and adjustment disorders. Another consideration is that in the setting of school closures students may spend a greater amount of time with their parents. While this phenomenon has certain benefits, without the support of schoolteachers, parents may become overwhelmed as the only caregivers, potentially exposing children to increased domestic violence, especially when parents have financial and mental health problems that may be exacerbated by the pandemic [2]. Virtual instruction also negatively impacts learning as children are taught best in hands-on learning, especially when learning to write [2]. Together, these factors illustrate some the hardships for children related to the pandemic and school closures.

For these reasons, it is important to implement in-person learning for children as part of early recovery. However, precautions should be effectively implemented and practiced, that may include social distancing, prevention of shared materials, ventilation of spaces, increased hand washing practices and sanitizing availability. Control measures include in-person learning could be started through alternating face-to-face and virtual learning scheduling to decrease density, the use of masks [2] and training of teachers in students in safety procedures [2].

5. The impact of the COVID-19 pandemic in children

The pandemic has affected children in great ways, impacting the way they grow, learn, play, and cope with their emotions [4, 60]. Younger children may be most at risk from the impacts of COVID-19, as lack of play, exercise, and interaction with peers [4, 60] can be affected. Additionally, other symptoms that affect brain development, such as stress, isolation, and depression [60], may develop if children witness friends and family members becoming infected or passing due to COVID-19. Children with psychiatric disorders face the greatest challenges, as 50% of psychiatric disorders [60] affect children by age 14. It is important to manage symptoms presented by these disorders as they may greatly affect child development.

Other symptoms children develop in this health crisis may include trouble sleeping and mental health problems. COVID-19 impacts the lives of children in various ways and include changing family-life circumstances. Parents might be working from home or become unemployed, increasing the risks for drug use and abuse in the home. These factors, as well as worries about their own physical health could cause children to have trouble sleeping. Additionally, if a child's mental health is affected, they are at risk for post-traumatic stress [60], depression [60], and suicide [4, 60].

Important factors for mental health in children include good physical health and a good education system. Schools are a valuable resource to provide adequate information and help children understand COVID-19. Schools with trained professionals can also help identify children with problems and develop therapeutic approaches to support them. Teaching children how to cope with their emotions, generate healthy behaviors, and allowing children to participate in activities they enjoy are some of the benefits that schools can provide to try and counteract problems caused by the pandemic.

6. Conclusion

In conclusion, the COVID-19 pandemic poses some unique challenges for child health and learning. In relation to child health, Multisystem Inflammatory Syndrome in Children (MIS-C) is a rare but severe complication of COVID-19 related to acquired immune responses that requires further research. Despite limited studies to date to define therapeutic guidelines in children, consensus recommendations from multiple organizations recommend the use of immunomodulatory therapies, anti-platelet and anti-coagulant therapies. Furthermore, considerations for safe return to the classroom such as strategies for optimized student to teacher ratios, hand washing, social distancing, sibling pairing and staged re-opening strategies may facilitate child learning in the setting of this evolving pandemic. Further research into efficacy of these proposed interventions will be necessary to inform evidence based guidelines for the prevention and management of COVID-19 in children.

Author details

Evelyn Mendoza-Torres[1], Franklin Torres[1], Wendy Rosales-Rada[2], Liliana Encinales[3], Lil Avendaño[4], María Fernanda Pérez[1], Ivana Terán[1], David Vergara[1], Estefanie Osorio-Llanes[2], Paige Fierbaugh[4], Wendy Villamizar[1], Aileen Y. Chang[4*] and Jairo Castellar-Lopez[5]

1 Faculty of Health Sciences, Universidad Libre, Barranquilla, Colombia

2 Faculty of Exact and Natural Sciences, Universidad Libre, Barranquilla, Colombia

3 Global Disease Research Colombia, Barranquilla, Colombia

4 George Washington University, Washington, DC, United States

5 Faculty of Exact and Natural Sciences, Grupo de Investigación Avanzada en Biomedicina, Universidad Libre Barranquilla, Barranquilla, Colombia

*Address all correspondence to: chang@email.gwu.edu

References

[1] Kabeerdoss J, Pilania RK, Karkhele R, Kumar TS, Danda D, Singh S. Severe COVID-19, multisystem inflammatory syndrome in children, and Kawasaki disease: immunological mechanisms, clinical manifestations and management. Rheumatol Int. 2021;41(1):19-32. Doi:10.1007/s00296-020-04749-4

[2] Fantini, M.P., Reno, C., Biserni, G.B., Savoia E., Lanari M. COVID-19 and the re-opening of schools: a policy maker's dilemma. Ital J Pediatr 46, 79 (2020). Doi:10.1186/s13052-020-00844-1

[3] Bhuiyan MU, Stiboy E, Hassan MZ, Chan M, Islam MS, Haider N, et al. Epidemiology of COVID-19 infection in young children under five years: A systematic review and meta-analysis. Vaccine. 2021;39(4):667-677. Doi:10.1016/j.vaccine.2020.11.078

[4] Bogiatzopoulou A, Mayberry H, Hawcutt DB, Whittaker E, Munro A, Roland D. et al. COVID-19 in children: what did we learn from the first wave?. Paediatr Child Health (Oxford). 2020;30(12):438-443. Doi:10.1016/j.paed.2020.09.005

[5] Park SE. Epidemiology, virology, and clinical features of severe acute respiratory syndrome -coronavirus-2 (SARS-CoV-2; Coronavirus Disease-19). Clin Exp Pediatr. 2020;63(4):119-124. doi:10.3345/cep.2020.00493

[6] Salvatori G, Luberto L, Maffei M, Aurisicchio L, Roscilli G, Palombo, F, et al. SARS-CoV-2 SPIKE PROTEIN: an optimal immunological target for vaccines. J Transl Med 18, 222 (2020). Doi:10.1186/s12967-020-02392-y

[7] Ou X, Liu Y, Lei X, Li P, Mi D, Ren L, et al. Characterization of spike glycoprotein of SARS-CoV-2 on virus entry and its immune cross-reactivity with SARS-CoV [published correction appears in Nat Commun. 2021 Apr 1;12(1):2144]. Nat Commun. 2020;11(1):1620. Published 2020 Mar 27. Doi:10.1038/s41467-020-15562-9

[8] World Health Organization. Questions and Answers About Coronavirus Disease (COVID-19) [Internet]. 2020. Available in: https://www.who.int/es/emergencies/diseases/novel-coronavirus-2019/advice-for-public/q-a-coronaviruses?gclid=CjwKCAiAjp6BBhAIEiwAkO9Wui6UTAQB2Py7L7Yf_mfrJL9aL2byMKpVpk9I6TV98ylNhgORJjRslxoC9AQQAvD_BwE [Access: 2020-Oct-12]

[9] Peng X, Xu X, Li Y, Cheng L, Zhou x, Ren B. Transmission routes of 2019-nCoV and controls in dental practice. Int J Oral Sci 12, 9 (2020). Doi:10.1038/s41368-020-0075-9.

[10] Kotfis K, Skonieczna-Żydecka K. COVID-19: gastrointestinal symptoms and potential sources of SARS-CoV-2 transmission. Anaesthesiol Intensive Ther. 2020;52(2):171-172. Doi:10.5114/ait.2020.93867

[11] Fu J, Zhou B, Zhang L, Srinivasa K, Wei C, Liu X et al. Expressions and significances of the angiotensin-converting enzyme 2 gene, the receptor of SARS-CoV-2 for COVID-19. Mol Biol Rep 47, 4383-4392 (2020). Doi:10.1007/s11033-020-05478-4

[12] Feldstein LR, Rose EB, Horwitz SM, Collins JP, Newhams MM, Son MBF, et al. Multisystem Inflammatory Syndrome in U.S. Children and Adolescents. N Engl J Med. 2020;383(4):334-346. Doi:10.1056/NEJMoa2021680

[13] Lokman SM, Rasheduzzaman M, Salauddin A, Barua R, Tanzina AY., Rumi M, et al (2020). Exploring the genomic and proteomic variations of SARS-CoV-2 spike glycoprotein: A

computational biology approach. Infection, genetics and evolution : journal of molecular epidemiology and evolutionary genetics in infectious diseases, 84, 104389. Doi:10.1016/j.meegid.2020.104389

[14] Cano, F., Gajardo, M., & Freundlich, M. (2020). Renin angiotensin axis, angiotensin converting enzyme 2 and coronavirus. Rev. Chil. de Pediatr., 91(3). Doi:10.32641/rchped.vi91i3.2548

[15] Zhang C, Gu J, Chen Q, Deng N, Li J, Huang L et al. Clinical and epidemiological characteristics of pediatric SARS-CoV-2 infections in China: A multicenter case series. PLoS Med. 2020;17(6):e1003130. Published 2020 Jun 16. Doi:10.1371/journal.pmed.1003130

[16] Valverde I, Singh Y, Sanchez-de-Toledo J, Theocharis P, Chikermane A, Di Filippo S, et al. Acute Cardiovascular Manifestations in 286 Children With Multisystem Inflammatory Syndrome Associated With COVID-19 Infection in Europe. Circulation. 2021;143(1):21-32. Doi:10.1161/CIRCULATIONAHA.120.050065

[17] Medicine, COVID Toes and Other COVID-19 Skin Conditions, 2020. Available at: https://weillcornell.org/news/covid-toe-and-other-covid-19-skin-conditions [Acceso: 2020- 07-09]

[18] Singh S, Jindal AK, Pilania RK. Diagnosis of Kawasaki disease. Int J Rheum Dis. 2018 ;21(1):36-44. Doi:10.1111/1756-185X.13224

[19] Verdoni L, Mazza A, Gervasoni A, Martelli L, Ruggeri M, Ciuffreda M et al. An outbreak of severe Kawasaki-like disease at the Italian epicentre of the SARS-CoV-2 epidemic: an observational cohort study. Lancet. 2020;395(10239):1771-1778. Doi:10.1016/S0140-6736(20)31103-X

[20] Blanco J. FUNDAMENTOS DE SALUD PÚBLICA. 3ª ed. Franco Silvana, editor. Medellín, Colombia; 2013. 0-227 p.

[21] Whittaker E, Bamford A, Kenny J, Kaforou M, Jones CE, Shah P et al. Clinical Characteristics of 58 Children with a Pediatric Inflammatory Multisystem Syndrome Temporally Associated with SARS-CoV-2. JAMA. 2020;324(3):259-269. Doi:10.1001/jama.2020.10369

[22] Cheung EW, Zachariah P, Gorelik M, Boneparth A, Kernie SG, Orange JS, Milner JD. Multisystem Inflammatory Syndrome Related to COVID-19 in Previously Healthy Children and Adolescents in New York City. JAMA. 2020 Jul 21;324(3):294-296. Doi: 10.1001/jama.2020.10374.

[23] Pain CE, Felsenstein S, Cleary G, Mayell S, Conrad K, Harave S, et al. Novel paediatric presentation of COVID-19 with ARDS and cytokine storm syndrome without respiratory symptoms. Lancet Rheumatol. 2020 Jul;2(7):e376-e379. Doi: 10.1016/S2665-9913(20)30137-5.

[24] Rafferty MS, Burrows H, Joseph JP, Leveille J, Nihtianova S, Amirian ES. Multisystem inflammatory syndrome in children (MIS-C) and the coronavirus pandemic: Current knowledge and implications for public health. J Infect Public Health. 2021 Apr;14(4):484-494. Doi: 10.1016/j.jiph.2021.01.008.

[25] Riphagen S, Gomez X, Gonzalez-Martinez C, Wilkinson N, Theocharis P. Hyperinflammatory shock in children during COVID-19 pandemic. Lancet. 2020 May 23;395(10237):1607-1608. Doi: 10.1016/S0140-6736(20)31094-1.

[26] Dufort EM, Koumans EH, Chow EJ, Rosenthal EM, Muse A, Rowlands J, et al; New York State and Centers for Disease Control and Prevention

Multisystem Inflammatory Syndrome in Children Investigation Team. Multisystem Inflammatory Syndrome in Children in New York State. N Engl J Med. 2020 Jul 23;383(4):347-358. Doi: 10.1056/NEJMoa2021756.

[27] Yáñez JA, Alvarez-Risco A, Delgado-Zegarra J. Covid-19 in Peru: from supervised walks for children to the first case of Kawasaki-like syndrome. BMJ. 2020 Jun 22;369:m2418. Doi: 10.1136/bmj.m2418. PMID: 32571770.

[28] DeBiasi RL, Song X, Delaney M, Bell M, Smith K, Pershad J, et al. Severe Coronavirus Disease-2019 in Children and Young Adults in the Washington, DC, Metropolitan Region. J Pediatr. 2020 Aug;223:199-203.e1. Doi: 10.1016/j.jpeds.2020.05.007

[29] Pediatric Intensive Care Society. PICS Statement: Increased number of reported cases of novel presentation of multi- system inflammatory disease. [April 27, 2020] Available at:

[30] World Health Organization. Multisystem inflammatory síndrome in children and adolescents temporally related to COVID-19, Scientific Brief. [15 May 2020] Available at: https://www.who.int/news-room/commentaries/detail/multisystem-inflammatorysyndrome-in-children-and-adolescents-with-covid-19.

[31] Belhadjer Z, Méot M, Bajolle F, Khraiche D, Legendre A, Abakka S, et al. Acute Heart Failure in Multisystem Inflammatory Syndrome in Children in the Context of Global SARS-CoV-2 Pandemic. Circulation. 2020 Aug 4;142(5):429-436. Doi: 10.1161/CIRCULATIONAHA.120.048360.

[32] Jones VG, Mills M, Suarez D, Hogan CA, Yeh D, Segal JB, et al. COVID-19 and Kawasaki Disease: Novel Virus and Novel Case. Hosp Pediatr. 2020 Jun;10(6):537-540. Doi: 10.1542/hpeds.2020-0123.

[33] Ouldali N, Yang DD, Madhi F, Levy M, Gaschignard J, Craiu I, et al; investigator group of the PANDOR study. Factors Associated With Severe SARS-CoV-2 Infection. Pediatrics. 2021 Mar;147(3):e2020023432. Doi: 10.1542/peds.2020-023432.

[34] Raisinghani M. Resumen OR 23-3. Poor diabetes control in children tied to high risk for COVID-19 complications, death. ENDO 2021. Available at: https://www.endocrine.org/news-and-advocacy/news-room/featured-science-from-endo-2021/poor-diabetes-control-in-children-tied-to-high-risk-for-covid19-complications-death. Presented on March 20, 2021.

[35] Organización Panamericana de la Salud / Organización Mundial de la Salud. Actualización epidemiológica: Enfermedad por Coronavirus (COVID-19). 15 de enero de 2021, Washington, D.C.: OPS/OMS; 2021.

[36] Shekerdemian LS, Mahmood NR, Wolfe KK, Riggs BJ, Ross CE, McKiernan CA, et al. Characteristics and Outcomes of Children With Coronavirus Disease 2019 (COVID-19) Infection Admitted to US and Canadian Pediatric Intensive Care Units. JAMA Pediatr. 2020 Sep 1;174(9):868-873. Doi: 10.1001/jamapediatrics.2020.1948.

[37] Ins.gov.co. 2021. Coronavirus Colombia. [online] Available at: <https://www.ins.gov.co/Noticias/paginas/coronavirus.aspx> [Accessed 9 May 2021].

[38] Consiglio CR, Cotugno N, Sardh F, Pou C, Amodio D, Rodriguez L, et al. The Immunology of Multisystem Inflammatory Syndrome in Children with COVID-19. Cell. 2020 Nov 12;183(4):968-981.e7. Doi: 10.1016/j.cell.2020.09.016.

[39] Shulman ST, Rowley AH. Kawasaki disease: insights into pathogenesis and

approaches to treatment. Nat Rev Rheumatol. 2015 Aug;11(8):475-82. Doi: 10.1038/nrrheum.2015.54.

[40] Diane Marie Del Valle, Seunghee Kim-Schulze, Hsin-Hui Huang, Noam Beckmann, Sharon Nirenberg, Bo Wang, et al. An inflammatory cytokine signature helps predict COVID-19 severity and death. medRxiv 2020.05.28.20115758; Doi: https://doi.org/10.1101/2020.05.28.20115758.

[41] McGonagle D, Sharif K, O'Regan A, Bridgewood C. The Role of Cytokines including Interleukin-6 in COVID-19 induced Pneumonia and Macrophage Activation Syndrome-Like Disease. Autoimmun Rev. 2020 Jun;19(6):102537. Doi: 10.1016/j.autrev.2020.102537.

[42] Tay MZ, Poh CM, Rénia L, MacAry PA, Ng LFP. The trinity of COVID-19: immunity, inflammation and intervention. Nat Rev Immunol. 2020 Jun;20(6):363-374. Doi: 10.1038/s41577-020-0311-8.

[43] Bonaventura A, Vecchié A, Dagna L, Martinod K, Dixon DL, Van Tassell BW, et al. Endothelial dysfunction and immunothrombosis as key pathogenic mechanisms in COVID-19. Nat Rev Immunol. 2021 May;21(5):319-329. Doi: 10.1038/s41577-021-00536-9.

[44] McFadyen JD, Stevens H, Peter K. The Emerging Threat of (Micro) Thrombosis in COVID-19 and Its Therapeutic Implications. Circ Res. 2020 Jul 31;127(4):571-587. Doi: 10.1161/CIRCRESAHA.120.317447.

[45] Nguyen A, David JK, Maden SK, Wood MA, Weeder BR, Nellore A, et al. Human Leukocyte Antigen Susceptibility Map for Severe Acute Respiratory Syndrome Coronavirus 2. J Virol. 2020 Jun 16;94(13):e00510-20. Doi: 10.1128/JVI.00510-20.

[46] Habel JR, Nguyen THO, van de Sandt CE, Juno JA, Chaurasia P, Wragg K, Koutsakos M, et al. Suboptimal SARS-CoV-2-specific CD8+ T cell response associated with the prominent HLA-A*02:01 phenotype. Proc Natl Acad Sci U S A. 2020 Sep 29;117(39):24384-24391. Doi: 10.1073/pnas.2015486117.

[47] Arad G, Levy R, Nasie I, Hillman D, Rotfogel Z, Barash U, et al. Binding of superantigen toxins into the CD28 homodimer interface is essential for induction of cytokine genes that mediate lethal shock. PLoS Biol. 2011 Sep;9(9):e1001149. Doi: 10.1371/journal.pbio.1001149. Epub 2011 Sep 13. Erratum in: PLoS Biol. 2015 Aug;13(8):e1002237.

[48] Li H, Llera A, Malchiodi EL, Mariuzza RA. The structural basis of T cell activation by superantigens. Annu Rev Immunol. 1999;17:435-66. Doi: 10.1146/annurev.immunol.17.1.435.

[49] Krakauer T. Staphylococcal Superantigens: Pyrogenic Toxins Induce Toxic Shock. Toxins (Basel). 2019 Mar 23;11(3):178. Doi: 10.3390/toxins11030178.

[50] Noval Rivas M, Porritt RA, Cheng MH, Bahar I, Arditi M. COVID-19-associated multisystem inflammatory syndrome in children (MIS-C): A novel disease that mimics toxic shock syndrome-the superantigen hypothesis. J Allergy Clin Immunol. 2021 Jan;147(1):57-59. Doi: 10.1016/j.jaci.2020.10.008.

[51] Fraser JD, Proft T. The bacterial superantigen and superantigen-like proteins. Immunol Rev. 2008 Oct;225:226-43. Doi: 10.1111/j.1600-065X.2008.00681.x.

[52] Cheng MH, Zhang S, Porritt RA, Noval Rivas M, Paschold L, Willscher E, et al. Superantigenic character of an insert unique to SARS-CoV-2 spike supported by skewed TCR repertoire in patients with hyperinflammation. Proc

Natl Acad Sci U S A. 2020 Oct 13;117(41):25254-25262. Doi: 10.1073/pnas.2010722117.

[53] Ellul MA, Benjamin L, Singh B, Lant S, Michael BD, Easton A, et al. Neurological associations of COVID-19. Lancet Neurol. 2020 Sep;19(9):767-783. Doi: 10.1016/S1474-4422(20)30221-0.

[54] Rosene KA, Copass MK, Kastner LS, Nolan CM, Eschenbach DA. Persistent neuropsychological sequelae of toxic shock syndrome. Ann Intern Med. 1982 Jun;96(6 Pt 2):865-70. Doi: 10.7326/0003-4819-96-6-865.

[55] Paediatric multisystem inflammatory syndrome temporally associated with COVID-19 (PIMS) - guidance for clinicians [Internet]. RCPCH. 2021 [cited 9 May 2021]. Available from: https://www.rcpch.ac.uk/resources/paediatric-multisystem-inflammatory-syndrome-temporally-associated-covid-19-pims-guidance

[56] Multisystem inflammatory syndrome in children and adolescents temporally related to COVID-19. [Internet]. Scientific Brief 2020. [cited 10 May 2021]. Available from: https://www.who.int/news-room/commentaries/detail/multisystem-inflammatory-syndrome-in-children-and-adolescents-with-covid-19

[57] Documento técnico para la vigilancia de casos probables y confirmados de Síndrome Inflamatorio Multisistémico en niños asociado a infección por SARS-Cov2, Versión 1 – 21 enero 2021. Instituto Nacional de Salud, Ministerio de Salud y Protección Social. https://www.ins.gov.co/Noticias/paginas/coronavirus.aspx

[58] Henderson, L.A., Canna, S.W., … Mehta, J.J., 2020. American College of Rheumatology Clinical Guidance for Multisystem Inflammatory Syndrome in Children Associated with SARS–CoV-2 and Hyperinflammation in Pediatric COVID-19: Version 1. Arthritis and Rheumatology 72, 1791-1805. doi:10.1002/art.41454

[59] Information for Healthcare Providers about Multisystem Inflammatory Syndrome in Children (MIS-C) [Internet]. Fact Sheet 2020. [cited 10 May 2021] https://www.cdc.gov/mis-c/hcp/

[60] Saavedra Trujillo C. Consenso colombiano de atención, diagnóstico y manejo de la infección por SARS-COV-2/COVID 19 en establecimientos de atención de la salud. Recomendaciones basadas en consenso de expertos e informadas en la evidencia ACIN-IETS. Infectio, Volumen 24, número 3 (suplemento COVID19), Mayo 2020.

[61] Infectious diseases society of America guidelines on the treatment and management of patients with covid-19. last updated March 18, 2021 and posted online at www.idsociety.org/covid19guidelines

[62] Shah K, Mann S, Singh R, Bangar R, Kulkarni R. Impact of COVID-19 on the Mental Health of Children and Adolescents. Cureus. 2020 Aug 26 ;12(8): e10051. Doi : 10.7759/cureus.10051.

[63] Honein MA, Barrios LC, Brooks JT. Data and Policy to Guide Opening Schools Safely to Limit the Spread of SARS-CoV-2 Infection. JAMA. 2021 ;325(9) :823-824. doi :10.1001/jama.2021.0374

[64] Viner, R. M., Bonell, C., Drake, L., Jourdan, D., Davies, N., Baltag, V., Jerrim, J., Proimos, J., & Darzi, A. (2021). Reopening schools during the COVID-19 pandemic: governments must balance the uncertainty and risks of reopening schools against the clear harms associated with prolonged

closure. Archives of disease in childhood, 106(2), 111-113; doi.org/10.1136/archdischild-2020-319963

[65] Phillips, B., Browne, D.T., Anand, M. et al. Model-based projections for COVID-19 outbreak size and student-days lost to closure in Ontario childcare centers and primary schools. Sci Rep 11, 6402 (2021). doi.org/10.1038/s41598-021-85302-6

[66] OECD Policy Responses to Coronavirus (COVID-19) - The impact of COVID-19 on student equity and inclusion: Supporting vulnerable students during school closures and school re-openings https://www.oecd.org/coronavirus/policy-responses/the-impact-of-covid-19-on-student-equity-and-inclusion-supporting-vulnerable-students-during-school-closures-and-school-re-openings-d593b5c8/

[67] OECD Policy Responses to Coronavirus (COVID-19) - Strengthening online learning when schools are closed: The role of families and teachers in supporting students during the COVID-19 crisis https://www.oecd.org/coronavirus/policy-responses/strengthening-online-learning-when-schools-are-closed-the-role-of-families-and-teachers-in-supporting-students-during-the-covid-19-crisis-c4ecba6c/

Chapter 6

Sexually Transmitted Infections in Pediatrics

Diana Coronel-Martínez and Luis Augusto Moya-Barquín

Abstract

Sexually transmitted diseases (STDs) disproportionately affect young people, with more than half of the infections occurring in 15- to 25-year-olds, although as an age group they constitute only 25% of the sexually active population. Adolescents have been considered as a key and vulnerable population; adolescents are considered as marginalized populations (i.e., poor access to adequate health services, social and parental acceptance, stigmatization, among others. Every year, 87 million new cases of gonorrhea are reported worldwide in the population from 15 to 49 years old. In 2016, the estimated global prevalence of CT in 15-to 49-year-old women was 3.8% and in men 2.7%, with regional values ranging from 1.5 to 7.0% in women and 1.2 to 4.0% in men. The worldwide prevalence of HSV-2 among 15–49-year old is 11.3% and for HSV-1 among 0–49-year-old is 67%. These numbers alert us about the increase in the frequency of these diseases among young populations; more open sexual behavior could be an important factor for this increase; the treatment of these diseases is challenging due to the difficulties with detection and treatment; in the case of gonorrhea, it could become a major public health problem due to the emerging antimicrobial resistance; in the case of Chlamydia, despite the effective treatment, reinfection is still a possibility and for genital herpes, the disease can be controlled but not cured. This chapter will describe the most important aspects of these three diseases for supporting the clinicians and researchers about the management of sexually transmitted diseases in the adolescent population.

Keywords: sexually transmitted diseases, chlamydia, genital herpes, HSV-1, HSV-2, gonorrhea

1. Introduction

Sexually transmitted diseases (STDs) disproportionately affect young people, with more than half of the infections occurring in 15- to 25-year-olds, although as an age group they constitute only 25% of the sexually active population [1]. Family physicians and pediatricians must be familiar with the context around STDs and mainly with the key clinical elements for diagnostic suspicion, always evaluating sexual abuse. More than 1 million sexually transmitted infections (STIs) occur every day and an estimated 376 million chlamydia, gonorrhea, syphilis, and trichomoniasis infections occur each year. STIs can have serious consequences beyond the immediate infection itself, through mother-to-child transmission of infections or conditions such as infertility and cervical cancer and some STIs can increase the risk of HIV acquisition three-fold or more. Adolescents have been considered as a key, vulnerable and marginalized population (i.e., poor access to adequate health services, social and parental acceptance, stigmatization, among others) [2]. In this chapter, we will be describing the major clinical features of Gonorrhea, Chlamydia Trachomatis, and Genital Herpes.

2. Gonorrhea

2.1 Epidemiology

Every year, 87 million new cases of gonorrhea are reported worldwide in the population from 15 to 49 years old (2016 incidence). The median cases rates per 100,000 men from 15 to 49 years old reporting urethral discharge are 82.5 (range: 1.1–6133.7) and gonorrhea are 16.9 (range 0.0–297.1); the highest case rates were reported from the African Region, followed by the European and Western Pacific regions. In the United States, the highest peak of gonorrhea has been reported in the 20–24 years of age (720.9/100,000 in men and 702.6/100,000 in women), the second group of age with the highest incidence is the group from 15 to 19 years old (320.5/100,000 in men and 548.1/100,000 in women) [3]. Latin American countries like Colombia, Peru, and Brazil have been reported an increase in the number of cases in 2000 [4]. The highest prevalence of gonorrhea has been detected in the African Region (1.7%) followed by the Western Pacific Region (around 1.5%) [5]. One of the biggest concerns about gonorrhea is the development of antimicrobial resistance (AMR); in 2016, 57 countries reported that ≥5% of N. gonorrhea (Ng) specimens had decreased susceptibility (including azithromycin and ciprofloxacin) [6].

2.2 The pathogen

Neisseria gonorrhea (Ng) is a diplococcal gram-negative microorganism and one of the two pathogenic Neisseria species pluralism (spp); this bacterium has 80–90% of similarity to Neisseria meningitidis. Ng genome was sequenced for the first time in 2003. Ng has a high degree of genetic plasticity that enables the rapid evolution of AMR [7].

Ng has evolved mechanisms for evading innate immunity and suppressing adaptive immune responses. Ng prevents complement activation, opsonization, and bacterial killing by binding to complement proteins, sialylating its lipooligosaccharide (LOS) to hide from the complement system. Ng can bind also to the Host factor H and C4b-binding protein (C4BP), becoming serum resistant by presenting as self and by shielding itself from complement recognition [8].

2.3 The disease

Ng is an obligated human pathogen that is primarily transmitted through genital, oral, and anal sexual contact, infecting mucosal surfaces at these sites leading to the various symptoms associated with gonorrhea. Transmission is highly efficient (a substantial proportion of people become infected after a single exposure); can be asymptomatic or symptomatic (all sites), both can lead to additional Sexual Reproductive Health (SRH) complications (infection itself or inflammatory response); it can be also transmitted to neonates from infected mothers during childbirth infecting the conjunctival mucosa [9].

The asymptomatic infection is frequently unrecognized and is accountable for the larger proportion of all infections, this is the most frequent presentation in women; the acute symptomatic syndrome is the most common presentation in men [8, 9].

In women, as already mentioned, most of the infections have no or mild symptoms like vaginal discharge, it is frequently mistaken for other reproductive conditions and the coinfection with Chlamydia trachomatis (CT) is common. In men, gonorrhea is presented as an acute lower genital tract infection with urethritis with purulent discharge or dysuria within 5 days of infection. Among both sexes, extragenital infections of the oropharynx and rectum are usually asymptomatic but can cause symptomatic pharyngitis and proctitis [8, 9].

Ng infections have potential adverse sexual reproductive health outcomes like pelvic inflammatory disease (PID), tubo-ovarian abscesses, infertility, epididymo-orchitis, ectopic pregnancy, chronic pelvic pain, urethral stricture in men, and adverse pregnancy outcomes. In the neonate can cause vision loss due by neonatal conjunctivitis. Ng also increases the risk of HIV, finally, the infection can be disseminated (i.e., arthritis, gonococcemia, endocarditis, and meningitis). Ng also generates important psychosocial consequences like stigmatization and negative effects on sexual relationships [7–10].

A recent increase in gonorrhea incidence has been reported, one of the main reasons is the change in sexual behavior in the era of antiretroviral treatment for HIV infection; it seems that people are less cautious and have sex with new and casual partners without condoms [7], this is of particular importance in the adolescent population that is considered a vulnerable group.

Gonorrhea infections are more common in adolescents, followed by neonatal infections; in children between these two periods, sexual abuse should be always considered [10].

2.4 Diagnosis

The most recent definition of a gonorrhea case is the one published by the Centers for Disease Control and Prevention (CDC). This definition includes laboratory criteria for diagnosis and case classification [11]. Observation of Ng in a urethral smear (gram-negative diplococci) from men or an endocervical smear from a female indicates Ng infection; also the isolation by culture can make the diagnosis; finally and more recently, the demonstration of Ng in a clinical specimen by detection of antigen or nucleic acid can also make Gonorrhea diagnosis. A case is confirmed when Ng is isolated by culture or N. gonorrhea is demonstrated in a clinical specimen by detection of antigen or detection of nucleic acid via nucleic acid amplification (e.g., PCR or hybridization with a nucleic acid probe).

For practical purposes, we can consider two types of diagnosis: Clinical gonorrhea defined by a confirmed case and clinical signs and symptoms; and asymptomatic gonorrhea, defined as a confirmed case without clinical signs and symptoms.

2.5 Gonorrhea in children and sexual abuse

In general, gonococcal infections in children and adolescents can occur in three different age groups [9]:

- In the newborn, in which the most frequent clinical manifestation is conjunctivitis; other manifestations include scalp abscess, disseminated disease, vaginitis, and urethritis. Infection in the newborn normally occurs due to vertical transmission.

- In children beyond this period, gonorrhea has been considered as "proof" of sexual abuse, vaginitis is the most common manifestation in pre-pubertal females. Sexual transmission should be considered always in these cases; it is mandatory to suspect and manage sexual abuse in the applicable legal and medical context [9, 10].

- In adolescents with active sexual life, in which the infection is often asymptomatic; in female adolescents the Fitz-Hugh-Curtis syndrome and be seen (perihepatitis).

2.6 Treatment

Since the discovery of the sulfonamides in the 1930's decade followed by Penicillin G, Spectinomycin, 3rd generation cephalosporins, macrolides, and finally fluoroquinolones; Ng has been developed evolutive mechanisms for antimicrobial resistance. The first Ng strain with high-level resistance to ceftriaxone was isolated in 2009 in Japan, same findings occurred in France and Spain 2 years later; other countries like Japan, China, Australia, Singapore, Canada, and Argentina also reported treatment failures with ceftriaxone. In 2014, the first failure of ceftriaxone–azithromycin dual therapy for gonorrhea was verified in the United Kingdom. Since 2015, an international spread of one ceftriaxone-resistant gonococcal strain, initially described in Japan, has been confirmed and the first strain with resistance to ceftriaxone plus high-level azithromycin resistance was isolated in 2018 in the UK and Australia [7–12].

2.6.1 Uncomplicated gonococcal infections treatment beyond the neonatal period and adolescents

Considering that older children normally acquire the infection through sexual abuse, it is very important to reduce the traumatic impact of treatment; in these cases, a single dose oral regimen is preferred [10]. The recommended regimens for Ng treatment depend on the location of the infection.

For uncomplicated vulvovaginitis, cervicitis, urethritis, proctitis, or pharyngitis, the primary recommendation is for children who weigh less than 45 kg: ceftriaxone 125 mg IM in a single dose; and for children who weigh 45 kg or more: 250 mg IM in a single dose plus azithromycin, 1 g orally in a single dose. In the case of uncomplicated infections that involve the anal region, dual treatment with cefixime (400 mg orally) and azithromycin may be used if ceftriaxone is not available. For infections located in the pharynx, the primary treatment recommended is ceftriaxone; cefixime should not be used [9, 13]. In the case of cephalosporin allergy, a consultation with a pediatric allergologist or an allergy expert consultation should be performed.

Tests-of-cure are not needed; these are recommended only for pharyngeal locations (test-of-cure 7–14 days after using NAAT or culture).

In the case of persistent infections, other causes must be considered: recurrent Ng infection can be seen among sexually active adolescents previously treated with gonorrhea mostly related to reinfection (i.e., sexual partners did not receive the treatment). It is recommended that this population that has been treated for Ng, should be retested 3 months after treatment [13–15].

2.6.2 Complicated gonococcal infections treatment beyond the neonatal period and adolescents

Complicated gonococcal infections include arthritis-dermatitis syndrome, meningitis, endocarditis, conjunctivitis, and epididymitis [9, 13–15].

- For disseminated infection, the recommendation is:

- In children who weigh less than 45 kg: Ceftriaxone (50 mg/kg/day; maximum 1 g/day, intravenous or intramuscular, once a day for 7 days) AND Erythromycin base or ethylsuccinate (50 mg/kg/day; maximum 2 g, orally divided into 4 doses every day for 14 days.

- In children who weigh 45 kg or more: Ceftriaxone (1 g, intravenous or intramuscular, once a day for 7 days) AND Azithromycin (1 g, orally in a single dose).

• For meningitis or endocarditis, the recommendation is:

- In children who weigh less than 45 kg: Ceftriaxone (50 mg/kg/day; maximum 2 g/day, intravenous or intramuscular, every 12–24 hours. For meningitis: 10 to 14 days. For Endocarditis: at least 28 days; AND Erythromycin base or ethylsuccinate (50 mg/kg/day; orally divided into 4 doses every day for 14 days.

- In children who weigh 45 kg or more: Ceftriaxone (1–2 g, intravenous or intramuscular, every 12–24 hours. For meningitis: 10–14 days. For endocarditis: at least 28 days; AND Azithromycin (1 g, orally in a single dose).

• For conjunctivitis, the recommendation is:

- In children who weigh less than 45 kg: Ceftriaxone 1 g, intramuscular in a single dose.

- In children who weigh 45 kg or more: Ceftriaxone, 1 g, intramuscular in a single dose; AND Azithromycin 1 g, orally in a single dose.

• For epididymitis the recommendation is:

- Ceftriaxone, 250 mg intramuscular in a single dose AND doxycycline, 100 mg orally twice daily for 10 days.

2.7 Prevention and patient counseling

The patient should be counseled about the importance of routine screening for gonorrhea to prevent reproductive health complications of untreated infections, especially in young women; the asymptomatic nature of most gonococcal infections in females, whereas males often present with symptoms; the importance of treating partners and the high risk of repeated infection; the need to abstain from intercourse after completion of treatment for both partners for at least 7 days and while symptomatic; and the risk reduction strategies, including consistent condom use [16].

3. Chlamydia Trachomatis

3.1 Epidemiology

Chlamydia trachomatis (CT) is one of the most reported diseases; however, case reports likely underestimate the burden of disease because most infections are asymptomatic and are neither diagnosed nor reported. Case report data are strongly influenced by screening activity, for these reasons, case report data are not reliable indicators of either population incidence or population prevalence [16]. In 2016 the estimated global prevalence of CT was 3.8% in women (95% UI: 3.3–4.5) and 2.7% in men (95% UI:1.9–3.7) in the group from 15 to 49-year-old [17]. A total of 1,758,668 cases of CT infection were reported in 2018 in the United States. Among females aged 15–24 years, the cases reported by chlamydia screening, increased 11.8% from 2014 to 2018; in men, the cases increased 37.8% from 2014 to 2018; this may reflect an increased number of men being tested and diagnosed due to increased availability of screening tests; this could also reflect increased transmission. Among sexually active women aged 16–24 years, CT screening has been increased [3].

3.2 The pathogen

CT is a gram-negative obligate intracellular bacterium; humans are its exclusive natural host. CT serovars include Agents of preventable blindness (serovars A–C), the most common bacterial sexually transmitted infections worldwide (serovars D–K), and lymphatic system infections (serovars L1–L3). Some distinctive features include its ability to avoid destruction by the host's innate and adaptive immune system. By autophagy, CT migrates to the upper genital tract and establishes a chronic infection. Without treatment, up to 50% of infected women continue to be infected for greater than 1 year [18, 19].

The life cycle of CT consists of 2 main phases, the elementary body (EB) and the reticulate body (RB). EBs are present in the semen from infected males and are also released from infected female genital tract epithelial cells. The EB represents the infectious extracellular form and the RB is the non-infectious replicative form; RBs can convert back to EBs as required. CT can enter the 3rd stage when it is exposed to certain stressors, like interferon-gamma, penicillin, or iron-depletion, the organism is metabolically active but does not divide and continues to increase in size [20].

3.3 The disease

In the pediatric population, CT is associated with several clinical conditions, these include conjunctivitis, nasopharyngitis, and pneumonia in young infants; and in the case of children and adolescents: genital tract infection, lymphogranuloma venereum, and trachoma.

Neonatal conjunctivitis is vertically transmitted, the neonate usually shows ocular congestion, edema, and discharge; these could last 1 to 2 weeks after birth. Pneumonia can be seen in young infants, normally occurs between 2 and 19 weeks after birth; could be afebrile and it is associated with hyperinflation of the lungs, nasal stuffiness, and otitis media; its presence could indicate immunosuppression.

Clinical manifestations in children and adolescents with genitourinary CT include vaginitis in prepubertal females and the post-pubertal females can present the Fitz-Hugh-Curtis syndrome (urethritis, cervicitis, endometritis, salpingitis, proctitis, and perihepatitis); also described for gonorrhea infections. In males, the most frequent manifestations are urethritis, epididymitis, and proctitis; also, Reiter syndrome can be seen (reactive arthritis, urethritis, and bilateral conjunctivitis) [20]. Lymphogranuloma venereum is another clinical manifestation of CT infection in adolescents; this is an invasion of the lymphatic nodes that generates an ulcerative lesion in the genital area plus inguinal or femoral or both lymphadenopathies, typically unilateral.

Young age is a strong predictor of CT infection, particularly prevalent in individuals younger than 25 years. CT infection is normally asymptomatic in both men and women (routine screening is essential for the detection); this situation increases the transmission between partners (rates are greater than 50%); also, it is important to highlight that transmission is more efficient from men to women. The incubation period ranges from 7 to 21 days after exposure. In the case of neonates, at least 60–70% acquire conjunctivitis when exposed to CT during passage through the birth canal [18]. The most common clinical presentations are described in **Figure 1**.

CT extra-genitourinary manifestations include rectal and oropharyngeal infections. Rectal infection is presented as proctitis; this can be acquired by sexual anal intercourse and due to autoinoculation in women. In the case of the oropharynx, the infection is usually asymptomatic, sometimes it can be presented as pharyngitis or cervical lymphadenopathy.

Finally, trachoma is a form of chronic keratoconjunctivitis, follicular with neovascularization of the cornea; blindness occurs in 1–15% of the affected population.

3.4 Diagnosis

Untreated CT infections can lead to complications like infertility (20%), life-threatening tubal pregnancy (9%), and debilitating chronic pain (18%). Currently, the best method for CT infection detection is the Nucleic acid amplification tests (NAATs). NAATs offer greatly expanded sensitivities of detection, usually well above 90%, while maintaining very high specificity, usually ≥99%. Currently, NAATs are the approved tests by international regulatory organisms for the detection of genital tract infections caused by CT in men and women with and without symptoms. Acceptable samples for NAATs are vaginal swabs in women and first catch urine from men. The performance of NAATs for overall sensitivity, specificity, and ease of specimen transport is better than that of any of the other tests available for the diagnosis of chlamydial infections NAATs are cost-effective in preventing sequelae due to CT [21].

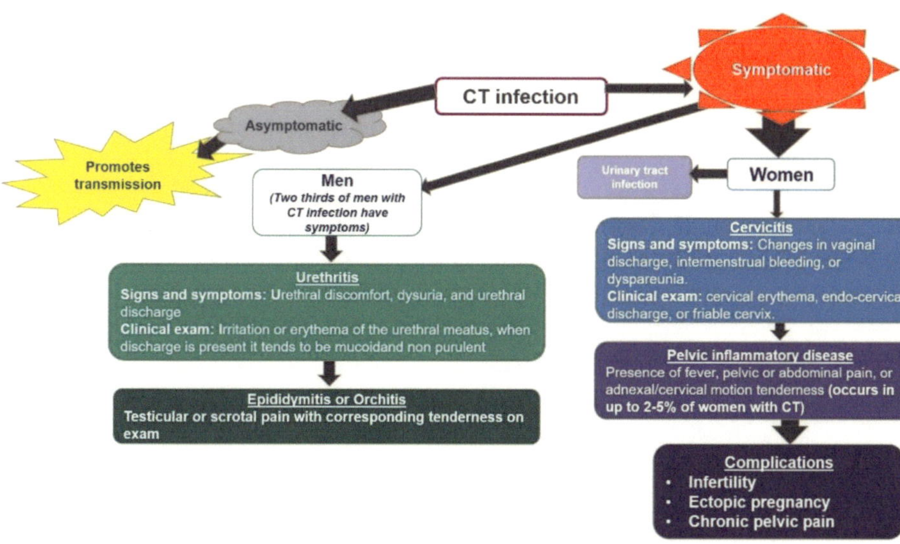

Figure 1.
Chlamydia trachomatis clinical manifestations and evolution.

3.4.1 Screening tests in the adolescent population

3.4.1.1 Genitourinary CT detection

As mentioned above, for female screening, samples from vaginal swabs are the preferred ones; these areas are sensitive as cervical swabs with similar specificity; for clinical and research settings it is also important to know that self-collected vaginal swabs are equivalent in sensitivity and specificity to those collected by health care personnel. Cervical samples could be done as part of pelvic examinations but not as routine tests; in general, cervical samples should be avoided; vaginal swabs should be preferred in all cases [21].

Currently, there are no specific recommendations for CT screening in heterosexual men. Recommendations are recommended only in specific settings such as sexually active heterosexual men in clinical settings with a high prevalence of C. trachomatis (i.e., sexually transmitted diseases clinics, adolescent clinics, detention and prisons, persons entering the armed forces. Etc).

3.5 Treatment

Treatment can be classified depending on the type of clinical manifestations that are frequently associated with the group of age. In infants with conjunctivitis or pneumonia, the treatment is oral erythromycin base or ethylsuccinate (50 mg/kg/day in 4 divided doses daily for 14 days) or with azithromycin (20 mg/kg, single daily dose for 3 days). When CT infection is detected in an infant, the mother and her sexual partner(s) must receive treatment. In the neonates, the presence of CT infection must alert the physician for also detecting Ng. Any infant younger than 6 weeks and treated with oral erythromycin or azithromycin must be monitored for any signs or symptoms of hypertrophic pyloric stenosis [20].

In adolescents with uncomplicated anogenital CT, the recommendation is doxycycline 100 mg, twice daily for 7 days; or azithromycin 1 g oral in a single dose. In affected children who weigh less than 45 kg the recommendation is oral erythromycin base or ethylsuccinate 50 mg/kg/day divided into 4 doses, daily for 14 days. For children younger than 8 years but weighing 45 kg or more, the recommendation is azithromycin 1 g orally in a single dose. In the case of 8 years and older children, the recommendation is azithromycin 1 g orally in a single dose; or doxycycline 100 mg orally 2 times a day for 7 days. Test of cure is not recommended; repeating the test 3 or 4 weeks after therapy to detect treatment failures can be done only if: adherence is in question, symptoms persist, or reinfection is suspected [17, 19, 20].

The treatment for lymphogranuloma venereum is with doxycycline 100 mg, orally twice daily for 21 days. Trachoma can be treated with oral azithromycin, a single dose of 20 mg/kg (maximum dose of 1 g) is recommended [20].

4. Genital herpes

4.1 Epidemiology

Genital herpes caused by HSV-2 and HSV-1 has been considered prevalent worldwide. The estimated global prevalence of these 2 pathogens is:

- HSV-2 among 15–49-year olds: 11.3% averaged across all ages [22]

- HSV-1 infection among 0–49-year-old: 67% averaged across all ages [23, 24]

A comparison between the most important epidemiological features is presented in **Figure 2**.

In several developed settings (e.g., the USA, Western Europe, Australia, and New Zealand) there is evidence that the proportion of first-episode genital herpes that is due to HSV-1 has increased, particularly among young people [25, 26]. Characteristics related to the first episode, latency site, viral shedding, and subsequent recurrence are presented in **Figure 3**.

Complications in HSV-2 are rare besides genital herpes; in HSV-1, the most common identified complications are sporadic encephalitis and ophthalmic disease in children and adults. HSV-2 rarely causes neonatal herpes, but these types of infections have a much more severe neurologic outcome. HSV-1 in the neonate, even rare can cause a devastating illness with high morbidity and mortality; when mothers shed genital HSV at delivery, HSV-1 may be more likely to be transmitted to the neonate [26].

4.2 The pathogen

Herpes simplex is a large DNA virus (150–200 nm) from the genus Simplex virus, subfamily Alphaherpesvirinae, and family Herpesviridae. It is a neurotropic virus with an envelope and depending on the protein coat, it can be named HSV-1 or HSV-2. HSV-2 shares>80% identity on the amino acid level with HSV-1. Both types can infect the oral or genital skin or mucosa and cause recurrent ulcerations.

	HSV-2	HSV-1
Age	Usually acquired through sexual contact; therefore, antibodies to virus are rarely found before ages of onset of sexual activity.	Occur during childhood and infection is never cleared
Most affected gender	Women	Women
Highly infectious	✓	✓
Primarily transmitted by	Almost entirely sexually transmitted, and is therefore most closely associated with genital herpes	Oral-oral contact (respiratory droplets or saliva, and most often by kissing) and causes orolabial herpes (notably "cold sores"). Potential to be transmitted through oral sex to cause genital infection
Worlwide highly prevalent and endemic	417 million ✓	3.7 billion ✓
Annual incidence (2012)	19 million ✓	118 million ✓

Figure 2.
Comparison between HSV-1 and HSV-2 in terms of age of onset, most affected gender, infectivity, transmission, prevalence, and incidence.

	HSV-2	HSV-1
First episode	Genital herpes, clinically indistinguishable	Oropharyngeal involvement occurs in the primary HSV-1 infection Primary infection is often more symptomatic and severe than reactivations Genital herpes, clinically indistinguishable
Latency site	Dorsosacral roots	Trigeminal Ganglia
Latency with reactivation periods	Normally benign, important feature of the infection.	
Viral shedding	Lifelong potential for symptomatic or asymptomatic viral shedding episodes	
Subsequent recurrences	**Severe and frequent**	**Milder and much less frequent.**

Figure 3.
Comparison between HSV-1 and HSV-2 based on the first episode, latency site, viral shedding, and subsequent recurrences.

The HSV genome consists of two covalently linked components, designated as L (long) and S (short). Each component is formed by unique sequences (UL and US, respectively) flanked by regions of repeated and inverted sequences that facilitate replication of the genome. The DNA molecular weight is estimated to be approximately 150 kbp, with a G + C content of 68% for HSV-1 and 69% for HSV-2. The viral composition is important for generating an immunogenic response, some of the most important proteins are in the capsid including VP5, VP19C, VP23, VP24, VP26, and the protein encoded by the UL6 gene. Another important component of the virion is the envelope, which consists of a lipid bilayer with approximately 11 viral glycoproteins, four of which (gB, gD, gH, and gL) are essential for virus entry into cells.

4.3 The disease

Once the virus replicates in the host, the intact virion is transported through a retrograde axonal flow to the sensory or autonomic ganglia, where the virus can remain in a latent form in the trigeminal ganglia for HSV-1 and the dorsosacral roots for HSV-2. Recurrences can occur when the latent virus is reactivated, being carried by anterograde axonal flow to the region of the primary infection. This reactivation is triggered by local stimuli (i.e., injury to the innervated tissue harboring latent HSV, systemic factors as physical or emotional stress, fever, exposure to ultraviolet light, menstruation, and hormonal imbalance).

Genital herpes is presented with one or more vesicles, or small blisters, on or around the genitals, rectum, or mouth. The average incubation period for an initial herpes infection is 4 days, ranging from 2 to 12 days after exposure. The vesicles then break leaving painful ulcers that may take 2–4 weeks to heal after the initial herpes infection; this is known as "outbreak" or genital herpes episode.

There are differences between the first and recurrent outbreaks. The first outbreaks have a longer duration of herpetic lesions, the viral shedding is increased (this makes HSV transmission more likely) and the patients experience more systemic symptoms like fever, body aches, swollen lymph nodes, or headache. In the case of the recurrent outbreaks, the duration is shorter and these episodes are less severe than the first outbreak; recurrent outbreaks are very common and normally have prodromal symptoms, either localized genital pain or tingling or shooting pains in the legs, hips, or buttocks, which occur hours to days before the eruption of herpetic lesions. The number of symptomatic recurrent outbreaks may decrease over time.

It is important to highlight that recurrences and subclinical shedding are much less frequent for genital HSV-1 infection than for genital HSV-2 infection.

Another important clinical manifestation in children and adolescents is HSV encephalitis, this can occur because of a primary or recurrent HSV-1 infection. The most common sign and symptoms include fever, alterations in the state of consciousness, personality changes, seizures, and other neurological symptoms. A form of self-limited aseptic meningitis has been associated with genital HSV-2 infection. HSV can cause other unusual central nervous system manifestations such as Bell's palsy, ascending and transverse myelitis, postinfectious encephalomyelitis, and recurrent meningitis.

4.4 Treatment

Currently, there is no treatment able to definitively cure genital herpes; some antiviral chemotherapy offers control and relief to the most symptomatic patients; also, recurrences can be reduced but not eradicated. For these patients, Acyclovir can be used for initial episodes, in the case of recurrences, 45, 52 and 63% of patients remain free of recurrences in the first, second and third year of treatment. Valacyclovir is also used for the initial episode and as suppressive therapy, it has been considered as the gold standard therapy; after 6 months of using valacyclovir almost 55% of the patients remain without recurrences and 34% one year after.

For a first episode, oral acyclovir is recommended 400 mg three times a day for 7–10 days or acyclovir 200 mg five times a day for 7–10 days or valacyclovir 1 g orally twice a day for 7–10 days. For suppressive treatment, valacyclovir can be used 1 g once daily; or acyclovir 400 mg orally twice a day.

5. Vaccines for Gonorrhea, Chlamydia trachomatis and genital herpes

In the last 10 years, several efforts have been done for developing vaccines for these pathogens. The most important challenges are related to the immunological pathways (i.e., local mucosal immunity involved, the need of cellular immune responses plus neutralizing antibodies induction); currently, there is new hope for the development of efficacious vaccines for these targets; mRNA technology and the recently discovered effectiveness against gonorrhea using Men B vaccines are showing some light at the end of the road.

Conflict of interest

Diana Leticia Coronel Martínez is a employee of Sanofi Pasteur.

Author details

Diana Coronel-Martínez[1*] and Luis Augusto Moya-Barquín[2]

1 Advanced Pediatrics Resuscitation Group, Mexico City, Mexico

2 San Juan de Dios General Hospital Pediatric Critical Care Unit Head, San Carlos de Guatemala University, Guatemala

*Address all correspondence to: dianacoronel75@gmail.com

References

[1] Gupta N. Sexually transmitted infections: Part I: Genital bumps and genital ulcers. Pediatrics in Review. 2020;**41**(9):455-468. DOI: 10.1542/pir.2018-0261

[2] World Health Organization Sexually Transmitted Infections. 2019. Available from: https://apps.who.int/iris/bitstream/handle/10665/329888/WHO-RHR-19.22-eng.pdf?ua=1 [Accessed: February 5, 2020]

[3] Sexually Transmitted Disease Surveillance 2018. Centers for Disease Control and Prevention. Atlanta: U.S. Department of Health and Human Services; 2019. DOI: 10.15620/cdc.79370.

[4] Korenromp EL, Ríos C, Apolinar ALS, et al. Prevalence and incidence estimates for syphilis, chlamydia, gonorrhea, and congenital syphilis in Colombia, 1995-2016. Revista Panamericana de Salud Pública. 2018;**42**:e118. DOI: 10.26633/RPSP.2018.118

[5] Newman L, Rowley J, Vander Hoorn S, et al. Global estimates of the prevalence and incidence of four curable sexually transmitted infections in 2012 based on systematic review and global reporting. PLoS One. 2015;**10**(12):e0143304. DOI: 10.1371/journal.pone.0143304

[6] Report on globally sexually transmitted infection surveillance, 2018. World Health Organization; 2018. Available from: https://apps.who.int/iris/bitstream/handle/10665/277258/9789241565691-eng.pdf?ua=1 [Accessed: February 5, 2020]

[7] Unemo M, Seifert HS, Hook EW 3rd, Hawkes S, Ndowa F, Dillon JR. Gonorrhoea. Nature Reviews. Disease Primers. 2019;**5**(1):79. DOI: 10.1038/s41572-019-0128-6

[8] Quillin SJ, Seifert HS. Neisseria gonorrhoeae host adaptation and pathogenesis. Nature Reviews. Microbiology. 2018;**16**(4):226-240. DOI: 10.1038/nrmicro.2017.169

[9] American Academy of Pediatrics. Gonococcal Infections. In: Kimberlin DW, Brady MT, Jackson MA, Long SS, editors. Red Book: 2018 Report of the Committee on Infectious Diseases. 31st ed. Itasca, IL: American Academy of Pediatrics; 2018. pp. 356-366

[10] Hammerschlang M. Chlamydial and gonococcal infections in infants and children. CID. 2011;**53**(Suppl 3):S99

[11] Gonorrhea (Neisseria gonorrhoeae) 2014 Case Definition. 2014. Available from: https://wwwn.cdc.gov/nndss/conditions/gonorrhea/case-definition/2014/#:~:text=Gonorrhea%20is%20a%20common%20sexually,at%20birth%20to%20a%20newborn [Accessed: February 6, 2020]

[12] WHO Preferred Product Characteristics for Gonococcal 1 Vaccines, Draft for Public Comment, 29-09-2020. 2020. Available from: https://www.who.int/immunization/research/ppc-tpp/Gonococcal_vaccine_PPCs_for-public-comment.pdf [Accessed: February 6, 2020]

[13] Sexually Transmitted Diseases Treatment Guidelines. Centers for Disease Control and Prevention; 2015. Available from: https://www.cdc.gov/std/tg2015/gonorrhea.htm [Accessed: February 6, 2020]

[14] St. Cyr S, Barbee L, Workowski KA, et al. Update to CDC's treatment guidelines for gonococcal infection. MMWR. Morbidity and Mortality Weekly Report. 2020;**69**:1911-1916. DOI: 10.15585/mmwr.mm6950a6

[15] Lemly D, Gupta N. Sexually transmitted infections Part 2: Discharge

syndromes and pelvic inflammatory disease. Pediatrics in Review. 2020;**41**(10):522-537. DOI: 10.1542/pir.2019-0078

[16] Lane AB, Decker CF. Chlamydia trachomatis infections. Disease-a-Month. 2016;**62**(8):269-273. DOI: 10.1016/j.disamonth.2016.03.010

[17] Witkin SS, Minis E, Athanasiou A, Leizer J, Linhares IM. Chlamydia trachomatis: The persistent pathogen. Clinical and Vaccine Immunology. 2017;**24**(10):e00203-e00217. DOI: 10.1128/CVI.00203-17

[18] Rowley J, Vander-Hoorn S, Korenromp E, Low N, Unemo M, Abu-Raddad LJ, et al. Chlamydia, gonorrhoea, trichomoniasis and syphilis: Global prevalence and incidence estimates, 2016. Bulletin of the World Health Organization. 2019;**97**:548-562P. DOI: 10.2471/BLT.18.228486

[19] Janssen KJH, Dirks JAMC, Dukers-Muijrers NHTM, Hoebe CJPA, Wolffs PFG. Review of Chlamydia trachomatis viability methods: Assessing the clinical diagnostic impact of NAAT positive results. Expert Review of Molecular Diagnostics. 2018;**18**(8):739-747. DOI: 10.1080/14737159.2018.1498785

[20] American Academy of Pediatrics. Chlamydia trachomatis. In: Kimberlin DW, Brady MT, Jackson MA, Long SS, editors. Red Book: 2018 Report of the Committee on Infectious Diseases. 31st ed. Itasca, IL: American Academy of Pediatrics; 2018. pp. 276-283

[21] Rapp JR, Schachter J, Gaydos CA, Van Der Pol B. Recommendations for the laboratory-based detection of Chlamydia trachomatis and Neisseria gonorrhoeae — 2014. MMWR. 2014;**63**(2):1-18

[22] Looker KJ, Magaret AS, Turner KME, Vickerman P, Gottlieb SL, et al. Global estimates of prevalent and incident Herpes Simplex Virus type 2 infections in 2012. PLoS One. 2015;**10**(1):e114989. DOI: 10.1371/journal.pone.0114989

[23] Looker KJ, Magaret AS, May MT, Turner KME, Vickerman P, Gottlieb SL, et al. Global and regional estimates of prevalent and incident Herpes Simplex Virus type 1 infections in 2012. PLoS One. 2015;**10**(10):e0140765. DOI: 10.1371/journal. pone.0140765

[24] Ayoub HH, Chemaitelly H, Abu-Raddad LJ. Characterizing the transitioning epidemiology of herpes simplex virus type 1 in the USA: Model-based predictions. BMC Medicine. 2019;**17**(1):57. DOI: 10.1186/s12916-019-1285-x

[25] Zendrini D, Faccin-Galhardi LG, Carvalho RE, Nozawa C. Herpesvirus: An underestimated virus. Folia Microbiologica. 2017;**62**:151-156. DOI: 10.1007/s12223-016-0482-7

[26] Whitley R, Baines J. Clinical management of herpes simplex virus infections: Past, present, and future. F1000Res. 2018;**7**:F1000 Faculty Rev-1726. DOI: 10.12688/f1000research.16157.1

Chapter 7

Chlamydial Infection

Dimitra Metallinou, Christina Nanou, Antigoni Sarantaki, Eleftheria Lazarou, Anastasia Liagkou and Katerina Lykeridou

Abstract

Chlamydial infection is one of the most common sexually transmitted infections worldwide, showing no decreasing trends in the incidence the last years. As a result, it presents a major burden of disease that impacts negatively people's sexual and reproductive health and may result in adverse perinatal outcomes. The aim of the chapter is to offer today's practitioners trustworthy guidance on the latest data in chlamydial infection. Thorough, up-to-date content on the epidemiology, pathophysiology, risk factors, clinical manifestations, diagnosis, treatment, prevention, prognosis and outcomes of infected infants, is presented. Data in children and adolescents that differ from infants, are also discussed. The chapter is organized consistently in order to help readers find information quickly and easily and thus, provide direct, optimal and evidence-based care to every pediatric patient.

Keywords: *Chlamydia trachomatis*, chlamydial infection, conjunctivitis, pneumonia, infant, children, adolescents

1. Introduction

More than 1 million sexually transmitted infections are acquired every day worldwide and chlamydial infection is the most common in the developed world, showing no decreasing trends in the incidence the last years [1]. As a result, chlamydial infection presents a major burden of disease that impacts negatively people's sexual and reproductive health and may result in adverse perinatal outcomes. As chlamydiae are largely asymptomatic and high rates of antibiotic resistance [2] have been shown, screening and treatment are the most crucial issues to reduce their impact globally.

Chlamydial infection can be transmitted to the infant during childbirth, resulting in conjunctivitis or pneumonia as a clinical disease. If present beyond the neonatal period in a child, may be a sign of sexual abuse. Sexually transmitted infection can occur in sexually active adolescents leading to a cascade of potentially serious inflammatory-induced sequelae.

2. Definition - background

"Chlamydiae", originate from the Greek word "chlamyda", meaning "cloak". They are Gram-negative obligate intracellular bacteria pathogenic to humans or animals and mainly transmitted through direct contact with infected tissue, including vaginal, anal or oral sex and can even be passed from an infected mother to the newborn during childbirth. Some species though, pathogenic to animals can be transmitted to humans also [3].

Chlamydiae have a unique biphasic developmental cycle which involves transition between two major morphologic forms: (1) the infectious forms, called elementary bodies convert into (2) non-infectious, reproductive forms, called reticulate bodies. This transition takes place within the host cell and differentiates the metabolically inactive elementary body into the metabolically active reticulate body. The reticulate body contains no cell wall and is detected as an inclusion in the cell. Chlamydiae contain DNA, RNA and ribosomes [4, 5].

There are four recognized species of Chlamydiae: Chlamydia trachomatis, Chlamydia psittaci, Chlamydia pneumoniae, and Chlamydia pecorum. Humans are the only natural host for *Chlamydia trachomatis (C. trachomatis)*. This bacterium has a distinct developmental cycle, approximately 48–72 hours, which only replicates inside eukaryotic host cells. It uses energy phosphate compounds from the host cell during its growth and replication [6]. Preferentially infects squamo-columnar epithelial cells of the eye and the genital tract. Its genome size is 1000 kB [7].

3. Pathophysiology

Although infection by C. trachomatis is a major sexually transmitted genital infection globally, eye infections may be also spread by personal contact and contaminated items which are touched or held by hands, such as towels, in areas with poor sanitation [8]. Repeated and chronic infections, usually in developing countries, can lead to trachoma, which is a chronic follicular keratoconjunctivitis that causes scarring and neovascularization of the cornea that can result in blindness [9].

In women, genital tract infections with by C. trachomatis are usually asymptomatic and that is why it is frequently characterized as the "silent epidemic" [10]. If left untreated though, it can lead to serious sequelae, including urethritis, bartholinitis, mucopurulent cervicitis, endometritis, salpigitis, and pelvic inflammatory disease which may subsequently compromise fertility or predispose to ectopic pregnancy. Additionally, several pregnancy complications have been linked to chlamydial infection, including chorioamnionitis, premature rupture of membranes, preterm labour and birth, low birth weight, intrauterine growth restriction and postpartum endometritis [11–15]. In males, (or men) may cause epididymitis, proctitis, prostatitis, urethritis and reactive arthritis [16].

In infants, C. trachomatis can cause conjunctivitis and/or pneumonia. More rarely, C. trachomatis occurs also in the vagina, urethra and rectum. Occasional C. trachomatis infection in children and adolescents (with no prior sexual activity) should be seen in the context of sexual abuse, especially when Chlamydiae are detected in the anorectal or genital region [17].

There are 18 serotypes of C. trachomatis. The genital strains belong to one of the serotypes D through K while trachoma strains to the serotypes A through C [18]. The most common genotype among infants is type E [19, 20].

4. Prevalence

Based on prevalence data from 2009 to 2016, the estimated pooled global prevalence of chlamydial urogenital infection in women and men, aged 15–49 years, was 3.8% and 2.7%, respectively [21]. Rates of infection among adolescent girls exceed 20% in many urban populations, but can be as high as 15% in suburban populations [22].

Worldwide, the prevalence of C. trachomatis in pregnant women varies from 1.0%–36.8%, while in high income countries it is estimated from 3%–14% [23]. Especially in European western countries, the prevalence of genital C. trachomatis infection in pregnant women based on nucleic acid amplification tests (NAAT) from either first void urine or a vaginal and/or endocervical swab, ranges from 3% to 6% [24]. However, prevalence may vary significantly during pregnancy among different continents [23] (**Figure 1**).

Approximately 50%–70% of infants exposed to an infected mother's genital flora during vaginal birth, will acquire chlamydia infection if no prophylaxis is given before or just after birth. More specifically, the 10%–20% of all infected infants will develop pneumonia and the 30%–50% conjunctivitis. Prevalence data of neonatal chlamydial conjunctivitis and pneumonia from several regions [25] are summarized in **Figure 2**.

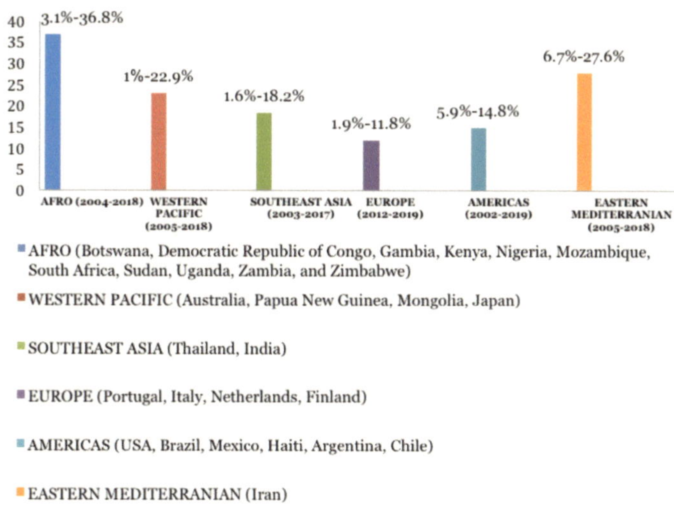

Figure 1.
Prevalence of C. trachomatis infection in pregnant women across all continents.

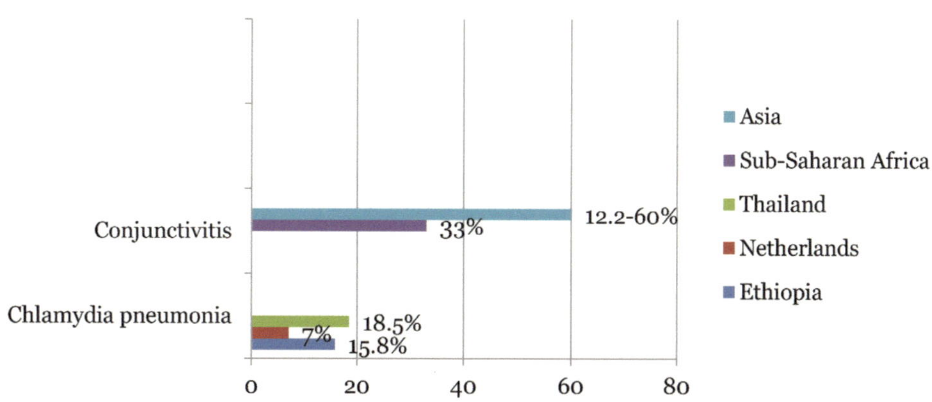

Figure 2.
Prevalence of chlamydial conjunctivitis and pneumonia in infants.

5. Risk factors

It seems that young women (<25 years old) are more prone to chlamydial infection due to anatomic differences in the cervix, such as cervical ectropion [16, 26]. In this condition, the glandular cells that line the endocervix are present on the ectocervix, leading to exposure of the glandular cells to the vaginal milieu and C. trachomatis has a preference for the glandular epithelium [5, 27].

Other factors associated with an increased risk of infection are numerous sexual partners, sexual intercourse with non-condom use, absence of barrier contraceptives, use of oral contraceptives, partner with concurrent partners or sexually-transmitted disease or non-gonococcal urethritis, non-gonococcal mucopurulent cervititis, sterile pyuria, other sexually transmitted diseases, unmarried status, nulliparity, African/American/Hispanic ethnicity and poor socio-economic condition [5, 23, 28].

Regarding infants, the main risk factor is vertical transmission (mother-to-child) after vaginal birth. Transmission after a cesarean section is unusual, unless premature rupture of the membranes of an infected mother is reported.

6. Clinical presentation

6.1 Conjunctivitis

Neonates exposed to C. trachomatis in an infected birth canal may develop conjunctivitis, sometimes referred to as "ophthalmia neonatorum", with transmission rate from 30%–50% [25]. Neonatal conjunctivitis caused by C. trachomatis has been reported as the most common infectious cause of neonatal conjunctivitis worldwide.

Conjunctivitis typically occurs between 5–14 days after delivery and can be unilateral or bilateral. It has a variety of clinical presentations in the infant. It is characterized by palpebral erythema and oedema, as well as eye discharge. Initially, the eye discharge is watery and later becomes purulent and copious. Moderate eye drainage and redness is common. Corneal opacification, chemosis and pseudomembranes may be present. Topical prophylaxis with erythromycin does not prevent but reduces the incidence of the chlamydial conjunctivitis [29–31].

Moreover, the 10%–20% of the infants with chlamydial conjunctivitis will develop pneumonia [25].

6.2 Pneumonia

The species C. psittaci, C. trachomatis and C. pneumoniae can all cause pneumonia in humans. Perinatal transmission of C. trachomatis has been reported to cause neonatal pneumonia with potentially a life-threatening severity. Usual age of presentation is at 3 weeks to 3 months of life [32]. In half of the cases concurrent or previous conjunctivitis is present and in one third of the cases otitis media is co-existing [33]. When C. pneumoniae is the cause, infection is predominantly asymptomatic or mild but can result in the development of acute upper and lower respiratory illness [34].

Upper and lower respiratory tracts may be directly infected intrapartum. C. trachomatis, which is the most common though, has been documented to be pathogen causing lower respiratory tract infection in children less than 6 months of age. Infants may present moderate symptoms, such as rhinitis, mucoid rhinorrhea together with cough and increased respiratory rate for 3 or more weeks before pneumonia. Most cases are afebrile. When pneumonia occurs, tachypnea, nasal obstruction and/or discharge, interstitial and peribronchiolar inflammation may exist, leading to significant morbidity manifested as low grade fever and paroxysmal staccato cough. Crepitant inspiratory rales often are heard on auscultation of the lungs, in contrast with expiratory wheezes which are distinctly uncommon. Hyperinflation of the lungs usually accompanies the diffused infiltrates observed on chest X-rays. Reticulonodular patterns and atelectasis have also been described. Eosinophilia may be also present [33, 35, 36].

In premature infants chlamydial pneumonia can be more serious. In the beginning, respiratory distress is observed which is followed later by worsening respiratory signs [37]. Apnea spells and respiratory failure may present as well [33, 38]. If chlamydial pneumonia is left untreated, infants are at high risk of developing later pulmonary dysfunction and possibly chronic respiratory disease, including mild to severe asthma [36]. Prophylaxis does not eliminate nasopharyngeal colonization or pneumonia.

It should be taken into consideration that C. trachomatis and C. pneumoniae are agents associated with community-acquired pneumonia in children and adolescents. They have not been associated with specific clinical syndromes among children and adolescents. Nevertheless, pharyngitis, bronchitis, and sinusitis may be present [38, 39].

6.3 Other clinical presentations in children and adolescents

In prepubertal girls, vaginitis may present, while in postpubertal girls, urethritis, bartholinitis, cervicitis, endometritis, salpingitis, proctitis, perihepatitis, are possible manifestations of the disease. Long-lasting infections may result in ectopic pregnancy, infertility or pelvic inflammatory disease [11, 13, 35]. In males, chlamydial infection may cause epididymitis, proctitis, prostatitis, urethritis and reactive arthritis. Lymphogranuloma venereum is extremely rare in children and adolescents below the age of 18 years old and is usually confined to HIV positive and homosexual men [35, 40].

Repeated and chronic chlamydial infection that affects eyes can lead to trachoma, a chronic follicular keratoconjunctivitis that causes scarring and neovascularization of the cornea and can even result in irreversible blindness [9]. It can be spread through contact with the eyes, eyelids, nose or throat secretions of infected people. Chlamydiae can be transmitted by contaminated handkerchiefs, towels, clothes or bed linen as well. Signs and symptoms of trachoma usually affect both eyes and may include: mild itching and irritation of the eyes and eyelids, eye discharge containing mucus or pus, eyelid swelling, light sensitivity (photophobia), eye pain, eye redness and vision loss. In areas where trachoma is endemic, usually poor and rural, active (inflammatory) trachoma is common among preschool-aged children, with prevalence rates which can be as high as 60–90% [8, 41].

7. Diagnosis

7.1 Laboratory studies

7.1.1 Tissue culture

For conjunctival specimens, any purulent exudate should be removed before collecting epithelial cells by rubbing a dry swab over the everted palpebral conjunctiva. The conjunctivae are often friable and may bleed after swabbing so great attention is needed. For suspected pneumonia, material should be obtained from nasopharyngeal aspiration or deep suctioning of the trachea.

Culture of the bacterium is considered as the gold standard for diagnosing neonatal conjunctivitis and pneumonia. Proficiency in specimen collection and transport is paramount to accuracy in diagnostic testing for Chlamydiae [5, 42]. Both the sensitivity and the specificity of culture is nearly 100% but is directly related to the adequacy of the specimen. For optimal isolation of the bacteria, specimens should be refrigerated immediately after collection at 2 to 8 °C and kept at this temperature during transport to the laboratory. The intervening period between collection and laboratory processing of specimens should ideally not exceed the 48 hours [42].

7.1.2 Nucleic acid amplification test (NAAT)

This method amplifies the nucleic acid sequences of chlamydiae. Non-viable bacteria can be detected contrary to cell culture. All relevant clinical materials can be analyzed by NAATs, including urethral, cervical, vulvo-vaginal, anorectal and ocular swabs, first void urine, sperm or tissues [43]. The test is recommended for routine use in adults and older children but data relating to infants are insufficient. The NAATs have not been approved by the US Food and Drug Administration (FDA) for testing of conjunctival specimens from infants with suspected C. trachomatis conjunctivitis or for testing of nasopharyngeal swab, tracheal aspirate or lung biopsy specimens from infants with suspected C. trachomatis pneumonia [33, 35].

7.1.3 Antigen detection tests

Antigen tests based on the detection of either chlamydial lipopolysaccharides (enzyme immunoassay, EIA) or direct fluorescent antibodies (DFA) have also been found to perform relatively well when used with conjunctival specimens. Sensitivity of nasopharyngeal samples is poor. Antigen tests are no longer recommended for chlamydia testing in infants due to insufficient diagnostic accuracy [43].

7.1.4 Serum anti-chlamydial antibody concentration

Chlamydial IgG antibodies detected from infants during the first months of life reflect maternally transferred antibodies and correlate with the levels of maternal serum antibodies. Maternal IgG antibodies do not protect infants from developing chlamydial infection and infants born to antibody positive mothers usually lose their maternally transferred IgG-antibodies by nine months of age [24]. In infants with chlamydial pneumonia a microimmunofluorescence serum titer of ≥1:32 is considered diagnostic for infection [31, 33]. The IgM antibodies have been observed to develop as early as five days after infection and to persist for three months. Their determination is difficult and availability limited [24].

7.1.5 Other tests

Obtaining lung biopsies is not a routine practise for confirming chlamydial pneumonia, since the course of the disease is rarely fatal, but when a biopsy is obtained the material should be examined for chlamydiae [44]. Additionally in pneumonia, eosinophilia in the peripheral blood is usual with white blood cell count being normal. Blood gas measurements reveal mild to moderate hypoxemia [33, 35, 36].

7.2 Imaging

In cases of chlamydial pneumonia, the most chest radiographs show bilateral hyperexpansion and diffuse infiltrates with a variety of radiographic patterns, including interstitial, reticular nodular, atelectasis, coalescence and bronchopneumonia. Pleural effusion and lobar consolidates are usually absent [33, 45]. Radiological findings alone are non-specific so it is almost impossible to determine by radiographic manifestations that a specie of clamydiae is the causative organism of the pneumonia.

8. Treatment

8.1 Conjunctivitis

Oral erythromycin base or ethylsuccinate is a usual treatment for conjunctivitis in the infant, although erythromycin has been reported as risk factor for infantile hypertrophic pyloric stenosis when administered the first 2 weeks of life. Thus, parents and physicians should observe infants closely for any signs of intestinal obstruction. Azithromycin is an acceptable alternative [30, 33, 35] which is also recommended by WHO in neonates with chlamydial conjunctivitis [46]. Dosages in the most preferable treatments are:

- Oral erythromycin 50 mg/kg/day in 4 divided doses for 14 days **or**
- Oral azithromycin 20 mg/kg/day for 3 days

8.2 Pneumonia

For children, the following regimens can be used for respiratory infection due to C. trachomatis and C. pneumoniae [47]:

Preferred therapy **intravenously**

- azithromycin 10 mg/kg on days 1 and 2 of therapy; transition to oral therapy if possible

Accepted alternatives are:

- erythromycin lactobionate 20 mg/kg/day every 6 hours
- levofloxacin 16–20 mg/kg/day in 2 doses for children 6 months to 5 years old and 8–10 mg/kg/day once daily for children 5 to 16 years old; maximum daily dose should not exceed the 750 mg

Preferred therapy **orally** [47, 48].

- azithromycin 10 mg/kg/once on day 1, followed by 5 mg/kg/day once daily for 2–5 days

Accepted alternatives are:

- clarithromycin 15 mg/kg/day for 10 days
- erythromycin 50 mg/kg/day for 10–14 days

- doxycycline 2–4 mg/kg/day in 2 doses for children with age greater than 7 years old
- levofloxacin 500 mg once daily or moxifloxacin 400 mg once daily for adolescents with skeletal maturity

Antibiotic resistance may diminish the overall efficacy of antibiotics, thus, it is strongly advised to follow-up patients to determine whether initial treatment was effective [33, 35, 39]. Clarithromycin is therapeutically equivalent to other antibiotics studied and is associated with a better bacteriological eradication and a lower risk for related adverse events in children [49]. In general, no isolation measures are necessary. Parents or mother and her sexual partner should be evaluated and treated if needed.

8.3 Uncomplicated genital chlamydial infection

For adolescents with uncomplicated genital chlamydial infection, guidelines relating to sexually transmitted diseases by WHO [46] suggest one of the following options:

- oral azithromycin 1 g as a single dose
- oral doxycycline 100 mg twice a day for 7 days

or one of the following alternatives:

- oral tetracycline 500 mg four times a day for 7 days
- oral erythromycin 500 mg twice a day for 7 days
- oral ofloxacin 200–400 mg twice a day for 7 days

Children with body weight < 45 kg, the recommended regimen is [35]:

- oral erythromycin base or ethylsuccinate, 50 mg/kg/day, divided into 4 doses daily for 14 days.

Children with body weight > 45 kg and age < 8 years old, the recommended regimen is [35]:

- oral azithromycin 1 g in a single dose

For children 8 years old and older, the recommended regimens are [35]:

- oral azithromycin 1 g in a single dose **or**
- oral doxycycline 100 mg twice a day for 7 days

8.4 Lymphogranuloma venereum (LGV)

In adolescents with LGV, it is suggested by WHO [46] the administration of doxycycline 100 mg orally twice daily for 21 days over azithromycin 1 g orally, weekly for 3 weeks.

9. Prevention

The most effective method of controlling perinatal chlamydial infection appears to be screening and treatment of pregnant women. The U.S. Centers for Disease Control and Prevention (CDC) recommend that "all pregnant women aged <25 years and older women at increased risk for infection should be routinely screened for C. trachomatis at the first prenatal visit and be retested during the third trimester to prevent maternal postnatal complications and chlamydial infection in the neonate" [44]. Healthcare professionals must cooperate closely to identify early the high-risk populations, educate and counsel the patients about sexual health and importance of screening and completing treatment.

According to recommendation of WHO [46], all neonates should be offered immediately after birth topical ocular prophylaxis to both eyes for the prevention of gonococcal and chlamydial ophthalmia neonatorum with one of the following options:

- tetracycline hydrochloride 1% eye ointment
- erythromycin 0.5% eye ointment
- povidone iodine 2.5% solution (water-based)
- silver nitrate 1% solution
- chloramphenicol 1% eye ointment

No vaccine is currently available for either trachoma or chlamydial genital infections. However, a first-in-human, randomized, double-blind, placebo-controlled, phase 1 trial was conducted between 2016–2017 to assess safety and immunogenicity of a chlamydial vaccine candidate [50].

As far as trachoma is concerned, a WHO-recommended elimination strategy summarized by the acronym"SAFE", is being implemented in endemic countries [41]. This consists of:

Surgery to treat the blinding stage.
Antibiotics to clear infection.
Facial cleanliness and.
Environmental improvement.

10. Prognosis

If proper treatment starts early, chlamydial infection should resolve without complications and with good prognosis, overall. Patients with mild symptoms usually recover within 7–10 days after initiation of the treatment. Dry cough and general weakness can persist after the disease, slowing complete remission from 1 week to 2 months. If neglected, serious complications may develop which can even lead to mortality [36].

11. Conclusion

Chlamydial infection is a significant worldwide public health problem, affecting both general and special populations. Early identification and management of high risk populations, with defined strategies, will eliminate crucially the burden of chlamydial infection. Obstetricians, gynecologists, midwives and pediatricians/neonatologists should be educated up-to-date and offered trustworthy guidance on the latest data in chlamydial infection. By applying scientific knowledge in clinical practice, these professionals can provide direct, optimal and evidence-based care to every pediatric patient.

Conflict of interest

The authors declare no conflict of interest.

Author details

Dimitra Metallinou[1*], Christina Nanou[1], Antigoni Sarantaki[1], Eleftheria Lazarou[2], Anastasia Liagkou[3] and Katerina Lykeridou[1]

1 Department of Midwifery, Faculty of Health and Care Sciences, University of West Attica, Athens, Greece

2 Iasis Private Hospital Paphos, Paphos, Cyprus

3 General Maternity and Gynecology Clinic"IASO," Athens, Greece

*Address all correspondence to: metallinoudimitra@gmail.com

References

[1] World Health Organization. Sexually transmitted infections (STIs) [Internet]. 2019. Available from: https://www.who.int/news-room/fact-sheets/detail/sexually-transmitted-infections-(stis) [Accessed 2021-01-30]

[2] Sandoz KM, Rockey DD. Antibiotic resistance in Chlamydiae.Future Microbiol. 2010;5(9):1427-1442. doi:10.2217/fmb.10.96

[3] Elwell C, Mirrashidi K, Engel J. Chlamydia cell biology and pathogenesis. Nat Rev Microbiol. 2016;14(6):385-400. doi:10.1038/nrmicro.2016.30

[4] Becker Y. Chlamydia. In: Baron S, editor. Medical Microbiology. 4th ed. Galveston (TX): University of Texas Medical Branch at Galveston; 1996.

[5] Malhotra M, Sood S, Mukherjee A, Muralidhar S, Bala M. Genital Chlamydia trachomatis: an update. Indian J Med Res. 2013;138(3):303-316

[6] Bastidas RJ, Elwell CA, Engel JN, Valdivia RH. Chlamydial intracellular survival strategies. Cold Spring Harb Perspect Med. 2013;3(5):a010256. Published 2013 May 1. doi:10.1101/cshperspect.a010256

[7] Stephens RS, Kalman S, Lammel C, et al. Genome sequence of an obligate intracellular pathogen of humans: Chlamydia trachomatis. Science. 1998;282(5389):754-759. doi:10.1126/science.282.5389.754

[8] Satpathy G, Behera HS, Ahmed NH. Chlamydial eye infections: Current perspectives. Indian J Ophthalmol. 2017;65(2):97-102. doi:10.4103/ijo.IJO_870_16

[9] Ubani U. Trachoma and Inclusion Conjunctivitis, Common Eye Infections. In: Chaudhry I, editor. Common eye infections. IntechOpen; 2013. doi: 10.5772/53861. Available from: https://www.intechopen.com/books/common-eye infections/trachoma-and-inclusion-conjunctivitis

[10] Okoror LE, Agbonlahor DE, Esumeh FI, Umolu PI. Prevalence of chlamydia in patients attending gynecological clinics in south eastern Nigeria. Afr Health Sci. 2007;7(1):18-24. doi:10.5555/afhs.2007.7.1.18

[11] Tsevat DG, Wiesenfeld HC, Parks C, Peipert JF. Sexually transmitted diseases and infertility. Am J Obstet Gynecol. 2017;216(1):1-9. doi:10.1016/j.ajog.2016.08.008

[12] Kacerovsky M, Romero R, Pliskova L, et al. Presence of Chlamydia trachomatis DNA in the amniotic fluid in women with preterm prelabor rupture of membranes [published online ahead of print, 2019 Jul 15]. J Matern Fetal Neonatal Med. 2019;1-12. doi:10.1080/14767058.2019.1640676

[13] Hussen S, Wachamo D, Yohannes Z, Tadesse E. Prevalence of chlamydia trachomatis infection among reproductive age women in sub Saharan Africa: a systematic review and meta-analysis. BMC Infect Dis. 2018;18(1):596. Published 2018 Nov 26. doi:10.1186/s12879-018-3477-y

[14] Menon S, Timms P, Allan JA, et al. Human and Pathogen Factors Associated with Chlamydia trachomatis-Related Infertility in Women. Clin Microbiol Rev. 2015;28(4):969-985. doi:10.1128/CMR.00035-15

[15] Cluver C, Novikova N, Eriksson DO, Bengtsson K, Lingman GK. Interventions for treating genital Chlamydia trachomatis infection in pregnancy. Cochrane Database Syst Rev. 2017;9(9):CD010485. Published

2017 Sep 22. doi:10.1002/14651858.CD010485.pub2

[16] Mohseni M, Sung S, Takov V. Chlamydia. In: StatPearls [Internet]. Treasure Island (FL): StatPearls Publishing; 2020. Available from: https://www.ncbi.nlm.nih.gov/books/NBK537286/

[17] Hammerschlag MR, Guillén CD. Medical and legal implications of testing for sexually transmitted infections in children. Clin Microbiol Rev. 2010;23(3):493-506. doi:10.1128/CMR.00024-09

[18] Vaulet LG, Entrocassi C, Corominas AI. et al. Distribution study of Chlamydia trachomatis genotypes in symptomatic patients in Buenos Aires, Argentina: association between genotype E and neonatal conjunctivitis. BMC Res Notes 3, 34. 2010. doi.org/10.1186/1756-0500-3-34

[19] Li Y, Xiong L, Huang Y, et al. The clinical characteristics and genotype distribution of Chlamydia trachomatis infection in infants less than six months of age hospitalized with pneumonia. Infect Genet Evol. 2015;29:48-52. doi:10.1016/j.meegid.2014.11.004

[20] Balla E, Petrovay F, Erdősi T, et al. Distribution of Chlamydia trachomatis genotypes in neonatal conjunctivitis in Hungary. J Med Microbiol. 2017;66(7):915-918. doi:10.1099/jmm.0.000523

[21] Rowley J, Vander Hoorn S, Korenromp E, et al. Chlamydia, gonorrhoea, trichomoniasis and syphilis: global prevalence and incidence estimates, 2016. Bull World Health Organ. 2019;97(8):548-562P. doi:10.2471/BLT.18.228486

[22] Hammerschlag M. Genital tract infections. In: Kliegman R, Stanton B, Geme J, Schor N, editors. Nelson textbook of pediatrics. 20th ed. Elsevier; 2016. p 1494

[23] Olaleye AO, Babah OA, Osuagwu CS, Ogunsola FT, Afolabi BB. Sexually transmitted infections in pregnancy – An update on Chlamydia trachomatis and Neisseria gonorrhoeae. European Journal of Obstetrics & Gynecology and Reproductive Biology. 2020;255: 1-12. doi:10.1016/j.ejogrb.2020.10.002.

[24] Honkila M. Chlamydia trachomatis infections in neonates and infants [thesis]. University of Oulu, Faculty of Medicine; 2018

[25] Adachi K, Nielsen-Saines K, Klausner JD. Chlamydia trachomatis Infection in Pregnancy: The Global Challenge of Preventing Adverse Pregnancy and Infant Outcomes in Sub-Saharan Africa and Asia. BioMed Research International, 2016; 9315757: 1-21. doi:10.1155/2016/9315757

[26] Lee V, Tobin JM, Foley E. Relationship of cervical ectopy to chlamydia infection in young women. J Fam Plann Reprod Health Care. 2006;32(2):104-106. doi:10.1783/147118906776276440

[27] Aggarwal P, Ben Amor A. Cervical Ectropion. In: StatPearls. Treasure Island (FL): StatPearls Publishing; November 17, 2020.

[28] Tiller CM. Chlamydia during Pregnancy: Implications and Impact on Perinatal and Neonatal Outcomes. Journal of Obstetric, Gynecologic & Neonatal Nursing. 2002; 31(1): 93-98. doi:10.1111/j.1552-6909.2002.tb00027.x.

[29] Makker K, Nassar GN, Kaufman EJ. Neonatal Conjunctivitis. In: StatPearls [Internet]. Treasure Island (FL): StatPearls Publishing; 2020. Available from: https://www.ncbi.nlm.nih.gov/books/NBK441840/

[30] Zikic A., Schünemann H., Wi Teodora, et al, Treatment of Neonatal Chlamydial Conjuctivitis: A Systemic Review and Meta-analysis, J Pediatric Infect Dis Soc,2018;7(3):e107-e115

[31] Darville T., Chlamydia trachomatis Infections in Neonates and Young Children, Seminars in Pediatric Infectious Diseases, 2005;16(4), 235-244

[32] Mishra KN, Bhardwaj P, Mishra A, Kaushik A. Acute Chlamydia trachomatis respiratory infection in infants. J Glob Infect Dis. 2011;3(3):216-220. doi:10.4103/0974-777X.83525

[33] Gomella T. Neonatology. 7th ed. McGraw Hill Education; 2013. p581–p583

[34] Porritt RA, Crother TR. Chlamydia pneumoniae Infection and Inflammatory Diseases. For Immunopathol Dis Therap. 2016;7(3-4):237-254. doi:10.1615/ForumImmunDisTher.2017020161

[35] American Academy of Pediatrics. Chlamydial infections. In: Kimberlin DW, Brady MT, Jackson MA, Long SS, editors. Red Book: 2015 Report of the Committee on Infectious Diseases. 30th ed. Elk Grove Village, IL: American Academy of Pediatrics, 2015:288-94

[36] Gautam J, Krawiec C. Chlamydia Pneumonia. [Updated 2020 Dec 15]. In: StatPearls [Internet]. Treasure Island (FL): StatPearls Publishing; 2020 Jan-. Available from: https://www.ncbi.nlm.nih.gov/books/NBK560874/

[37] Bekler C, Kultursay N, Ozacar T, Sayiner A, Yalaz M, Akisu M. Chlamydial infections in term and preterm neonates. Jpn J Infect Dis. 2012;65(1):1-6.

[38] Davies HD. Community-acquired pneumonia in children. Paediatr Child Health. 2003;8(10):616-619. doi:10.1093/pch/8.10.616

[39] Leung AKC, Wong AHC, Hon KL. Community-Acquired Pneumonia in Children. Recent Pat Inflamm Allergy Drug Discov. 2018;12(2):136-144. doi:10.2174/1872213X12666180621163821

[40] Cole MJ, Field N, Pitt R, et al. Substantial underdiagnosis of lymphogranuloma venereum in men who have sex with men in Europe: preliminary findings from a multicentre surveillance pilot. Sex Transm Infect. 2020;96(2):137-142. doi:10.1136/sextrans-2019-053972

[41] World Health Organization. Trachoma. Fact sheet [Internet]. 2020. Available from: https://www.who.int/news-room/fact-sheets/detail/trachoma [Accessed 2021-01-30]

[42] Watson EJ, Templeton A, Russell I, et al. The accuracy and efficacy of screening tests for Chlamydia trachomatis: a systematic review. J Med Microbiol. 2002;51(12):1021-1031. doi:10.1099/0022-1317-51-12-1021

[43] Meyer T. Diagnostic Procedures to Detect Chlamydia trachomatis Infections. Microorganisms. 2016;4(3):25. Published 2016 Aug 5. doi:10.3390/microorganisms4030025

[44] Centers for Disease Control and Prevention. Sexually Transmitted Diseases Treatment Guidelines [Internet]. 2015. Available from: https://www.cdc.gov/std/tg2015/chlamydia.htm. [Accessed 2012-01-31]

[45] Radkowski MA, Kranzler JK, Beem MO, Tipple MA. Chlamydia pneumonia in infants: radiography in 125 cases. AJR Am J Roentgenol. 1981;137(4):703-706. doi:10.2214/ajr.137.4.703

[46] World Health Organization. Guidelines for the Treatment of

Chlamydia trachomatis. Geneva; 2016 [Internet]. Available from: https://www.ncbi.nlm.nih.gov/books/NBK379708/ [Accessed 2021-01-31]

[47] Bradley JS, Byington CL, Shah SS, et al. The management of community-acquired pneumonia in infants and children older than 3 months of age: clinical practice guidelines by the Pediatric Infectious Diseases Society and the Infectious Diseases Society of America. Clin Infect Dis. 2011;53(7):e25-e76. doi:10.1093/cid/cir531

[48] Kohlhoff SA, Hammerschlag MR. Treatment of Chlamydial infections: 2014 update. Expert Opin Pharmacother. 2015;16(2):205-212. doi:10.1517/14656566.2015.999041

[49] Gutiérrez-Castrellón P, Mayorga-Buitron JL, Bosch-Canto V et al. Efficacy and safety of clarithromycin in pediatric patients with upper respiratory infections: a systematic review with meta-analysis. Rev Invest Clin. 2012;64(2):126-135.

[50] Abraham S, Juel HB, Bang P, et al. Safety and immunogenicity of the chlamydia vaccine candidate CTH522 adjuvanted with CAF01 liposomes or aluminium hydroxide: a first-in-human, randomised, double-blind, placebo-controlled, phase 1 trial. Lancet Infect Dis. 2019;19(10):1091-1100. doi:10.1016/S1473-3099(19)30279-8

Section 3

Maternal Health in Primary Care

Chapter 8

The Effects of Multivitamin Use in Pregnancy on Mother and Fetus Health

Neda Taner and Gülden Zehra Omurtag

Abstract

Pregnancy and birth method are the key factors to boost healthy new generations. Pregnancy may be a special period during which ladies have lived several process. During this period, for the protection of maternal and fetus health enhanced energy and nutrition demand supply is needed. Sufficient intake of nutrients and correct weight gain has necessary effects on each the mother's and the developing fetal health. it's also important to guard against short and long run complications. Nutrition is very important before and once pregnancy yet as throughout pregnancy. During this study, the intake of macro and micro nutrient items moving maternal and ve fetal health issues absolutely during pregnancy is detailed. As macro nutrition items carbohydrate, protein and fat examined. Adequate protein is important during pregnancy. Fats are important nutrients that provide essential fatty acids for the development of the brain and central nervous system of the fetus. Micro nutrition items water soluble and oil soluble as 2 cluster examined. The consequences of minerals during pregnancy were also examined.

Keywords: Maternal and fetus health, nutrition, pregnancy, mineral, vitamin supplementation

1. Introduction

In order for the species to be preserved over time, genetic data must be transferred from generation to generation [1]. Reproduction, which takes place so as to take care of the continuity of the lineage, starts with the fertilization stage at the start and continues with the pregnancy method [2].

The feminine body undergoes several physiological, anatomical and biochemical changes in order to adapt to the pregnancy process [3, 4]. Though the prevalence of those changes throughout pregnancy is taken into account physiological, occurrence outside of pregnancy is considered a pathological condition [4]. Pregnancy covers a period of nine months and ten days or 280 days or forty weeks from the primary day of the last menstrual day of the expectant mother [2, 5].

The main symptoms that occur during this process are as follows: interruption of the menstrual cycle, tenderness within the breasts, nausea-vomiting, frequent urination, augmented vaginal discharge, tiredness, cittosis and feeling baby movements [6, 7]. Throughout pregnancy, the bond between mother and fetus is maintained by the placenta shaped in the 1st month of pregnancy. Providing the development of the fetus by carrying the nutrients taken by the mother to the fetus, and also the passage of the wastes in the fetus to the mother' circulation happens through placental circulation [6, 8].

The importance of nutrition during pregnancy is extremely necessary in terms of fetus development, and this issue has attracted loads of attention in recent years [8]. So as for kids to turn healthy and for the protection of mothers' health, among the most necessities are a property healthy fetal development method throughout pregnancy, stimulation of milk production, enlarged would like for nutrients, and accordingly, adequate and balanced nutrition [5]. Inadequate or excessive intakes during nutrition during pregnancy cause several health issues similar to inborn disorders, preterm or miscarriage, mental biological process delays [9]. Variations in social and cultural values, errors in preparation, storage and cooking within the foods that pregnant ladies can consume, failure of addition to the daily diet in response to the increasing would like of the mother, economic inadequacies, alcohol, cigarettes and drug use by the pregnant girl are often counted among the most reasons for organic process issues throughout pregnancy [10]. The mother' weight at the start of pregnancy is very important in terms of the number of weight she ought to gain during the full pregnancy. Throughout pregnancy, one among the foremost important problems in terms of maintaining maternal and fetal health is body weight gain during pregnancy. Gaining adequate body weight is possible by providing energy at suggested levels and taking macro and micronutrients throughout pregnancy [11].

2. Carbohydrates

macromolecules: Carbohydrates are organic compounds consisting of carbon (C), element (H) and atomic number 8 (O) [1]. Carbohydrate demand varies betting on the energy requirement for acceptable pregnancy weight [12]. The specified energy would like depends on the individual' age, gender, physically activeness and, if any, their special condition [13]. 60% of the overall daily energy ought to be met from carbohydrates [12]. 1 g of carbohydrates provides a median of four calories of energy [13]. The daily carbohydrate intake need for pregnant ladies is 170 g/day, and the daily macromolecule intake for non-pregnant ladies is 130 g/day [14].

3. Proteins

Proteins, that are the building blocks of cells, are the littlest a part of the body and incorporates amino acids [13]. They're one among the most nutrients that has got to be taken for growth and development. 10–11% of daily energy would like is met from supermolecules [13]. 1 g of protein offers four kcal of energy. Proteins are the body' highest energy store once fatty tissue [1]. Throughout pregnancy, proteins are functionally needed for fetal growth, placental development, formation of amnionic fluid, increase of maternal blood volume and growth of maternal tissues. Therefore, the supermolecule demand will increase throughout pregnancy [15]. The order of protein requirement for tissue building and repair is as follows: fetus (42%) followed by female internal reproductive organ (17%), blood (14%), placenta (10%), and breast enlargement (8%). Throughout pregnancy, the uterus and maternal blood are comparatively wealthy in protein instead of fat or macromolecule [15]. Despite the decrease in total protein and albumin during pregnancy, there's no downside within the protein requirement for the fetus since the protein taken in the diet is employed additional effectively. Studies have shown that the organic compound concentration is higher in the fetal compartment than within the maternal one. This higher concentration is usually regulated by the placenta. The placenta not solely concentrates amino acids in the fetal circulation, however is additionally liable for supermolecule synthesis, oxidation, and transamination of some non-essential amino acids [15]. Whereas the number of protein that non-pregnant ladies ought to take is 0.8 g/kg/day, this figure is 1.1 g/kg/day throughout pregnancy [14].

4. Lipids

Fats are organic compounds composed of fatty acids and glycerol. Fatty acids are named in step with the amount of carbon atoms in the molecule and also the number of double bonds between carbons. Those while not double bonds are referred to as saturated fatty acids, and those with double bonds are called unsaturated fatty acids [13]. Fats are necessary as a result of the surplus energy within the body is hold on as fat tissue. One gram of fat provides a median of nine calories of energy [13]. Fat demand varies betting on the energy requirement needed for correct weight gain. Roughly 20–30% of daily energy ought to be provided from fats [12]. Additionally to providing energy, fats modify the utilization of fat-soluble vitamins (A, D, E and K) in the body [12]. In addition, the intake of some fatty acids with food, that are enclosed within the composition of fats and do not seem to be created by the body, gains importance for growth and skin health [14]. Fats are necessary nutrients that offer essential fatty acids necessary for the event of the brain and central system of the fetus [12].

5. Vitamins

Vitamins are essential organic substances that are necessary for the traditional prevalence of metabolic events in the body and for maintaining a healthy state. Lack of any creates a selected disorder and damage. Vitamins are taken outwardly with most plant or animal foods. Some vitamins, on the opposite hand, are often partially synthesized within the body, albeit in lean amounts, or they are infatuated food [16]. They're not the fundamental artifact in the human organism; however, they need totally different operates for the regulation and continuity of body functions. Vitamins do not offer energy like different body parts similar to carbohydrates, proteins, and lipids. Their main function is to act as a catalyst in the energy-releasing reactions of carbohydrates, proteins and lipids [17]. In some western countries such as the United States and England, the "recommended daily ration (RDA)" value for every vitamin has been determined as a basis for evaluating food things as nutrients and control the daily diet. This determination was supported a daily food intake of 2000 kilocalories [16]. A diet with foods that contain adequate amounts of main nutrients similar to carbohydrates, supermolecule and fat, and particularly from numerous sources provides enough vitamins for the body' daily would like, aside from some special cases [16]. Pregnant women, lactating women, children, athletes, smokers, the elderly, those that are underneath stress and who are sick from sickness have a better need for vitamins [17]. Vitamins are divided into two main teams as fat soluble and water soluble. This solubility property determines the pharmacokinetic properties of vitamins and a few of their qualities relating to their use. They're divided into fat-soluble vitamins (A, D, E, and K) and soluble vitamins (group B and vitamin C) [14]. These are summarized in **Table 1**:

Water soluble vitamins	Fat soluble vitamins
• Vitamin B_1 (Thiamin)	• Vitamin A
• Vitamin B_2 (Riboflavin)	• Vitamin D
• Vitamin B_3 (Niacin)	• Vitamin E
• Vitamin B_5 (Pantothenic acid)	• Vitamin K
• Vitamin B_6 (Pyridoxin)	
• Vitamin B_7 (Biotin)	
• Vitamin B_9 (Folic acid)	
• Vitamin B_{12} (Cyanocobalamin)	
• Vitamin C	

Table 1.
Water and fat soluble vitamins.

Since water-soluble vitamins cannot be hold on much within the body, they have to be taken frequently in enough quantities to fulfill the daily demand [1, 16]. They're additionally straightforward to expel from the body. Since fat-soluble vitamins are generally hold on in the liver, they are doing not cause vitamin deficiency symptoms though they are taken in lean amounts for a while, if they are taken in enlarged amounts later on. Urinary excretion of fat-soluble vitamins is mostly limited. Therefore, high-dose treatments with these vitamins carry a risk of toxicity [18]. One among the foremost common useful properties of soluble vitamins is their incorporation into specific enzymes as cofactors. In contrast, a minimum of 2 of the fat-soluble vitamins (vitamins A and D) act as hormones and act with specific receptors in their target tissues [1]. The necessity for micronutrients throughout pregnancy will increase thanks to physiological changes, and vitamin supplements applied during this era became customary [19]. The expansion and development of the fetus depends on the essential nutrients and vitamins taken by the mother [18]. Since several micronutrients are passed from mother to baby, maternal deficiency causes deficiency in fetus and newborn [20]. In some studies, vitamin deficiency during pregnancy could end in megaloblastia, ectoblast defects, placental and fetal defects, low birth weight, and premature birth [18]. Since several micronutrients are passed from mother to baby, deficiency within the mother causes deficiency in the fetus and newborn. The mechanism of passage through the placenta differs between micronutrients, so some micronutrients are at larger risk of not being transferred to the fetus than others [20].

5.1 Use of vitamin a in pregnancy

Since vitamin A cannot be synthesized in the body while not a precursor, it's a vitamin that has got to be taken outwardly [21]. It's a lipid-soluble inhibitor [22]. It's hold on in the liver [8]. Fat-soluble vitamin is taken into the body in 2 totally different forms, that are necessary for the living body. The foremost common and necessary within the body is antiophthalmic factor [23]. Fat-soluble vitamin plays a basic role in retinoid metabolism and visual functions, cellular differentiation relating to embryonic development, respiratory organ maturation and system development [8]. The most pathological conditions related to vitamin A deficiency throughout pregnancy are declared as preterm birth, low birth weight and low infant liver vitamin A storage cases. Low vitamin A level in newborns seems to be an element that will increase the chance of bronchopulmonary abnormal condition and infection [24]. Fat-soluble vitamin supplementation does not result on the chance of maternal mortality, perinatal death, infant death, stillbirth, neonatal anemia, preterm birth and having a low birth weight baby. However, studies on vitamin A supplementation have shown a reduced maternal risk of visual disorder [25]. Associate early and necessary symptom of vitamin A deficiency is night blindness [8]. High-dose vitamin A supplementation includes an agent effect and will increase the risk of abnormalities within the central nervous system, urinary organ system and vessel systems in the newborn [18]. Each lean and excessive intake of vitamin A will cause issues in fetal growth and development, thus vitamin A sources ought to be adequate and reliable throughout pregnancy [24]. Several pregnant ladies will get the specified quantity of vitamin A from their daily diet while not the necessity for extra vitamin supplements [18]. It's celebrated that vitamin A supplementation will increase the birth weight and growth of the kid born to HIV-infected women, however excessive use should be avoided [11]. Fat-soluble vitamin is believed to cross the placenta by straightforward diffusion [18]. throughout pregnancy, a daily vitamin A intake of 770 mcg is important, and vitamin A intake on top of 3000 mcg is not suggested [14].

5.2 Use of vitamin D in pregnancy

Calciferol is taken into account a pre-hormone in steroid structure [1]. It's 2 sources: D_3 (cholecalciferol), that is synthesized within the skin by daylight, and vitamin D_2 (ergocalciferol), which is taken through diet and dietary supplements [26]. They are often hold on in the liver in the body [27]. It's the foremost poisonous of the fat-soluble vitamins [28]. Calciferol is provided by dietary intake and also the result of sunlight on the skin. Therefore, vitamin D deficiency develops thanks to inadequate diet, living inside or in unsunny climates, and sporting sun-proof covering [18]. Vitamin D regulates Ca and phosphorus metabolism alongside hormone and thyrocalcitonin [14]. It will increase calcium resorption and decreasing calcium excretion by taking part in a task in maintaining bone balance [24]. It also has results on the nervous system, heart and clotting mechanism [14]. There also are studies showing that it's necessary for immune operate concerning aldohexose regulation, fetal brain development, and female internal reproductive organ contractions at birth [12]. As a results of clinical studies on the effect of calciferol on pregnancy outcomes, it's been determined that vitamin D deficiency is also related to preeclampsia, pregnancy diabetes, low birth weight, preterm delivery, cesarean section and enlarged risk of infectious diseases [26]. Calciferol deficiency throughout pregnancy is that the most significant risk issue for vitamin D deficiency in newborns and infancy. Since maternal vitamin D deficiency is common in Turkey, it's declared that vitamin D deficiency is liable for symptom in early infancy [24].

5.3 Use of vitamin E in pregnancy

Use of vitamin E in pregnancy is important for tissue development, cell membrane structure, and red blood cell integrity. However, its most important physiological result is its being inhibitor [18]. It's the smallest amount poisonous of the fat-soluble vitamins. Once taken over necessary, it's excreted in excreta and urine. Terribly high doses can cause nausea and symptom [28]. The necessity for vitamin E will increase throughout pregnancy and particularly within the trimester [12]. The most finding in its deficiency is anemia. However, additionally to this, muscle and system disorders and muscle fatigue also can be seen. Though its use is controversial, premature newborns are ordinarily supplemented with vitamin E to stabilize erythrocytes and haemolytic anemia is prevented [28]. Maternal level of vitamin E increases during pregnancy. It peaks around thirty seven weeks and returns to pre-pregnancy levels shortly once birth. The rationale for this increase throughout pregnancy are often attributed to the enlarged would like thanks to fetal growth [18]. Pre-eclampsia is a vital pregnancy-related complication and is related to each maternal and fetal problems. it's thought that preeclampsia symptoms can be reduced by inhibitor support in early pregnancy. Vitamin E additionally plays a task in reducing preeclampsia in pregnancy due to its antioxidant properties [24]. The suggested intake for vitamin E during pregnancy is fifteen mg per day, and also the most quantity to be taken is a 1000 mg per day [14].

5.4 Use of vitamin K in pregnancy

Vitamin K exists in nature in two forms, K_1 and K_2. fat-soluble vitamin K_1 is synthesized within the leaves of inexperienced plants. The well-liked variety of drugs is fat-soluble vitamin K_1 sort. Vitamin K_2 is of microbic origin. It's synthesized by microorganism bacterium settled in the small intestine and colon in humans and by another bacteria. The synthetically derived type is vitamin K_3 [16, 28]. Though the foremost important operate of vitamin K is anticoagulant, it additionally has a vital result on bone health [28]. Vitamin K has been shown to repair bone deformation and forestall bone loss caused by corticosteroids [14]. In newborns, the symptom of fat-soluble vitamin deficiency throughout the amount once microorganism is not shaped is manifested as a bent to bleeding. Breast milk is poorer in vitamin K than ready-made formulas. Therefore, the very fact that the baby is fed solely with breast milk could cause low vitamin K levels. If vitamin K is not given to the baby at birth, disorders within the action mechanism may occur. Therefore, for prophylaxis, administration of vitamin K straightaway once delivery is suggested [28]. If high doses of artificial vitamin K (K_3) are administered to the newborn for a long time, poisonous effects are seen, leading to anemia and jaundice [28]. High doses of vitamins A and E intake could interfere with the viscus absorption of fat-soluble vitamin [18]. Like all fat-soluble vitamins, overdoses of vitamin K accumulate within the body and are toxic. However, the traditional average diet provides over adequate amounts of vitamin K and does not need routine supplementation throughout pregnancy. However, vitamin K supplementation is suggested for a few sure indications [18]. With a traditional average diet, the necessity for vitamin K is more than met. There's no need for routine supplementation during pregnancy. The daily dose needed for non-pregnant ladies and pregnant women is that the same and this value is 90 mcg. [14].

5.5 Use of vitamin B_1 in pregnancy

Though vitamin B_1 is not used directly within the body, it takes half in several mechanisms. It's used as a molecule in the synthesis of acetylcholine, that is concerned in neurotransmission [14]. Vitamin B_1 is required for aldohexose chemical reaction in the body for hormone production from exocrine gland cells and cell growth [18]. It additionally plays a vital role in macromolecule metabolism [29]. Daily supplementation of vitamin B_1 in pregnant women prevents low birth weight, ensures intrauterine growth and will increase aldohexose tolerance [18]. Higher intake of vitamin B_1 than the most needed dose could cause nausea, vomiting, lethargy, and eating disorder [18]. The number of vitamin B_1 that a pregnant girl ought to take daily is 1.4 mg.

5.6 Use of vitamin B_2 in pregnancy

Riboflavin acts as a molecule in chemical reaction and reduction reactions, in tissues that manufacture energy through respiration [18]. Vitamin B_2 is important for the formation of red blood cells and production of antibodies, that are a vital a part of the body' defense system. it's also accountable for getting energy from supermolecule associated fats [14]. Whereas the number that an adult girl ought to take daily is 1.1 mg, the daily amount that a pregnant woman should take is 1.4 mg [14].

5.7 Use of vitamin B3 in pregnancy

Vitamin B_3 is a vital element of 2 enzymes in metastasis and tissue respiration [18]. It's concerned within the structure of hydrogen-carrying coenzymes similar to NAD and NADP. These molecules play a task in chemical reaction and reduction events in the body [14]. It's focused in the erythrocytes in the blood. It is often found in muscle and kidney tissue, particularly within the liver [28]. In studies, vitamin B_3 deficiency was seldom encountered, and it absolutely was disregarded that vitamin B_3 given to pregnant ladies in low or high amounts had any result [14]. As a results of the rise in estrogen throughout pregnancy, vitamin B_3 is synthesized so as to stay the hormones in restraint [12]. The daily dose that a pregnant girl ought to take is 18 mg. The most dose to be taken during pregnancy is decided as 35 mg [14].

5.8 Use of vitamin B5 in pregnancy

It takes half in carbohydrate, supermolecule and cholesterol metabolism and aerophilous chemical process reactions. Since vitamin B5 is wide found in nature and synthesized by the viscus flora, its deficiency is not seen in humans. Vitamin B_5 in pregnant ladies has not been determined with certainty [28].

5.9 Use of vitamin B_6 in pregnancy

It's the beginning material within the biogenesis of the most molecule of supermolecule metabolism. The breakdown of all amino acids in protein metabolism and also the synthesis of non-essential amino acids occur in the presence of coenzymes of vitamin B_6 [28]. Therefore, vitamin B_6 has to be enlarged in parallel with the rise in the amount of supermolecule within the diet throughout pregnancy [16]. At identical time, vitamin B_6 helps the event of the central system [12]. Nausea and innate reflex are one among the foremost common and necessary symptoms in pregnant women, occurring in the early stages of pregnancy [28]. Vitamin B_6 is employed as an alternate treatment to forestall nausea and vomiting during pregnancy [30]. At the same time, vitamin B_6 is of interest as a result of the preservation of the placental tube-shaped structure bed [18]. Clinical manifestations of vitamin B_6 deficiency are epilepsy-like convulsions and dermatitis [28]. An awfully high dose (2–6 g/d) is needed for toxicity in dults. This toxicity happens at mega doses given for the treatment of carpal tunnel syndrome and preeclampsia. No fetal effects are reportable thanks to dose [18]. Whereas the number of vitamin B_6 that an adult girl ought to take daily is 1.3 mg, this amount is 1.9 mg in a pregnant woman [11]. The most dose that a pregnant woman should take is 100 mg [14].

5.10 Use of vitamin B9 in pregnancy

Vitamin B_9 plays a vital role within the construction of latest cells by serving to the assembly of desoxyribonucleic acid (DNA) and ribonucleic acid (RNA), that management cell proliferation within the body [12]. It additionally facilitates biological processes as a compound for enzymes involving polymer and RNA synthesis [31]. In addition, it works in conjunction with cobalamin to create hemoglobin in erythrocytes [12]. It should be infatuated food, and also the totally different forms it enters to be used in the body are usually referred to as 'folate' [28]. All defects that occur throughout pregnancy occur in the 1st 28 days of pregnancy, largely once the expectant mother does not apprehend she is pregnant yet. The foremost common of those is NTD (Neural Tube Defect). It is one among the common and severe malformations among inborn malformations. All of the malformations similar to anencephaly, encephalocele, meningocele, myelocele, meningomyelocele and myelosis, which are caused by the neural tube during which the brain and neural structure develop, stay open once it ought to be closed till the tip of the fourth week of intrauterine life, are all serious congenital anomalies and are expressed underneath the name of 'neural tube defect' [31]. It's suggested to begin vitamin B_9 supplementation with four hundred mcg with the design of pregnancy and three months before, and to continue it throughout the primary trimester of pregnancy [32]. So as to be shielded from NTD, 600 mcg vitamin B_9 supplement ought to be taken daily. The most quantity of folic acid that a pregnant girl should take daily is a thousand mcg [14].

5.11 Use of vitamin B12 in pregnancy

In contrast to different soluble vitamins, up to four mg of vitamin B_{12} is hold on within the body. Therefore, vitamin deficiency is not determined for several years. Those with deficiency are additional doubtless to be strict vegetarians [28]. Vitamin B_{12} may be a molecule essential for organic process and lipid, protein, and macromolecule metabolism. It is synthesized within the liver and is named extrinsic factor. Though it acts on all cells, it plays a serious role in the bone marrow, gastrointestinal system and central nervous system. It acts as a compound for polymer synthesis in the bone marrow. Though we have got little information on the necessity for vitamin B_{12} throughout pregnancy, in step with some studies, body fluid vitamin B_{12} values decrease in the advancing weeks of pregnancy. Tries to interchange this decline in pregnancy are unsuccessful. This fact supports the idea that serum vitamin B_{12} level is freelance of diet and this decrease will not necessitate a decrease in maternal aliment stores [18]. Vitamin B_{12} is very important for the continuity of cell division. In its deficiency, methylcobalamin cannot be shaped and polymer synthesis cannot be made of quick growing tissues throughout pregnancy. As a result, megaloblastic anemia, inborn anomalies and issues within the system develop. Low plasmic vitamin B_{12} concentration was found to be related to high plasmic homocysteine level, pre-eclampsia and preterm birth risk all told age groups. It's been reportable that maternal insufficiencies cause NTD and spina bifida. Vitamin B_{12} is infatuated foods of animal origin. In humans, viscus bacterium also can synthesize vitamin B_{12} [28]. The number of vitamin B_{12} that an adult girl ought to take daily is 2.4 mcg. This dose will increase to 2.6 mcg in an exceedingly pregnant woman [11]. There aren't any adequate resources for the most daily intake throughout pregnancy [14].

5.12 Use of calcium in pregnancy

Calcium is an inorganic element that's the foremost superabundant and essential mineral element within the human body. Ca metabolism is regulated by hormones similar to vitamin D, parathyroid gland hormone, and calcitonin. Oral calcium is absorbed from the intestines by the result of vitamin D. Parathyroid gland hormone, on the opposite hand, will increase viscus Ca absorption and bone calcium mobilization by increasing calciferol synthesis within the kidneys [14]. The fullness of iron stores together with calcium is very important for bone and red blood cell development [33]. Enlarged calcium intake throughout pregnancy is important for the health of mother and baby. Throughout this period, the utilization of calcium supplements reduces preeclampsia. At identical time, once enough calcium is not taken during pregnancy, the necessity is met by retreating calcium from the bones. Frequent births, lack of movement and lean use of daylight cause bone softening and tooth decay. Adequate vitamin D intake is important to facilitate Ca absorption [33]. It's wrong to assume that dental caries happens thanks to calcium deficiency throughout pregnancy which each pregnancy causes a tooth loss. Changes within the composition of spittle during pregnancy accelerate the progression of pre-pregnancy caries and also the gums bleed easily. Despite harm gums, teeth ought to be brushed regularly. All types of dental treatment (tooth symptom treatment, tooth extraction) are often done during pregnancy. Long-run treatments (such as passage treatment) can be delayed for once six months [6]. Whereas the number of calcium that girls would like during pregnancy is a 1000 mg, the most quantity to be taken is 2500 mg [14].

5.13 Use of iron in pregnancy

Iron is a component within the structure of heme, that has the power to simply exchange electrons, rework into ferric (Fe+2) and ferrous (Fe+3) forms. It's additionally needed for the assembly of haemoprotein and plenty of different enzymes. However, as a results of the conversion of peroxide into free ion radicals, it's the ability to break plasma membrane protein and DNA. Iron-protoporphine (heme) and iron sulfide compounds act as enzyme-cofactors [14]. The fullness of Ca stores together with iron is important for bone and red blood cell development [33]. Iron balance within the body is extremely delicate, and iron deficiency or excess is one among the foremost common diseases in humans [14]. Pregnancy, lactation, adolescence, rapid growth periods, factors that increase iron need, increase iron loss, decrease iron intake, absorption or use are among the most causes of iron deficiency [30]. Anemia, besides being a vital pathological state which will have an effect on the pregnancy method and also the quality of lifetime of the newborn, will increase its importance even additional because it is preventable. Therefore, the general public ought to learn regarding the explanations for mistreatment vitamin and iron medicine throughout pregnancy and nutrition [3, 10]. Iron deficiency ends up in enlarged preterm birth, low birth weight, and mortality within the 1st 2 trimesters of pregnancy. Enlarged plasma volume during pregnancy, increased iron demand of the fetus, quantity of vitamin C taken by the mother orally or with food, antacid use, excessive dietary intake of cereals with phytate content that have an effect on iron absorption, viscus parasites, consumption of tea and coffee, affect iron absorption and cause iron deficiency anemia [14]. However, the necessity for iron during pregnancy will increase particularly during the 3rd trimester [34]. Aspect effects associated with iron use are typically dose-dependent. Aspect effects similar to epigastric discomfort, nausea, vomiting, symptom or constipation could develop. Whereas the incidence of those side effects is reduced in low-dose use, they are seen in roughly 1/3 of cases in high-dose use [35]. Whereas the number of iron to be taken daily is eight mg in associate adult girl, a pregnant woman ought to take twenty seven mg of iron daily [11]. The most amount of iron a pregnant woman should take daily is 45 mg [14].

5.14 Use of iodine in pregnancy

Iodine, that is concerned within the production of thyroid hormones, is an element necessary for traditional growth and development, and brain and body functions. In relevance the iodine content of the soil and water, the number of iodine we have a tendency to take with food varies. Iodine infatuated food and water is excreted within the body waste once it's employed in the assembly of thyroid hormone. Since iodine is not hold on in the body, a sufficient amount of iodine should be taken into the body a day [36]. Pregnant and lactating women are in the risk group for iodine deficiency. Among the most cases seen in iodine deficiency throughout pregnancy are miscarriage, stillbirths, inborn anomalies, increase in perinatal deaths and infant mortality rate, psychological feature dysfunction, infertility, deafness, abnormal condition (diplopia), psychomotor disorders, and hypothyroidism disorder [11]. Iodine deficiency within the fetus throughout pregnancy adversely affects particularly cerebral development. The foremost essential period of time is between the trimester and also the age of three, once cerebral development is basically completed. The foremost important reason behind correctable backwardness is iodine deficiency [14]. The typical daily iodine intake of fertile women is between 10 and 20 mcg. Daily iodine intake during pregnancy and nursing mothers ought to be 220 mcg. With breastfeeding, 100 mcg/day of iodine is transferred to baby. Body waste iodine concentration should be 10–20 mcg/day or 100–200 mcg/L throughout pregnancy. If daily iodine intake falls below 100 mcg during pregnancy, iodine deficiency is mentioned [37]. The most quantity of iodine that ought to be taken daily during pregnancy is 1100 mcg [14].

5.15 Use of magnesium in pregnancy

Since it cannot be made by the body, it must be obtained through food. Magnesium is found in soil and sea water. There are magnesium reserves in our body that has got to be perpetually replenished, that is, it must be taken unendingly so as to satisfy its functions. The most reservoir of metal is bones, 60% of that is found here alongside Ca and phosphate. However, the most operate of magnesium is not within the bones, however in the blood and muscle systems, wherever 40% is found. It plays a vital role in strengthening muscles, supermolecule synthesis and protein system activity, growth and regeneration of cells. Magnesium is that the fourth ion among the cations found in the body, whereas it's the second cation once atomic number 19 in the cell. In things similar to stress, pregnancy and breastfeeding, the body' would like for magnesium will increase [17]. Once fetal characteristics such as birth weight associated height were examined, magnesium supplementation was found to possess positive results [14]. At identical time, magnesium additionally has the effect of preventing vital sign rise in pregnancy [12]. Whereas the number of magnesium that an adult girl ought to take daily is 320 mg, the amount that a pregnant woman should take is 350 mg [14].

6. Conclusion

Nutrition is important before and after pregnancy as well as during pregnancy. The intake of macro and micro nutrient items affecting maternal and fetal health problems positively during pregnancy. Vitamin A plays a fundamental role in retinoid metabolism and visual functions, cellular differentiation related to embryonic development, lung maturation and immune system development of fetus. Vitamin D regulates calcium and phosphorus metabolism together with parathyroid hormone and calcitonin. It increases calcium reabsorption and decreasing calcium excretion by playing a role in maintaining bone balance. It also has effects on the nervous system, heart and blood clotting mechanism. Vitamin E is important and the main finding of Vitamin E deficiency, is hemolytic anemia. However, in addition, muscle and nervous system disorders and muscle fatigue can also be seen with its deficiency. The most important function of vitamin K is anticoagulation; If vitamin K is not given to the baby at birth, disorders in the coagulation mechanism may occur. Therefore, for prophylaxis, intramuscular administration of vitamin K immediately after delivery is recommended. Vitamin K has also an important effect on bone health. Vitamin B_6 is used as an alternative treatment to prevent nausea and vomiting during pregnancy. At the same time, vitamin B_6 is of interest because of the preservation of the placental vascular bed. Folic acid works in conjunction with vitamin B12 to form hemoglobin in erythrocytes. Deficiency leads to NTD in newborn. Vitamin B12 deficiency result with megaloblastic anemia, congenital anomalies and problems in the nervous system of the fetus. Increased calcium intake during pregnancy is important for the health of mother and baby. During this period, the use of calcium supplements reduces preeclampsia. Ca is necessary for dental health. On the other hand, Iron deficiency or excess is one of the most common diseases in humans. Pregnant and lactating women are in the risk group for iodine deficiency. The most important cause of correctable mental retardation of newborn is iodine deficiency.

Conflict of interest

The authors have not any conflict of interest to declare.

Author details

Neda Taner[1]* and Gülden Zehra Omurtag[2]

1 Department of Clinical Pharmacy, School of Pharmacy, İstanbul Medipol University, İstanbul, Turkey

2 Department of Toxicology, School of Pharmacy, İstanbul Medipol University, İstanbul, Turkey

*Address all correspondence to: ntaner@medipol.edu.tr

References

[1] Sencer E, Orhan Y. Nutrition, Istanbul Medical Publishing, I. Edition, Istanbul, 2005.

[2] Aydemir H, Uyar Hazar H. Low Risk, Risky, High-Risk Pregnancy and the Midwife's Role, Gümüşhane University Journal of Health Sciences 3(2), 2014.

[3] Ozdincerler Arzu R. Anatomy & Physiology, Istanbul Medicine Bookstores, 1st Edition, Istanbul, 2015.

[4] Guven S. Iron Deficiency Anemia Due to Nutritional Habits During Pregnancy and Investigation of Antioxidant Values, Yüzüncü Yıl University Health Sciences Institute Master's Thesis, Van, 2014.

[5] Akan LS. Determination of Dietary Patterns, Diet Quality Index and Healthy Eating Index of Pregnant Women, Ankara University, Institute of Science, Doctoral Thesis, Ankara, 2015.

[6] Sen C, Yayla M. Turkish Perinatology Society, 1st Edition, ISBN:975-93267-2-8, 2006

[7] Mete S, Okumus H. Preparation for Birth, ISBN: 978-975-8882-31-1, 2008.

[8] Garipoglu G. Investigation of the Effect of Nutritional Status on Breast Milk Lipid Content and Fatty Acid Composition during Pregnancy, Gazi University Institute of Health Sciences Master Thesis, Ankara, 2010.

[9] Karaoglu N, Eroglu Samur G. Mother and Child Nutrition, Pegem Academy, 4th Edition, Ankara, 2015.

[10] Tas EE, Ustuner I, Ozdemir H, Dikec A, Avsar AF. Evaluation of Nutritional Status of Pregnant Women, Bidder Journal of Medical Sciences, Vol: 2, No:1, p.7-12, 2010.

[11] Uzdil Z, Ozenoğlu A. Effects of Consumption of Various Nutrients in Pregnancy on Infant Health, Balıkesir Journal of Health Sciences, Vol: 4, Issue:2, p.117-121, 2015.

[12] Haklı G. Evaluation of Nutritional Status and Newborn Weight in Adolescent Pregnants, Ankara University Institute of Science Doctoral Thesis, Ankara, 2015.

[13] Aydin GE. Basic Nutrition Handbook for Healthy Individuals, Turkish Kidney Foundation, 2017.

[14] Arslan E. The Effect of Supportive Therapy in Pregnancy on Maternal and Fetal Health, Istanbul Medipol University, Istanbul, 2017.

[15] Akgun N. The Relationship between Maternal Body Mass Index and Follow-up of Body Weight Gain in Pregnancy with Perinatal Outcomes, Hacettepe University Institute of Health Sciences Master Thesis, Ankara, 2015.

[16] Kayaalp O. Medical Pharmacology, Feryal Printing, p.1301-1356, Ankara, 2005.

[17] Gormuş ZS, Ergene N. Clinical Significance of Magnesium, Journal of General Medicine, 12(2):69-75,2003.

[18] Erata Yakup E, Guclu S. Vitamin Supplement in Pregnancy, Journal of Perinatology, Vol: 11, Issue:1-2, 2003.

[19] Arlı M, Sanlıer N, Küçükkömürler, Yaman M. Mother and Child Nutrition, Pegem Academy, 8th Edition, Ankara, 2011.

[20] Figo Adolescent, Pre-Pregnancy and Maternal Nutrition Recommendations, International Journal of Gynecology and Obstetrics,131: Suppl 4, 2015.

[21] Otleş S, Atlı Y. The Importance of Carotenoids for Human Health, Journal of Engineering Sciences, Vol:3, Issue:1, P.249-254, 1997.

[22] Eren A. The Effect of Vitamin A (Retinol Level), Vitamin D, Vitamin B12 Levels on Disease Severity and Treatment in Chronic Viral Hepatitis C Patients, Mustafa Kemal University Tayfur Ata Sökmen Medical Faculty Specialization Thesis, Hatay, 2015.

[23] Bilber O. Optimization of the Simultaneous Determination Method of Water and Fat-Soluble Vitamins in Some Foods, Selcuk University, Institute of Science, Master's Thesis, Konya, 2010.

[24] Kabaran S, Ayaz A. Effects of B12, Folic Acid, Vitamins A, D, E and C on Maternal and Fetal Health, Turkish Journal of Hygiene and Experimental Biology, 70(2): 103-112, 2013.

[25] Mecdi M, Rathfisch G. Evidence-Based Practices in Pregnancy Disorders, F.N. Hem Journal, Vol:21, Issue:2:129-138, 2013.

[26] Kurklu SN, Ayaz A. Vitamin D and Gestational Diabetes, Gümüşhane University Journal of Healthy Science, 4(3), 2005.

[27] Ozen S, Haspolat K. Vitamin D, Calcium, Bone Metabolism and Psychiatric Disorders, Clinical Psychiatry, 6:102-113, 2003.

[28] Konukoglu D, Basic and Clinical Biochemistry, p.164-188, Istanbul, 2016.

[29] Tulum Y. B Complex Vitamins and Biochemistry, Ege University Faculty of Medicine Graduation Thesis, İzmir, 2007.

[30] Ozdemir SE. Comparison of Hemogram, Iron, Total Iron Binding Capacity, Ferritin, Vitamin B12 and Folic Acid Values and Cord Blood Values of Pregnants in Labor, Dr. Lütfi Kırdar Kartal Training and Research Hospital Family Medicine Specialization Thesis, Istanbul, 2008.

[31] Aksu H, Sevil U, Yurtsev E, Guvendiren G, Neural Tube Defects and Folic Acid, Maltepe University Journal of Nursing Science and Art, Vol:2, Issue:3, 2010.

[32] Arslan T, Beşgul Yigitler A. Current Approaches in Pregnancy Follow-up, Turkish Family Physcian, Vol: 3, Issue:2. 2012.

[33] Arınkan Sevcan A, Donmez Emin E, Butun Z, Bilgic Mehmet T, Muhcu M, The Effect of Multivitamin Use in Pregnancy on Birth Weight, Perinatal Journal, 2017.

[34] Demir C, Kocaman EC, Dilek I. Serum Ferritin Levels in Pregnancy, 2009.

[35] https://www.uptodate.com/contents/search/2021

[36] Ertas T. Iodine Deficiency and Goiter, Medical Geology Symposium Book with International Participation, ISBN: 978-975-7946-33-5, p:94-95, 2008.

[37] Yılmaz M, Importance of Iodine in Biological System, Toxicity and Analysis Methods, Erciyes University Faculty of Pharmacy Dissertation, Kayseri, 2013.

Chapter 9

Anemia during Pregnancy and Its Prevalence

Sehar Zulkifal, Shumaila Sarwar, Madiha Saddique, Khalida Yaqoob, Arshia Muneer, Aisha Fatima, Ayesha Kabir, Muhammad Asad Mangat, Laiba Mateen, Zeeshan Javed and Maleeha Manzoor

Abstract

Anemia is a serious health issue throughout the world affecting both sexes of any age group. This nutritional disease is more common among the pregnant women of developing countries, where it is a major cause of maternal death and negative outcome of pregnancy. Among all anemic types, IDA is most prevalent one and is comprises of about 95% of all anemic cases around the world. In many developing countries it is more common in women of low socio-economic background and with no record of antenatal checkup. There is need for further health educational programs to overcome anemia especially for pregnant females.

Keywords: iron deficiency anemia, pregnancy outcomes, iron supplements

1. Introduction

Anemia is a common nutritional deficiency condition in which the number of healthy red blood cells (the cells which can carry adequate oxygen to all tissues of the body) or the level of hemoglobin within the red blood cells is less than that of normal. Hemoglobin is required to transport oxygen and if a person does not have a normal number of healthy red blood cells, or does not have sufficient hemoglobin then there will be a decreased competence of the blood to take oxygen to all tissues of the body. Some of the ordinary and frequent causes of anemia include nutritional deficiencies including the deficiencies of vitamins and minerals, particularly deficiency of iron, folic acid deficiency, and deficiency of cobalamin or vitamins B12 [1].

Globally Anemia is a deceptive health issue that is especially affecting youngsters and women during pregnancy. World health organization has estimated that about 42% of children with an age less than 5 years and 40% of the women during the 2nd and 3rd trimester of their pregnancy are anemic all over the world. The rate of iron deficiency anemia in pregnant women is very high because of the high demands of iron and blood during pregnancy [2].

It is a worldwide occurring universal problem with more than 2000 million people around the globe of different ages [3]. And it is more customary in pregnant women of economically developed nations and affects both the mother's and fetus's health [4]. Globally its prevalence is 35% for women who are not pregnant and 51% for women who are pregnant and 3–4 times higher in developed nations [5].

2. Types of anemia

2.1 Iron-deficiency anemia

In case of iron deficiency anemia, the blood lacks an adequate number of normal red blood cells for carrying oxygen to the body tissues. Iron is one of the most plentiful elements on the surface of the earth. It participates in redox reactions which are crucial for numerous elementary organic processes such as cellular respiration and digestion. Therefore, it is not starling that iron contributes an important role in nearly all animal's lives. In *Homo sapien* iron is assimilated into proteins as an important constituent of heme (e.g., globin's, proteins, oxidases, and synthetases). These iron-containing proteins are essential for carrying out vital cellular and organismal functions including oxygen transport, mitochondrial respiration, nucleic acid replication and repair, host defense, and cell signaling. About 4 grams of iron is present in an adult human body. More than 75% of total body iron is correlated with hemoglobin, which is accountable for transporting oxygen (**Figure 1**). Deficiency of iron in the body decreases the production of the iron-containing heme group, which is a prosthetic group of hemoglobin protein that in turn limits the production of hemoglobin and decreases the synthesis of red blood cells (RBCs) from stem cells in the bone marrow which results in anemic conditions [6].

Pregnancy is one of the major reasons for iron-deficiency anemia because during the 2nd and 3rd trimester of pregnancy the iron demands of the body increase incredibly. The other major causes of iron deficiency anemia are heavy menstrual periods, pregnancy, bleeding from the gut, bleeding from the kidney, lack of certain

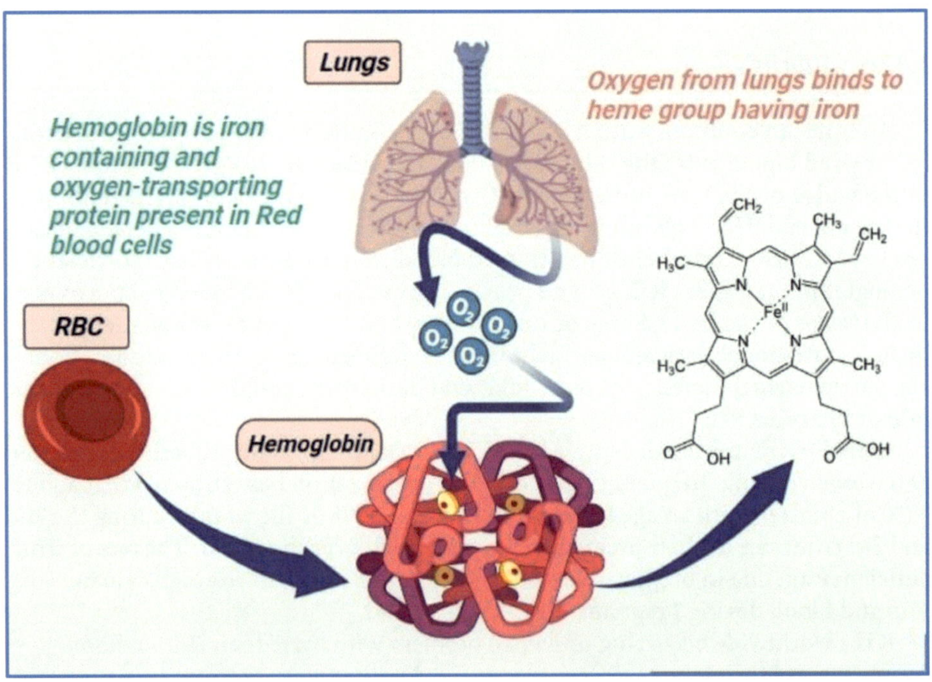

Figure 1.
Hemoglobin in RBC'S carrying oxygen from lungs.

vitamins, and problems with bone marrow [7]. Apathy, inactiveness, feeling feeble, faded and weak, panting, becoming exhausted and puffed easily, asymmetrical and disorderly heartbeats, fatigue and weariness, taste disturbances, smarting mouth are some common symptoms of iron-deficiency anemia.

Besides this, anemia during pregnancy can increase the risk of premature delivery and premature babies suffering from other health issues including low birth weight and neural tube defects to death. In developing countries, this premature birth is one of the main causes of death of an infant before his or her first birthday and this risk can be reduced by taking iron supplements during pregnancy [8].

2.1.1 Treatment

Due to the astounding effect of iodine deficiency anemia on maternal and fetal wellbeing, iron treatment is emphatically suggested. The adequacy of iron enhancement for the treatment of iron insufficiency is recorded by clinical preliminaries including pregnant ladies. The utilization of liposomal iron may address a promising technique of oral iron treatment in pregnant ladies with IDA. This compound shows high gastrointestinal retention and bioavailability and a low rate of results. Hence, liposomal iron presents great bearableness and favors preferable consistency over iron salts [9].

During pregnancy, a continuous elective treatment to oral iron, when it is not demonstrated, is IV iron. The new details of IV iron treatment advance a higher, just as quicker, increment of Hb focus and SF levels than oral iron supplementation, as was at that point appeared in changed studies in contrast with oral iron, ICM ensures a faster rectification of frailty and an apparent improvement of value existence with a slower pace of side effects like weariness and sorrow. It likewise presents higher bearableness and, thusly, more noteworthy consistency than oral iron. As the carb moiety ties the essential iron all the more firmly, high dosages of FCM (around 1000 mg in a solitary organization with a short implantation time) are permitted, in this way ensuring an improvement in consistency and a decrease of expenses because of rehashed organizations [10].

2.2 Pernicious anemia

Pernicious Anemia is an autoimmune disorder that affects the gastric mucosa of the stomach causing the lower and inadequate absorption of dietary Cobalamin or vitamin B12. It is essential for the proper functioning and forming of red blood cells. Vitamin B12 is also essential for the proper and normal functioning of the central nervous system and peripheral nervous system. The food or products which are enrich with protein such as beef, mutton, chicken, pork, fish, (dried fish, tilapia, halibut, tuna, salmon, carps, and shrimps), cereal, milk, yogurt, cheese, egg white, and other dairy products are major sources of vitamin B12 [11].

Vitamin B12 is separated from the proteins in the stomach through the action of hydrochloric acid. After this separation, vitamin B12 become incorporated with a protein called intrinsic factor in parietal cells of the stomach and is absorbed through villi which is present on the inner wall of the small intestine through which it is either computed into the blood circulation for the formation of red blood cells or stored in the liver (**Figure 2**). In the stomach, the parietal cell synthesizes intrinsic factor (IF) and secretes it, as well as hydrochloric acid into the gastric cavity of the stomach. The inability of parietal cells to secrete the intrinsic factor leads to failure of efficient vitamin B12 absorption into the blood. This inability is due to autoimmune antibody-mediated devastation of parietal cells of the gastric lumen which critically reduces the amount of intrinsic factor secreted in the

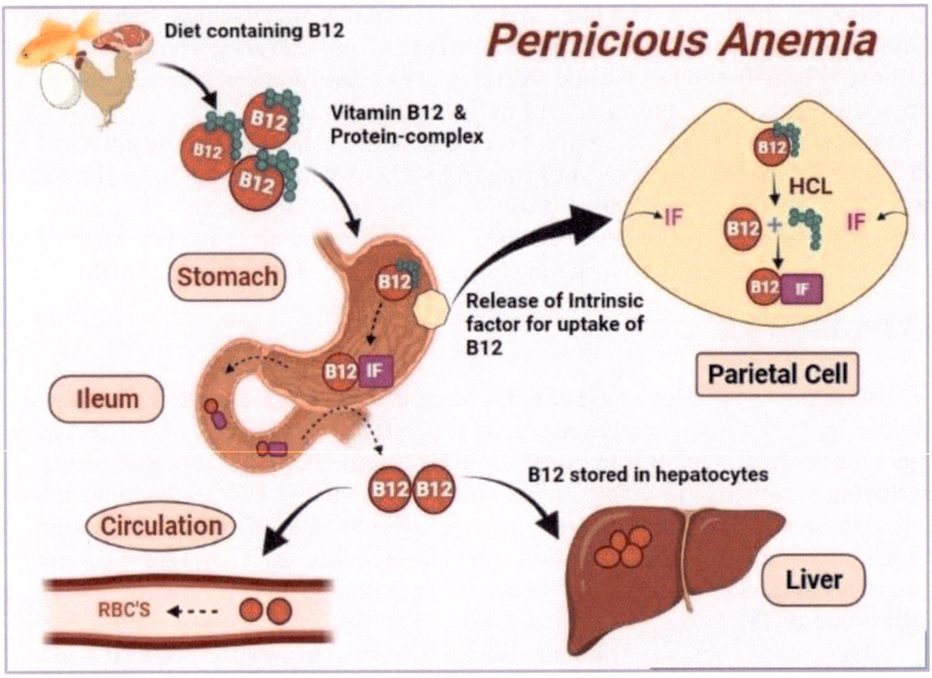

Figure 2.
Metabolic pathway for vitamin B12 absorption.

stomach. The antibodies attack and block the active site on intrinsic factors where vitamin B12 binds. This blockage of IF and inhibition of vitamin B12 binding will inhibit the formation of intrinsic factor-vitamin B12 complex. Without the formation of this complex, blood circulation cannot take up vitamin B12 and this will lead to the decrease in the level of red blood cells because vitamin B12 is an essential component in the synthesis of RBC'S. These blocking antibodies have been found in blood-serum or gastrointestinal fluid of 90% of patients suffering from pernicious anemia [12].

The major causes of pernicious Anemia are either the deficiency of vitamin B12 in diet or the inability of the stomach to absorb vitamin B12 from the diet. Vitamin B12 is also stored in the body. This stored vitamin B12 can last for years. When this is eventually depleted, pernicious anemia begins to develop. The amount of vitamin B12 required to fulfill the demands of a body depends on age [13]. The most serious outcome of B12 deficiency is diminished development and function of neurological processes throughout the lifecycle. Low maternal plasma vitamin B12 may result in pregnancies affected by anencephaly that is a type of neural tube defect (NTDs) [14].

Hypotonic muscles, failure to thrive, cerebral atrophy, and developmental regression are general outcomes of deficiency of vitamin B12. Folic acid supplemented pregnant women with negative B12 balance have increased risk for adverse maternal and infant outcomes (e.g., increased cardiometabolic disease risk) while pregnant women with Low B12 and a normal-to-high range of folate have high insulin resistance and adiposity in the offspring at 5 years of age [15].

2.2.1 Treatment

Folate lack is promptly treated with oral folic acid substitution. Folic acid supplementation (≥0.4 mg) is prescribed for multi-month before origination and for the initial 12 weeks of pregnancy as this is has been appeared to lessen the danger of fetal neural cylinder defects. High portion (5 mg) folate is suggested for ladies at high danger of neural cylinder surrenders (for example past pregnancy with a neural cylinder deformity) or in danger of malabsorption. To medicate B_{12} deficiency usually proton pump inhibitor, histamine H_2-receptor antagonists and metformin used [16].

2.3 Hemolytic anemia

Hemolytic anemia is the destruction of red blood cells (RBCs) before their normal 120-day life span. The process of destruction of red blood cells is called hemolysis. There are three types of hemolysis:

i. Intravascular hemolysis

When the RBCs are destroyed in the blood vessel itself, it is called intravascular hemolysis. Intravascular hemolysis is very dramatic because free hemoglobin is released into the plasma leading to hemoglobinuria. In the case of intravascular hemolysis, certain enzymes such as glucose-6-phosphate dehydrogenase (G6PD) or immune-mediated enzymes can be defective.

ii. Extravascular hemolysis

Extravascular hemolysis usually occurs due to more subtle RBC destruction, typically with chronic splenic enlargement and jaundice. In Extravascular hemolysis, RBC membrane disorders such as hereditary spherocytosis can also occur [17].

iii. Antibody-mediated hemolysis

Antibodies are the proteins that are synthesized by the immune system. These proteins normally attach to the surface of any foreign invaders such as bacteria and viruses and destroy them. In the case of antibody-mediated hemolysis, the body makes antibodies against its red blood cells. These antibodies target red blood cells and kill them before completion of their life cycle (**Figure 3**). It depends on the duration and the rate of hemolysis, whether the anemia may or may not occur. If the degree of hemolysis is moderate and the erythropoietic response of the bone marrow is completely compensating for the decreased RBC lifespan, then the hemoglobin concentration may remain normal. If the erythropoietic response is not sufficient to completely compensate for decreased RBCs lifespan, then anemia will occur [18].

Anemia has multi-factorial etiology in pregnancy. There is a rare chance of maternal complication due to Pregnancy-induced hemolytic anemia that occurs during pregnancy and resolves later on delivery. The absence of any identifiable immune mechanism or intracorpuscular or extracorpuscular defects despite the use of specific and sensitive complement-fixation techniques and an assay of all red blood cell (RBC) enzymes are the characteristics of this problem. It is necessary to rule out other causes of non-immune hemolytic anemia including broad etiologies such as congenital, mechanical, toxic agents, medications, infection, lymphoproliferative disorder, etc. to embark on the diagnosis of idiopathic hemolytic anemia. A rare entity called Coomb's negative hemolytic anemia of pregnancy may be life-threatening, and for an optimum maternal-fetal outcome it desires a tireless diagnostic and appropriate treatment approach [19].

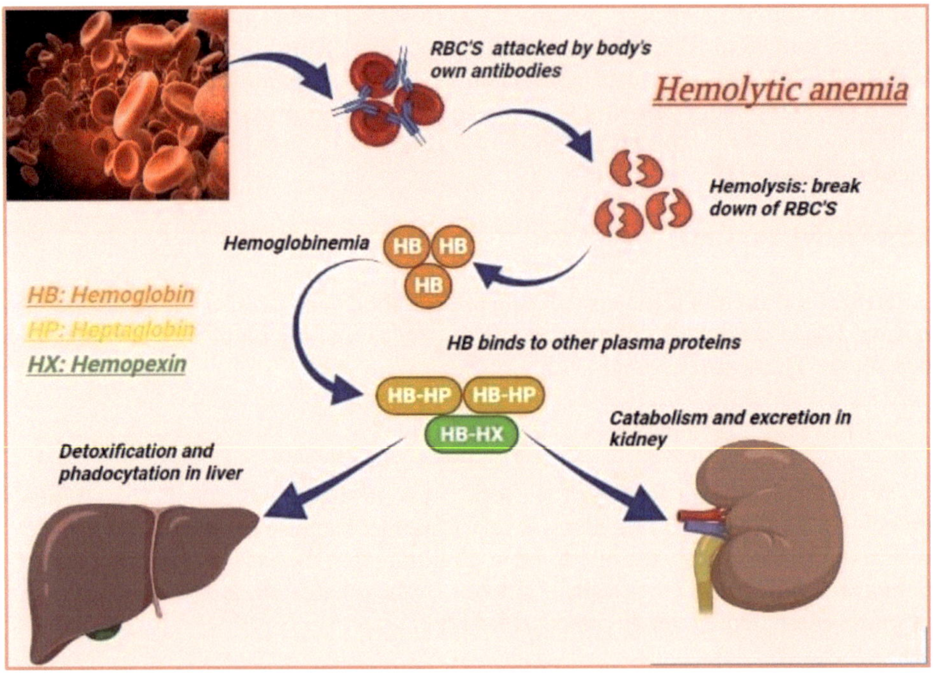

Figure 3.
Antibody-mediated hemolysis of red blood cells.

2.3.1 Treatment

They are challenging to treat, given distinct treatments. The basic treatment for TTP and complement-mediated HUS is the exchange of plasma. Delivery is the basic treatment for other pregnancy-related thrombotic microangiopathies (HELLP and preeclampsia) that occur during the third trimester [20].

2.4 Aplastic anemia

Aplastic anemia (AA) is a non-cancerous disorder in which the stem cells in the bone marrow (the cells responsible for making all mature blood cells) are attacked and destroyed by the patient's immune system. Aplastic Anemia can be mild or severe; it can develop suddenly at very early stages of life or slowly at later stages of life [21].

If the parents have defective genes which are constructing antibodies against their stem cells, then this disorder can be inherited into the offspring through parents. The other causes of this disorder can be the usage of some medicines and certain toxins in the environment. An individual who has a record of certain infectious diseases, such as AIDS, HIV, hepatitis, viral diseases, Epstein–Barr, or having a record of consuming several medicines, such as antibiotics and anticonvulsants can also develop aplastic anemia. Subjection to certain toxins and heavy metals such as cadmium, mercury, lead, and thallium can cause aplastic anemia. Exposure to radiation and a history of having an autoimmune disorder, such as lupus are some other major causes of aplastic anemia [22].

Aplastic anemia is a rare disease that occurs due to the destruction of pluripotent stem cells in the bone marrow. Significant factors including extremely low platelet counts, low bone marrow cellularity, and late disease presentation result in severe Aplastic anemia during pregnancy [23]. In pregnancies with Aplastic anemia, Low hemoglobin concentration and platelet counts may be the primary risk factors for obstetric complications. Premature labor, gestational diabetes, pre-eclampsia, acute heart failure, postpartum hemorrhage, and severe postpartum infection are the major maternal complications [24].

2.4.1 Treatment

The principle of aplastic anemia treatment is to know about the cause and treatment of cytopenias and minimize the side effects of therapy for mother and fetus. Abortion is also preferred in case of severe pancytopenia. It is also treated by the transplantation of hemopoietic stem cells and by using immunosuppressive regimens. Hemopoietic stem cell transplantation (HSCT) is done after the delivery and it may lead to reduced fertility so the patient is asked before the treatment [25].

Antithymocyte globulin (ATG) is also used for the treatment. ATG is a safe medication but it may cause allergic reactions, vein irritation, nausea, vomiting, and diarrhea. It does not cause any drug toxicity but in pregnant women, it may cause low birth weight. Corticosteroids are also used for aplastic anemia treatment. As they cannot cross the placenta so it reduces fetal brain exposure but it also may lead to glucose intolerance, gestational diabetes, and premature rupture of membranes.

Transfusion of blood products is the basic treatment for aplastic anemia. It also causes some complications such as hemochromatosis and HLA alloimmunization. Alloantibodies may cause platelet-transfusion refractoriness (PTR). They are challenging to treat, given distinct treatments. The basic treatment for TTP and complement-mediated HUS is the exchange of plasma. Delivery is the basic treatment for other pregnancy-related thrombotic microangiopathies (HELLP and preeclampsia) that occur during the third trimester.

2.5 Sickle-cell anemia

In normal conditions, the body produces red blood cells which are round and flexible and can flow easily through the blood vessels. But in the case of sickle cell anemia, the body forms sickle-shaped or C-shaped red blood cells which become rigid, sticky and these irregularly sickle-shaped cells become stuck in small blood vessels, which can slow down or inhibit the flow of blood and supply of oxygen to all parts of the body (**Figure 4**). The average life of every red blood cell is 120 days which means that after 120 days red blood cells are replaced with new ones in the circulation. But in the case of sickle cell anemia red blood cells usually die within 10 to 20 days, causing a red blood cell deficiency that leads to Anemia and cannot supply oxygen properly throughout the body [26].

Pregnancy and sickle cell disease have reciprocal impacts on each other and it's a risky situation. The risk of infection becomes significantly higher during pregnancy in sickle cell anemia. The risk of low birth weight increases by 4 times than in the general population in homozygous sickle cell disease. The presence or conjunction of several risk factors including chronic fetal distress, vasculorenal syndrome, acute vaso occlusive crisis, or pelvic dystocia due to bone lesions of the pelvis explains the high cesarean rate in sickle cell women [27].

In the postpartum period, nearly half of women with sickle cell disease experienced a vasoocclusive crisis. Actually, it's a period at high risk of decompensation of sickle cell disease that combines maternal fatigue, intense pain in the absence of epidural analgesia, fasting with dehydration, a state of metabolic acidosis linked to uterine muscle work, and respiratory alkalosis. All of these factors result in a vaso occlusive accident [28].

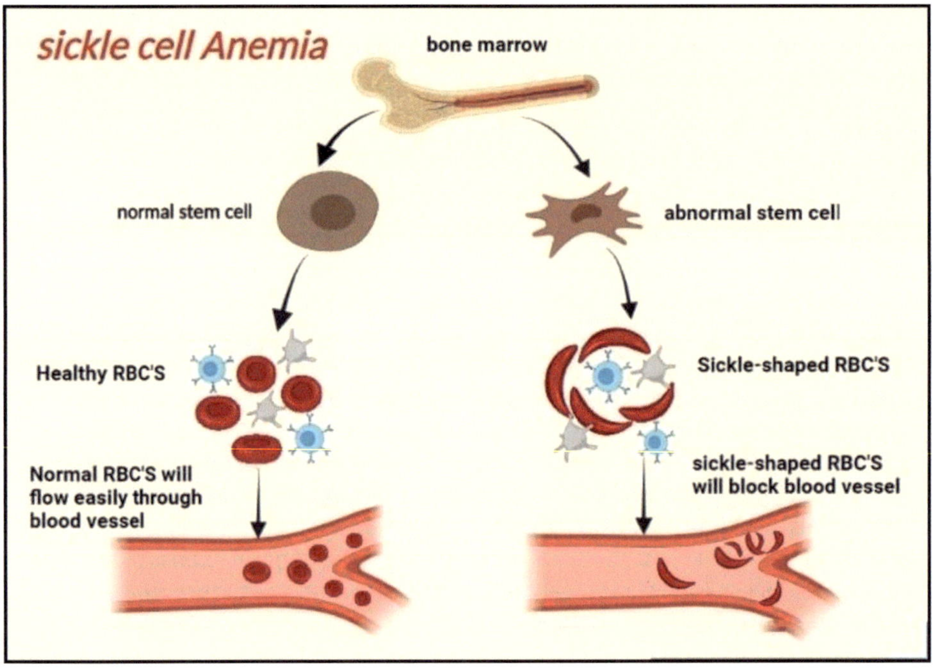

Figure 4.
Formation of sickle-shaped RBC'S blocking the blood vessels.

2.5.1 Treatment

Enough perinatal care should be given during pregnancy. During severe symptoms, pregnant women should be hospitalized. For pain relief narcotics analgesic and paracetamol should be given. To treat acute chest pain antibiotics, oxygen support, hydration, analgesics should be given. If required blood transfusion should also be done so the risk of stroke and the coronary syndrome is reduced [29].

3. Global prevalence of anemia

Anemia is a universal problem with billions of people around the globe, and it is more common in pregnant women. According to WHO, during pregnancy, less than 110 g/l of Hb level in blood is a sign of anemia and it became severe if Hb level is <70 g/l.

4. Effect on young ones and effect on mother

Anemia is a serious and most common nutritional disorder, the main population who is suffering from anemia are children under 5 years, mostly in the first 24 months of their age. Worldwide 47.4% of patients suffering from anemia are children. Anemia leads to the impairment of physical growth as well as cognitive and motor growth. The consequences of anemia, even if it is treated in later childhood are irreversible. Hence, it is important to recognize and treat anemia, frequently among the young ones because they are more susceptible to it [30]. Anemia also causes a decrease in the performance of school-going children, work productivity in adulthood, personal satisfaction of a person [12].

Anemic children have lower blood concentration than normal and have less motor and cognitive development which affects the output rate of work in adulthood [31]. In developing countries, the frequency of anemia in children of age 5 is 39% and in children from 5 to 9 age the frequency is 48%. The reason for low hemoglobin Hb level in the children are, lack of awareness among the mothers, nutrition and harmful eating habits and other parasitic infections are the factors leading to anemia [32].

In developing countries, anemia is the major cause of maternal death and negative outcomes of pregnancy. There are major nutritional deficiencies (vitamin B12 deficiency, folic acid, or riboflavin deficiency) in developing countries that lead to anemia and other chronic infections, malaria which is a serious parasitic infection, and hemoglobinopathies. Women experience anemia during their maternal periods which increases the risk of low birth weight of the newborn, premature birth of the children, before and after birth mortality of the newborn [33].

Despite the presence of symptoms, patients with Iron deficiency-anemia should be treated as early as possible because they are in danger of organ ischemia, and if not treated further worsening anemia until the fundamental reason for the disease is not revealed and refill the bone marrow with iron [34]. Similarly, children with iron deficiency-anemia alone should be treated because it may lead to sideropenia in children is related to neurocognitive disabilities, affect their learning abilities and capacity, impaired motor function as well. Most frequently, people with anemia may also get Febrile seizures, breath-holding spells, and a restless leg syndrome shown much more in anemic people [22].

During childhood, anemia may be involved in the growth delay of the children such as height, they are more vulnerable to infections, their poor cognitive growth such as mental development and growth from childhood to adulthood, poor motor development which results in low work productivity in the future [35]. Normally 500–800 mg of blood is consumed from a mother during the pregnancy. In premenopausal women mostly have less iron stored or iron deficiency ID in them, they may get anemia or are without anemia, they are mostly belonging to less developed areas of the world. Maternal iron deficiency has a huge complex impact on a child. One report stated that the woman was diagnosed with schistosomiasis when she was pregnant, maternal iron deficiency appears in a child at an age of six months. Iron deficiency in the mother results in the abnormal cognitive development of a child [36]. When severe iron deficiency occurs in the mother, placenta hypertrophy occurs and the risk of the premature birth of the child increases. Maternal iron deficiency also causes low-weight birth of the child and death of the newborn. Sometimes in the first trimester, iron deficiency anemia is related to the low birth weight of the child but the development of anemia later is not involved. Maternal anemia or iron deficiency may occur due to less parental care or eating unhealthy food, which may cause similar effects [37].

The newborn may create paleness because of low iron stores in the body [38]. During pregnancy, anemia can cause serious complications maternal as well as in newborn childlike unexpected labor and post-pregnancy anxiety. Anemic mothers, particularly during the early trimester of pregnancy, can be considered as a danger factor for pregnancy results [23].

Iron deficiency in infants leads to serious and major behavior problems. There are uncertain effects of micronutrient deficiency in the middle of childhood. Vitamin B12 deficiency leads to psychological symptoms such as depression, loss of memory, major nervous problems, and structural changes in some parts of the brain that are important in the development of a child in solving behavioral problems that are basal ganglia, hippocampus, the amygdala. Severe anemic conditions may result in brain damage or nerve damage may occur [39].

Anemia with sickle cell disorder is the most common inherited disease, it results in an increased risk of complications and mortality rate. Sickle cell anemia affects pregnancy and increases maternal and perinatal complexities and early labor pain. The most common sign are pale skin, tiredness, vision changes, hand, and feet swelling, and include some bacterial infections [29]. Maternal anemia directly increases perinatal mortality, low weight of the child at the time of birth, stillbirth, and abortion [40]. In pregnancy, anemia lessens the chances of tolerance to blood loss, which results in heart failure or other abnormal functions of the body [41].

5. Preventive measures

In pregnancy, anemia is a major health problem especially in developing countries and it is also a common nutritional deficiency disease globally, approximately affecting two-fifths of pregnant women worldwide. During pregnancy, if anemia becomes severe it can lead to maternal and paternal harmful effects like preterm labor, low birth weight, and intrauterine fetal death. One of the leading causes is maternal mortality due to anemia. In order to prevent anemia during pregnancy preventive measures are required [42].

Multifactorial and nutritional deficiencies of iron, folate, and vitamin B_{12} are the leading causes of anemia in developing countries. Moreover, malaria and intestinal parasitic infections also contribute to anemia in pregnancy. The causes which contribute to anemia in pregnant women vary greatly by geographical location, season, and dietary practice. Iron deficiency anemia (IDA) is the most common type of anemia all around the world. According to the study, 75% of cases of anemia are due to iron deficiency [43]. Iron deficiency anemia (IDA), often coexists with a deficiency in other important micronutrients, that make it more harmful for fetal growth [44].

5.1 Supplements

Iron intake and folic acid supplements are the keystones for the prevention of anemia in pregnancy. In earlier times these are the initial preventive measures suggested to the women in pregnancy to avoid anemia. The normal level of folic acid in approximately 25% of pregnant women is not sufficient to avert megaloblastic changes in the bone marrow. In developing countries, women in pregnancy should receive 40 mg daily supplementation of folic acid. 100 mg iron and 350 μg folate are present in fefol, women in pregnancy can take this supplement as standard oral preparation for prevention of anemia.

Due to physiological changes in pregnancy iron intakes are several times higher than in nonpregnant women [42]. To maximize iron intake and absorption all women should be given dietary information in pregnancy. 100-200 mg elemental iron should be suggested to women with iron deficiency anemia (IDA) [45].

The amount of iron in the diet, its bioavailability, and physiological requirements in pregnancy are some of the factors that contribute to iron absorption. Pregnant women should eat well-balanced meals that are rich in iron. Heme iron and non-heme iron are the 2 types of iron that are present in our meal or food.

5.2 Dietary advice

Animal flesh like red meat, poultry, and seafood contain dietary heme iron. Non-heme iron absorption is two to three-fold less than that of the heme iron. The meat in which organic compounds like peptides are present promotes the absorption of iron from non-heme iron sources which are less bioavailable. It is difficult to absorb non-heme iron than heme iron but still non-heme iron forms about 95% of dietary iron intake. Iron absorption from non-heme sources can significantly increase by the use of Ascorbic acid. By the fermentation and germination of cereals and legumes, we can increase the bioavailability of non-heme iron in pregnancy. This results in the decline of phytate content, a component of food that hampers iron absorption. The use of tea and coffee shortly after a meal or with the meal hinders iron absorption because of the presence of tannins. Therefore, Pregnant women should avoid it.

The bioavailability of non-heme iron is enhanced by germination and fermentation of cereals and legumes which results in a decrease in the phytate content, a food constituent that hinders iron absorption. Tannins in tea and coffee hinder iron absorption on consumption with or shortly after a meal [42].

5.3 Oral supplements

In pregnancy, once women are subjected to iron deficiency anemia (IDA), it is very difficult to correct iron deficiency anemia through dietary changes alone. Therefore, oral supplements are necessary to replenish iron deficiency. An effective, inexpensive, and safe way to ensure replenish of iron is oral iron [46]. The inefficiency of absorption or iron ferrous salts show only marginal differences between each other. Ferrous fumarate, ferrous sulphate, and ferrous gluconate are the available ferrous salts. Serum ferritin should be checked in women with known haemoglobinopathy. If the ferritin ˂30 μg/l then women should offer therapeutic iron [45]. If it is possible women should avoid proton pump inhibitors because they decrease the production of gastric juice. Gastric juice helps with iron absorption by converting the ferric to ferrous salt. But in some cases, oral iron is not tolerated and patients may develop side effects like nausea, abdominal pain, and epigastric discomfort.

5.4 Intravenous iron source (IV)

So, in order to maintain hemoglobin concentration in pregnancy intravenous iron (IV), sources are now recommended. Sodium ferric gluconate (Ferrlecit), iron sucrose (Venofer), iron (III)-hydroxide dextran complex (Cosmofer), ferric carboxymaltose (Ferinject), and iron (III) isomaltoside 1000 (Monofer) are now available forms of IV [47]. In order to combat anemia in pregnancy nutritional education or awareness is the main objective [42].

5.5 Counseling in pregnancy

Proper counseling should be given to pregnant women as to how to take iron supplements correctly. In case of severe anemia, secondary care should be considered. 200 mg elemental iron daily should be starting dose in these types of cases [45]. Moreover, doctors should suggest family planning and control of birth spacing as a preventive measure for anemia [42].

Author details

Sehar Zulkifal, Shumaila Sarwar[1], Madiha Saddique, Khalida Yaqoob, Arshia Muneer, Aisha Fatima, Ayesha Kabir, Muhammad Asad Mangat, Laiba Mateen, Zeeshan Javed and Maleeha Manzoor*
Faculty of Life Sciences, Department of Zoology, Government College University, Faisalabad, Pakistan

*Address all correspondence to: maleehamanzoor@gcuf.edu.pk

References

[1] Wouters, H. J., van der Klauw, M. M., de Witte, T., Stauder, R., Swinkels, D. W., Wolffenbuttel, B. H., & Huls, G. (2019). Association of anemia with health-related quality of life and survival: a large population-based cohort study. Journal of Haematologica, 104(3): 468.

[2] WHO (1992). Maternal Health and safe Motherhood Programme. The prevalence of Anemia in women. A tabulation of available information. 2nd ed. World Health Organization, Geneva, Switzerland.

[3] Ayensu, J., Annan, R., Lutterodt, H., Edusei, A., & Peng, L. S. (2020). Prevalence of anaemia and low intake of dietary nutrients in pregnant women living in rural and urban areas in the Ashanti region of Ghana. Joural of Plos one, 15(1): e0226026.

[4] UNCF (2001). Iron deficiency anaemia: assessment, prevention, and control. A guide for programme managers. United Nations Children's Fund, United Nations University, World Health Organization. Geneva.

[5] Khalil, A., Jabbar, T., Akhtar, S., & Mohyuddin, S. (2007). Frequency and types of anemia in an antenatal clinic in the third trimester of pregnancy. Pakistan Armed Forces Medical Journal, 57(4): 273-278.

[6] Dev, S., & Babitt, J. L. (2017). Overview of iron metabolism in health and disease. Hemodialysis International, 21: S6-S20.

[7] Fishbane, S., & Spinowitz, B. (2018). Update on anemia in ESRD and earlier stages of CKD: core curriculum 2018. American Journal of Kidney Diseases, 71(3): 423-435.

[8] Yanovich, R., Merkel, D., Israeli, E., Evans, R. K., Erlich, T. et al. (2011). Anemia, iron deficiency and stress fractures in female combatants during 16 months. J Strength Cond Res., 25: 3412-3421.

[9] Elstrott, B., Khan, L., Olson, S., Raghunathan, V., DeLoughery, T., & Shatzel, J. J. (2020). The role of iron repletion in adult iron deficiency anemia and other diseases. European journal of haematology, *104*(3): 153-161.

[10] Iqbal, S., Ekmekcioglu, C. (2019). Maternal and neonatal outcomes related to iron supplementation or iron status: a summary of meta-analyses. J Matern Fetal Neonatal Med., 32:1528-1540.

[11] Carmel, R., & Agrawal, Y. P. (2012). Failures of cobalamin assays in pernicious anemia. The New England journal of medicine, 367(4); 385-386.

[12] Nederstigt, C., Uitbeijerse, B. S., Janssen, L. G. M., Corssmit, E. P. M., de Koning, E. J. P., & Dekkers, O. M. (2019). Associated auto-immune disease in type 1 diabetes patients: a systematic review and meta-analysis. European journal of endocrinology, 180(2): 135-144.

[13] Kesbeh, Y., & Pakbaz, Z. (2019). Pernicious anemia: a myelodysplastic syndrome look-alike. Journal of community hospital internal medicine perspectives, 9(3): 240-243.

[14] Molloy, A. M., Kirke, P. N., Brody, L. C., Scott, J. M., and Mills, J. L. (2008). Effects of folate and vitamin B12 deficiencies during pregnancy on fetal, infant, and child development. Food and nutrition bulletin, *29*(2): S101–S115.

[15] Siddiqua, J. T., Allen, H. L., Raqib, R., and Ahmed, T. (2014). Vitamin B12 Deficiency in Pregnancy and Lactation: Is there a Need for Pre and Postnatal Supplementation. J Nutr Disorders

Ther, 4: 142. doi:10.4172/2161-0509.1000142

[16] Shand, A., Austin, K., Nassar, N., and Kidson-Gerber, G. (2020). Pharmacological management of anaemia in pregnancy: a review. J Pharm Pract Res., 50: 205-212.

[17] Grossi, F., Shum, M. K., Gertz, M. A., Roman, E., Deschatelets, P., Hamdani, M., & Francois, C. G. (2018). Inhibition of C3 with APL-2 results in normalisation of markers of intravascular and extravascular hemolysis in patients with autoimmune hemolytic anemia (AIHA). *Blood, 132(supplement 1),* 1989134: 3623-3623.

[18] Brodsky, R. A. (2019). Warm autoimmune hemolytic anemia. New England Journal of Medicine, 381(7): 647-654.

[19] Gupta, M., Kala, M., Kumar, S., Singh, G., Chhabra, S., and Sen, R. (2015). Idiopathic Hemolytic Anemia of Pregnancy: A Diagnostic Dilemma. Journal of Hematology, 3(4):118-120.

[20] Felemban, A. A., Rashidi, Z. A., Almatrafi, M. H., and Alsahabi, J. A. (2019). Autoimmune hemolytic anemia and ovarian dermoid cysts in pregnancy. Saudi medical journal, 40(4): 397-400.

[21] Shallis, R. M., Ahmad, R., & Zeidan, A. M. (2018). Aplastic anemia: etiology, molecular pathogenesis, and emerging concepts. European journal of haematology, 101(6): 711-720.

[22] Schoettler, M. L., & Nathan, D. G. (2018). The pathophysiology of acquired aplastic Anemia: current concepts revisited. Hematology/ Oncology Clinics, 32(4): 581-594.

[23] Stibbe, K. J., Wildschut, H. I., and Lugtenburg, P. J. (2011). Management of aplastic anemia in a woman during pregnancy: a case report. Journal of medical case reports, 5: 66.

[24] Bo, L., Mei-Ying, L., Yang, Z., Shan-Mi, W., and Xiao-Hong, Z. (2016). Aplastic anemia associated with pregnancy: maternal and fetal complications. The journal of maternal-fetal & neonatal medicine : the official journal of the European Association of Perinatal Medicine, the Federation of Asia and Oceania Perinatal Societies, the International Society of Perinatal Obstetricians, *29*(7): 1120-1124.

[25] Zdanowicz, J. A., and Surbek, D. (2019). Patient blood management in obstetrics - Review. Transfus Apher Sci., 58:412-415.

[26] Mburu, J., & Odame, I. (2019). Sickle cell disease: Reducing the global disease burden. International journal of laboratory hematology, 41: 82-88.

[27] Means, R. T. (2020). Iron deficiency and iron deficiency anemia: implications and impact in pregnancy, fetal development, and early childhood parameters. Nutrients, *12*(2): 447.

[28] Mirza, F. G., Abdul-Kadir, R., Breymann, C., Fraser, I. S., & Taher, A. (2018). Impact and management of iron deficiency and iron deficiency anemia in women's health. Expert review of hematology, 11(9): 727-736.

[29] Molloy, A. M., Kirke, P. N., Brody, L. C., Scott, J. M., and Mills, J. L. (2008). Effects of folate and vitamin B12 deficiencies during pregnancy on fetal, infant, and child development. Food and nutrition bulletin, 29(2): S101–S115.

[30] Muñoz, M., Stensballe, J., Ducloy-Bouthors A. S. et al. (2019). Patient blood management in obstetrics: prevention and treatment of postpartum haemorrhage. Blood Transfus, 17:112-136.

[31] Onyeneho, N. G., I'Aronu, N., Chukwu, N., Agbawodikeizu, U. P., Chalupowski, M., & Subramanian, S. V. (2016). Factors associated with compliance to recommended

micronutrients uptake for prevention of anemia during pregnancy in urban, peri-urban, and rural communities in Southeast Nigeria. Journal of Health, Population and Nutrition, *35*(1): 1-17.

[32] Pavord, S., Daru, J., Prasannan, N., Robinson, S., Stanworth, S., Girling, J., & BSH Committee. (2020). *UK guidelines on the management of iron deficiency in pregnancy*. Br J Haematol, *188*(6): 819-830.

[33] Rahmati, S., Delpishe, A., Azami, M., Ahmadi, M. R. H., & Sayehmiri, K. (2017). Maternal Anemia during pregnancy and infant low birth weight: A systematic review and Meta-analysis. International journal of reproductive biomedicine, *15*(3): 125.

[34] Robinson, S. L., Marín, C., Oliveros, H., Mora-Plazas, M., Richards, B. J., Lozoff, B., & Villamor, E. (2018). Iron deficiency, anemia, and low vitamin B-12 serostatus in middle childhood are associated with behavior problems in adolescent boys: Results from the Bogotá school children cohort. The Journal of nutrition, 148(5): 760-770.

[35] Shaban, L., Al-Taiar, A., Rahman, A., Al-Sabah, R., & Mojiminiyi, O. (2020). Anemia and its associated factors among Adolescents in Kuwait. Scientific reports, 10(1): 1-9.

[36] Shallis, R. M., Ahmad, R., & Zeidan, A. M. (2018). Aplastic anemia: etiology, molecular pathogenesis, and emerging concepts. European journal of haematology, 101(6): 711-720.

[37] Shand, A., Austin, K., Nassar, N., and Kidson-Gerber, G. (2020). Pharmacological management of anaemia in pregnancy: a review. J Pharm Pract Res., 50: 205-212.

[38] Siddiqua, J. T., Allen, H. L., Raqib, R., and Ahmed, T. (2014). Vitamin B12 Deficiency in Pregnancy and Lactation: Is there a Need for Pre and Postnatal Supplementation. J Nutr Disorders Ther, 4: 142.

[39] Szudzik, M., Starzyński, R. R., Jończy, A., Mazgaj, R., Lenartowicz, M., & Lipiński, P. (2018). Iron supplementation in suckling piglets: An ostensibly easy therapy of neonatal iron deficiency anemia. Pharmaceuticals, 11(4): 128.

[40] Taylor, S., & Rampton, D. (2015). Treatment of iron deficiency anemia: practical considerations. POLSKIE ARCHIWUM MEDYCYNY WEWNETRZNEJ-POLISH ARCHIVES OF INTERNAL MEDICINE. 7624.

[41] UNCF (2001). Iron deficiency anaemia: assessment, prevention, and control. A guide for programme managers. United Nations Children's Fund, United Nations University, World Health Organization. Geneva.

[42] WHO (1992). Maternal Health and safe Motherhood Programme. The prevalence of Anemia in women. A tabulation of available information. 2nd ed. World Health Organization, Geneva, Switzerland.

[43] Wiegersma, A. M., Dalman, C., Lee, B. K., Karlsson, H., & Gardner, R. M. (2019). Association of prenatal maternal anemia with neurodevelopmental disorders. JAMA psychiatry, 76(12): 1294-1304.

[44] Wouters, H. J., van der Klauw, M. M., de Witte, T., Stauder, R., Swinkels, D. W., Wolffenbuttel, B. H., & Huls, G. (2019). Association of anemia with health-related quality of life and survival: a large population-based cohort study. Journal of Haematologica, 104(3): 468.

[45] Wouters, H. J., van der Klauw, M. M., de Witte, T., Stauder, R., Swinkels, D. W., Wolffenbuttel, B. H., & Huls, G. (2019). Association of anemia with health-related quality of life and

survival: a large population-based cohort study. Journal of Haematologica, 104(3): 468.

[46] Zavaleta, N., & Astete-Robilliard, L. (2017). Effect of anemia on child development: Long-term consequences. Revista peruana de medicina experimental y salud publica, 34(4): 716-722.

[47] Zdanowicz, J. A., and Surbek, D. (2019). Patient blood management in obstetrics - Review. Transfus Apher Sci., 58:412-5.

Section 4

Adult and Elderly Health in Primary Care

Chapter 10

Managing Polypharmacy and Deprescribing in Elderly

Çiğdem Apaydın Kaya

Abstract

The increase in the number of medications used may result many negative consequences for patients and health system. Elderly patients are more likely to encounter these health problems associated with polypharmacy. Deprescribing, the process of tapering, withdrawing, discontinuing, or stopping medications, is important in reducing polypharmacy, adverse drug effects, inappropriate or ineffective medication use, and costs. Deprescribing in elderly patients in accordance with the evidence based guidelines has many positive outcomes in older people such as decrease in the risk of falls, improvement in cognition, and improvement in patients' global health status. Therefore, each visit of an elderly patient should be considered as an opportunity to evaluate the unnecessary use or harms of the prescribed or nonprescribed medications. Clinicians should decide to deprescription process by individualized care goals in line with current guidelines. Beers Criteria, STOPP/START and The Medication Appropriateness Index-MAI can be used to assit clinicians to identify unnecessary or potentially inappropriate drugs and reduce the number of medications in older patients. But, a balance is required between over and under prescribing. In conclusion, prevention of polypharmacy and withdrawing unneccesary and inappropriate medications may be the best clinical decision for family physicians who follow the elderly in primary care.

Keywords: polypharmacy, deprescription, elderly, older adults, aging, drug use, advers drug events, primary care

1. Introduction

Although lacking a consensus definition, the concurrent use of two or more medications is described polypharmacy [1]. However, in many researches investigating the use of multiple medications and their effects, the concurrent use of 5 or more drugs is defined as "polypharmacy" [2–4]. The concurrent use of 2 or 3 medications does not cause a significant problem if they are chosen correctly, but the use of 4 or more medications carries a significant risk. Although polypharmacy is seen in all age groups, it is more common with increasing age. Nearly half of the older people use at least 1 drug even though it is not necessary [5, 6]. One of the most important causes for the increase in the number of medications used in the elderly is the coexistence of more than one chronic disease.

IntechOpen

2. Polypharmacy in elderly

Increase in the number of medications used may cause many health problems. As the metabolism and elimination of drugs will be affected by the decrease in kidney and liver functions with increasing age, the older people are more susceptible to the negative effects of polypharmacy. In addition, with increasing age, the onset of amnesia, decreased visual acuity, and the onset of physical disabilities cause the elderly, who already use many drugs, to make mistakes in the use of drugs. As a result, the elderly are more likely to encounter many health problems caused by the use of multiple drugs. Therefore, polypharmacy is accepted as one of the geriatric syndromes.

Apart from increasing age and the presence of chronic disease, other risk factors for polypharmacy are listed below [7, 8]:

- Follow-up of patients by more than one physician and lack of communication between physicians
- Patients' drug expectations for their illness
- Medical guidelines specific to diseases, not to patients
- Pharmaceutical advertisements
- Recent hospitalization
- Over-the-counter drug sales
- Prescribing medication for symptoms rather than diagnosis
- Failure to adequately explain the medication changes to the patients by the doctors
- Residing in long-term care facilities
- Prescription cascade (addition of new medications to counter adverse drug reactions or drug side effects. For example, addition of an antitussive agent to relieve cough caused by angiotensin converting enzyme inhibitors, or addition of an antihypertensive due to increased blood pressure with NSAID use.

The increase in the number of medications used may result many negative consequences for patients and health system. For example, overall, 30% of hospital admissions are related in some way to medications in people aged over 65 years and half of these could be prevented [9]. Also, with increasing age, compliance to drug usage declines due to increase in the number of the drugs used, the beginning of memory loss, weakness of vision and the onset of physical incapabilities. The most common health problems reported in the elderly people associated with polypharmacy are listed below [10–15]:

- Increase risk of:
    - Drug interactions
    - Advers drug events

- Morbidity and mortality
- Physical and cognitive dysfunction
- Falls and associated harms (hip fracture, etc)
- Prescribing cascade

- Increase in use of the health care system and hospitalizations
- Decreased compliance to medication use
- Increased treatment cost
- Increased need of residing in long-term care facilities

As can be seen above, most of the problems caused by polypharmacy can be prevented. Visits for prescribing the medications used regularly, health maintanece and control visits are the convenient opportunities for physicians to evaluate drug interactions. In addition, while making a differential diagnosis for a new complaint or symptom, polypharmacy and drug interactions, should be evaluated and kept in mind that changes in the patient's condition may be associated with drug interactions or an adverse effect of a medication.

Although polypharmacy is referred to prescribed medications, the number of over-the-counter and herbal/dietary supplements used should be also considered. It should be noted that beside the all medications used by the patient, over-the-counter drugs with dietary or herbal supplements should be evaluated in terms of interactions. For example, garlic or *Ginkgo biloba* extract taken with warfarin may cause an increased risk of bleeding. St. John's wort taken with atorvastatin or diltiazem, may increase the advers effects of atorvastatin or diltiazem in older adults [16, 17].

Even not recommended by a physician, elderly people self-medicate more than the other age groups. This leads to an increased risk of adverse events and side effects. For example, the use of non-steroidal anti-inflammatory drugs, which are used common nonprescription, may lead to hypertension, decreased effect of the antihypertensives or a gastrointestinal bleeding.

There are many web-based applications developed for the physicians to control drug interactions. The addresses of some free applications that can be easily used on smartphones and tablets are listed below:

- http://www.drugs.com/drug_interactions.html
- http://reference.medscape.com/drug-interactionchecker?cid=med
- http://www.webmd.com/interaction-checker
- http://www.micromedex.com
- https://online.epocrates.com/interaction-check
- http://cpref.goldstandard.com/inter.asp?r=8084

Probably most of the medications used by the patients were prescribed and clinically indicated. However, some medications may be unnecessary or cause harm over time due to physiological changes occur with aging or added health problems. These physiological changes that occur with aging affect the sensitivity of drugs mainly by causing changes in the pharmacokinetics of the drug. Pharmacodynamic changes also play a role, although to a lesser extent. The changes in the number and sensitivity of the receptors due to aging or some diseases that occur with aging, and the change of post-receptor events are the main reasons for the changes in pharmacodynamic responses of the medications. In general, these changes cause the effect of the drug to occur more or less and the emergence of drug toxicity and adverse drug reactions. Because of all these changes, the beneficial effects of drug use and the potential harmful effects of drug use should be evaluated together. The decrease in body functions, which occurs with aging is not the same in people of the same age. Therefore, the concept of "*patient centered assessment*" becomes even more important in the older age groups. Avoiding over-prescription and inappropriate drugs in elderly patients is the other important point in preventing adverse health problems caused by polypharmacy and changes due to aging. There are a few tools can be used to assit clinicians to identify unnecessary or potentially inappropriate drugs for older patients. Beers Criteria, Screening Tool of Older Person's Potentially Inappropriate Prescriptions (STOPP), Screening Tool to Alert to Right Treatment (START) and The Medication Appropriateness Index-MAI are some of them [18–20]. These tools allow the comparison of the patient's medications in terms of duplications, interactions, and potencially inappropriateness and to check for medication adjustments required for certain disease states, such as renal impairment.

Another problem encountered with the polypharmacy in the elderly is the use of narrow therapeutic index drugs. As a result of interaction of these drugs with other drugs the therapeutic dose can be easily increased to the toxic dose due to reduction in metabolism, increase in absorption or decrease in elimination. So, the medications with narrow therapeutic index may cause death even use in therapeutic doses. Small changes in the dosage of narrow therapeutic index drugs can lead to significant changes in pharmacodynamic response, particularly in elderly patients with comorbidities or using multiple medications. Therefore, recognizing the narrow therapeutic index drugs is very important issue in terms of preventing serious problems. Narrow therapeutic index drugs commonly used are shown in **Table 1**.

In the light of these information, each visit of an elderly patient should be considered as an opportunity to evaluate the unnecessary use or harms of the prescribed or nonprescribed medications. Studies showed that reducing the number of medications has many positive outcomes in older people such as decrease in the risk of falls, improvement in cognition, and improvement in patients' global health

- Amiodarone
- Carbamazepin
- Cyclosporine
- Digoxin
- Gentamicin
- Levothyoxine
- Lithium carbonate
- Morfin
- Phenytoin
- Tacrolimus
- Theophylline
- Valproic acide
- Warfarin

Table 1.
Common narrow therapeutic index drugs.

status [21–23]. Moreover, approxymately, over half of the people over 70 years of age medicines could be discontinued [24].

In some cases, it is necessary to use multiple drugs for therapeutic purposes at once. For example, concomitant use of aspirin, beta-blockers, ACE inhibitors and lipid-lowering drugs is inevitable in cardiovascular diseases. For this reason, what needs to be done is to try to keep the number of drugs as few as possible by making a risk–benefit assessment by considering the personal treatment goals [25, 26].

In addition to the unnecessary and excessive use of drugs in the elderly, another important problem is that some drugs are not prescribed by physicians or are not used by patients, even though they are necessary. For example, it has been reported that only half of the patients take an anticoagulant in atrial fibrillation, although the guidelines suggest. It has also been reported that inhaled anticholinergic bronchodilators in COPD, SSRIs in depression, ACE inhibitors in the presence of diabetes mellitus and hypertension are not prescribed although necessary [27]. The other medications that are often underprescribed in the elderly include those used to Alzheimer disease, pain (eg, opioids), heart failure, post-MI (β-blockers), glaucoma, and incontinence. In addition to the medications, vaccines are not prescribed as recommended.

3. Deprescription process

Deprescribing, the process of tapering, withdrawing, discontinuing, or stopping medications, is important in reducing polypharmacy, adverse drug effects, inappropriate or ineffective medication use, and costs [28]. The first step in deprescription is the identifing the patients with risk. To identifying the patients with risk, a comprehensive geriatric assessment should be necessery. Comprehensive geriatric assessment is a systematic evaluation of older people by a multidisciplinary health professionals to determine the medical, psychological and functional capabilities and develop a coordinated and integrated personalized follow up plan. Comprehensive geriatric assessment of the elderly patient in primary care should include multimorbidity, cognitive changes, functional status changes, frailty, risk of falling, medication nonadherence, polypharmacy, transitions in care setting, unexplained weight loss, and family concerns for safety [29]. Although comprehensive geriatric assessment expected to be performed by a multidisciplinary health professionals, family physicians have a central role in comprehensive geriatric assessment and coordinating the care. Comprehensive geriatric assessment can be performed in over time with regularly scheduled visits in primary care. During each visit, it should be targeted at least one domain and evaluation of polypharmacy risk and polypharmacy related problems prioritized. Periodic evaluation of a patient's drug regimen and risk of polypharmacy and adverse drug events is an essential component of comprehensive geriatric assessment. Patients need to be specifically told to bring all of the over-the-counter products, ointments, vitamins, ophthalmic preparations, or herbal medicines, used by them to the visit.

It should be aimed to reduce the number of drugs, particularly in those use 7 or more drugs, a history of adverse drug reactions or falls, develope confusion or lethargy as a new symptom, worsen general health status, transfered to nursing homes, have multiple care providers or cared by more than one institutions. Anticipation of polypharmacy and inappropriate drug use is a part of deprescription process. Approximately one-fifth of the drugs used in elderly people are inappropriate drugs [30].

To reduce the number of medications used in older patients, Beers Criteria, Screening Tool of Older Person's Potentially Inappropriate Prescriptions (STOPP),

Screening Tool to Alert to Right Treatment (START) and The Medication Appropriateness Index-MAI can be used by the physicians [18–20]. The STOPP/START guideline contributes to the recognition of potentially inappropriate drugs for use in elderly patients and to drug selection in common diseases with evidence-based recommendations. The Beers Criteria is a guide to identify the inappropriate drugs that should be avoided in the elderly. The criteria include three categories: those that should always be avoided (regardless of disease or condition (eg, diphenhidramine, benzodiazepines); those that are potentially inappropriate in older adults with particular health conditions or syndromes; and those that should be used with caution (eg, carbamazepines, SSRIs) [19]. Medical Appropriateness Index, contributes to the evaluation of each medications in terms of indication, efficacy, appropriate dose and correct use, drug interactions, presence of medications with similar effect, appropriate treatment duration and cost [20].

It can be predicted that polypharmacy and unnecessary drugs may be used by the patients recently discharged from the hospital. It is known that medications used temporarily during hospitalization are also continued to use after discharge by the patients. Therefore, after discharge from the hospital, medications used by the patients should be reviewed. Additionally, increasing age, female gender, higher levels of education, cognitive dysfunction, general poor health, having cardiovascular disease, hypertension, asthma, diabetes or using high-risk drugs (antithrombotic agents, insulin, oral hypoglycaemic agents, cardiovascular and central nervous system drugs, anticolinergics) are the risks for polypharmacy and adverse drug events.

After the risk identification, the physician should prepare the patient and their closers to deprescribing. Asking the elderly and caregivers, which medications they prefer to use, and getting their opinion will make it easier for the physician. Because the passion of the elderly to some drugs can be an obstacle in the process of deprescribing, and the insistent attitude of the physician to discontinue the drug may reduce the trust to the doctor. Moreover, learning the patients' and caregivers' preferences are the first step of shared decision making process, that be very important in patient centered approachment in primary care.

Prioritization of the medicines to cease or doses to reduce is the second step of deprescription [31, 32]. For this, it should be checked the medications in terms of there is still a valid indication and benefit, presence of adverse drug reactions or new symptoms and risky drugs eg. anticholinergic and sedating drugs.

If there is a medication that is not preferred by the patient among the medications considered for discontinuation, deprescription can be started by discontinuing this medication.

If any adverse drug reaction or new symptom are suspected, the suspected drug should be discontinued first, and the next target medication to discotinue should be anticholinergic and sadative drugs. Because elderly patients are particularly susceptible of anticholinergic and sedating drugs advers effects. Adverse effects associated with anticholinergic use in older adults include memory impairment, confusion, hallucinations, dry mouth, blurred vision, constipation, nausea, urinary retention, impaired sweating, and tachycardia [33, 34]. Moreover, it was reported an association between anticholinergic use and risk of community acquired pneumonia [35]. Presence of these symptoms should be a warning to the physician. Some examples of anticholinergic drugs are shown in **Table 2**.

Discontinuation of the drugs with similar effects is another step in reducing the number of drugs. Then, the presence of drugs that can be used in combination among the drugs used should be reviewed, and if possible, the number of drugs should be reduced by prescribing the medications in combination.

- Anti-arrhythmic drugs
  - Procainamide
  - Disopyramide
- Antihistamines
  - Chlorphenamine
  - Diphenhydramine
  - Cyproheptadine
  - Hydroxyzine
  - Promethazine
- Antidepressants
  - Amitriptyline
  - Dosulepin
  - Doxepin
  - Clomipramine
  - Imipramine
  - Nortriptyline
- Antipsychotics
  - Chlorpromazine
  - Clozapine
  - Olanzapine
- Bronchodilators
  - Ipratropium
  - Tiotropium
- Drugs for urinary frequency, enuresis and incontinence
  - Flavoxate
  - Oxybutynin
  - Tolterodine
  - Darifenacin
  - Trospium
- Antiparkinson drugs
  - Trihexyphenidyl (benzhexol)
  - Orphenadrine
  - Amantadine
- Mydriatics and cycloplegics
  - Atropine
  - Cyclopentolate
  - Tropicamide
- Antispasmodics
  - Dicycloverine
  - Hyoscine butylbromide
- Antiemetics
  - Hyoscine hydrobromide
  - Prochlorperazine
- Skeletal muscle relaxants
  - Methocarbamol
  - Antidiarrhoeals
  - Diphenoxylate

Table 2.
Anticholinergic drugs.

Physicians should assess whether treatment goals have changed for the patient at each visit. In updated guidelines, treatment goals may change based on new evidence or depending on the patient's age or other intervening disease. For example, after recognizing that strict targeting for hemoglobin A1c and blood pressure values was harmful in the elderly, the guidelines were updated on this issue [36, 37]. In addition to goals of care, the patients' life expectancy also considered in deprescription process. The patient's life expectancy may have been decrease by an intervening cancer or other serious illness. In this case, some medications that are expected to show their effects in long term (eg statins), can be discontinued.

• Risk identification and anticipation • Defining inappropriate or unnecessary medicine use • Preparation of patient and their closers to deprescription • Learning patient and caregivers preferences • Prioritization of the medicines to cease or doses to reduce • Checking valid indication and benefit of the medications • Checking adverse drug reactions or new symptoms • Identification anticholinergic and sedating drug use • Identification of medications with similar effects • Reviewing the presence of drugs that can be used in combination • Assessing whether treatment goals have changed • Considering non-pharmacologic options

Table 3.
The steps of deprescription.

Clinicians should decide to discontinuation process by individualized treatment goals in line with current guidelines.

It is known that non-pharmacological treatments are even more effective than drug treatment in several chronic diseases. Therefore, while prescribing, non-pharmacologic treatment options should always be considered first [26]. If the patient can apply non-pharmacologic options, it will be easier to reduce the number of drugs. For example, in many patients, hypertension can be controlled only by sodium restriction or weight loss. In diabetes mellitus patients the number and dose of the medications can be reduced by low glycemic index diet and exercise.

The steps of deprescription process was shown in **Table 3**.

If it is not possible to cease of medications, it should be considered whether it is possible to reduce their dose. Because, many adverse drug reactions are dose-related. While prescribing it is important to use the minimal dose required to obtain clinical benefit.

3.1 Points to consider when reducing the number of medications

- A comprehensive geriatric assessment should be necessery to detect the risk of polypharmacy, polypharmacy related problems, possibility to reduce the number of medications and anticipate the consequences of withdrawal. Although consern of withdrawal reactions may be a barrier to deprescription, withdrawal reactions are seen rare when discontinuation is carried slowly and carefully [38].

- While reducing the number of drugs, it is very important that some drugs should be discontinued by tapering over time. Anticonvulsants, benzodiazepines, corticosteroids, antidepressants, beta blockers, levodopa, opiates, proton pump inhibitors, and gabapentin are the examples of drugs that should not be stopped abruptly. Abrupt discontinuation of these drugs may cause withdrawal syndrome and a rebound effect.

- Only stop or reduce one medicine at a time.

- Possible problems that may occur in case of discontinuation of the drug should be anticipated.

- Drug interactions should also be considered while reducing the number of drugs. For example, when using warfarin with omeprazole, discontinuation of omeprazole, the INR may decrease because omeprazole had been inhibiting the metabolism of warfarin.

- In cases where it cannot be decided which medication should be discontinued, a collaboration with other physicians following the patient should be established.

- The necessity of drug discontinuation should be explained to the patient and their closers with an appropriate communication language.

- Effort should be made to improve communication in transition of the patients between health care centers or caregivers. Sharing the medication lists used by the patients or planned to withdrawal, between health providers at the time of care transition may be help to prevent adverse drug events.

- After the drug is withdrawal, warning messages about the discontinuation of the medications should be given to the patients in writing, a follow-up appointment should be planned, and should be informed about when to consult a doctor [39].

- Patients and their closers should be informed about the monitoring of blood parameters that may change after drug withdrawal.

- While trying to prevent polypharmacy and polypharmacy-related problems in elderly patients and to reduce unnecessary and inappropriate drug use, care should be taken not to discontinue the drugs that the patient really needs. START criteria is developed to help the identify potential prescribing omissions in older patients can be used in this regard [18].

- If treatment is indicated, the current regimen with a higher probability of adverse effects can be replaced with a safer alternative medication. As an example, acetaminophen instead of NSAID.

4. Conclusion

The patient's condition and goals of care changed over time are the key principles to be considered in deprescription. A comprehensive geriatric assessment should be necessery to detect the risk of polypharmacy, polypharmacy related problems, possibility to reduce the number of medications and anticipate the consequences of withdrawal. Avoiding from over-prescribing and inappropriate medications in older patients is the key step to prevent negative health problems due to polypharmacy. It should be kept in mind that in addition to over-prescribing, under-prescribing appropriate medications is also of concern in older patients. Therefore, a balance is required between over- and under-prescribing.

It should be kept in mind that reducing the number of drugs in the elderly patients in accordance with the evidence based guidelines can be carried without any serious problems and this situation can improve the health parameters of the older patients. In conclusion, prevention of polypharmacy and withdrawing unneccesary and inappropriate medications may be the best clinical decision in older patients.

Author details

Çiğdem Apaydın Kaya
School of Medicine, Marmara University, İstanbul, Turkey

*Address all correspondence to: cigdemapaydin@yahoo.com

References

[1] Bjerrum L, Rosholm J, Hallas J, Kragstrup J. Methods for estimating the occurance of polypharmacy by means of a prescription database. Eur J Clin Pharmacol 1997;53:7-11.

[2] Junius-Walker U, Theile G, Hummers-Pradier E. Prevalence and predictors of polypharmacy among older primary care patients in Germany. Fam Pract 2007; 24:14-19.

[3] Linjakumpu T, Hartikainen S, Klaukka T, et al. Use of medications and polypharmacy are increasing among the elderly. J Clin Epidemiol. 2002;55: 809-817.

[4] Rankin A, Cadogan CA, Patterson SM, et al. Interventions to improve the appropriate use of polypharmacy for older people. Cochrane Database Syst Rev. 2018;(9): CD008165.

[5] Hajjar ER, Hanlon JT, Sloane RJ, et al. Unnecessary drug use in frail older people at hospital discharge. J Am Geriatr Soc. 2005;53:1518.

[6] Steinman MA, Hanlon JT. Managing medications in clinically complex elders: "There's got to be a happy medium". JAMA 2010;304:1592.

[7] Green JL, Hawley JN, Rask KJ. Is the number of prescribing physicians an independent risk factor for adverse drug events in an elderly outpatient population? Am J Geriatr Pharmacother 2007;5:31.

[8] Halli-Tierney AD, Scarbrough C, Carroll D. Polypharmacy: Evaluating risks and Deprescribing. Am Fam Physician. 2019;100(1):32-38.

[9] Roughead, E. E., Semple, S. J. Medication safety in acute care in Australia: Where are we now? Part 1: a review of the extent and causes of medication problems 2002-2008. Australia and New Zealand Health Policy 2009;6:18.

[10] Field TS, Gurwitz JH, Avorn J, et al. Risk factors for adverse drug events among nursing home residents. Arch Intern Med. 2001;161:1629.

[11] Wimmer BC, Cross AJ, Jokanovic N, et al. Clinical outcomes associated with medication regimen complexity in older people: A systematic review. J Am Geriatr Soc 2017;65:747.

[12] Lai SW, Liao KF, Liao CC, et al. Polypharmacy correlates with increased risk for hip fracture in the elderly: A population-based study. Medicine (Baltimore) 2010;89:295

[13] Leipzig RM, Cumming RG, Tinetti ME. Drugs and falls in older people: A systematic review and meta-analysis: II. Cardiac and analgesic drugs. J Am Geriatr Soc. 1999;47(1):40-50.

[14] Rochon PA, Gurwitz JH. Optimising drug treatment for elderly people: The prescribing cascade. BMJ 1997;315:1096.

[15] Lu WH, Wen YW, Chen LK, Hsiao FY. Effect of polypharmacy, potentially inappropriate medications and anticholinergic burden on clinical outcomes: A retrospective cohort study. CMAJ 2015;187:E130

[16] Fugh-Berman A. Herb-drug interactions. Lancet 2000; 355:134.

[17] Andrén L, Andreasson A, Eggertsen R: Interaction between a commercially available St John's wort product (Movina) and atorvastatin in patients with hypercholesterolemia. Eur J Clin Pharmacol. 2007;63:913–916.

[18] Brunetti E, Aurucci ML, Boietti E, et al. Clinical Implications of Potentially

Inappropriate Prescribing According to STOPP/START Version 2 Criteria in Older Polymorbid Patients Discharged From Geriatric and Internal Medicine Wards: A Prospective Observational Multicenter Study. J Am Med Dir Assoc. 2019;20(11):1476.e1-1476.e10.

[19] By the 2019 American Geriatrics Society Beers Criteria Update Expert Panel. American Geriatrics Society 2019 updated AGS Beers criteria for potentially inappropriate medication use in older adults. J Am Geriatr Soc. 2019 Apr;67(4):674-694.

[20] Hanlon JT, Schmader KE. The medication appropriateness index at 20: Where it started, where it has been, and where it may be going. Drugs Aging. 2013;30(11):893-900.

[21] Sönnichsen A, Trampisch SU, Rieckert A, et al. Polypharmacy in chronic diseases – Reduction of inappropriate medication and adverse drug events in older populations by electronic decision support (PRIMA-eDS): Study protocol for a randomized controlled trial. Trials 2016;17:57.

[22] van der Velde N, Stricker BH, Pols HA, van der Cammen TJ. Risk of falls after withdrawal of fall-risk-increasing drugs: A prospective cohort study. Br J Clin Pharmacol. 2007;63(2): 232-237.

[23] Graves T, Hanlon JT, Schmader KE, et al. Adverse events after discontinuing medications in elderly outpatients. Arch Intern Med. 1997;157:2205-2210.

[24] Garfinkel D, Mangin D. Feasibility study of a systematic approach for discontinuation of multiple medications in older adults: Addressing polypharmacy. Arch Intern Med. 2010 Oct 11;170(18):1648-1654.

[25] Pesante-Pinto JL. Clinical pharmacology and the risks of polypharmacy in the geriatric patient. Phys Med Rehabil Clin N Am. 2017;28 (4):739-746.

[26] Burt J, Elmore N, Campbell SM, et al. Developing a measure of polypharmacy appropriateness in primary care: Systematic review and expert consensus study. BMC Med. 2018;16(1):91.

[27] Wright RM, Sloane R, Pieper CF, et al. Underuse of indicated medications among physically frail older US veterans at the time of hospital discharge: Results of a cross-sectional analysis of data from the Geriatric evaluation and management drug study. Am J Geriatr Pharmacother. 2009;7(5):271-280.

[28] Gnjidic D, Le Couteur DG, Kouladjian L, et al. Deprescribing trials: Methods to reduce Polypharmacy and the impact on prescribing and clinical outcomes. Clinics in Geriatric Medicine 2012;28(2):237-253.

[29] Tatum Iii PE, Talebreza S, Ross JS. Geriatric Assessment: An office-based approach. Am Fam Physician. 2018 Jun 15;97(12):776-784.

[30] Curtis LH, Østbye T, Sendersky V, et al. Inappropriate prescribing for elderly americans in a large outpatient population. Arch Int Med. 2004;164 (15):1621-1625.

[31] Endsley S. Deprescribing unnecessary medications: A four-part process. Fam Pract Manag. 2018;25(3): 28-32.

[32] Jansen J, Naganathan V, Carter SM, et al. Too much medicine in older people? Deprescribing through shared decision making. BMJ 2016;353:i2893.

[33] Carrière I, Fourrier-Reglat A, Dartigues JF, et al. Drugs with anticholinergic properties, cognitive decline, and dementia in an elderly general population: The 3-city study. Arch Intern Med. 2009;169:1317

[34] Salahudeen MS, Hilmer SN, Nishtala PS. Comparison of anticholinergic risk scales and associations with adverse health outcomes in older people. J Am Geriatr Soc. 2015;63:85.

[35] Paul KJ, Walker RL, Dublin S. Anticholinergic medications and risk of community-acquired pneumonia in elderly adults: A population-based case-control study. J Am Geriatr Soc. 2015;63: 476.

[36] Action to Control Cardiovascular Risk in Diabetes Study Group, Gerstein HC, miller ME, Byington RP, et al. effects of intensive glucose lowering in type 2 diabetes. New England Journal of Medicine. 2008;358 (24):2545-2559.

[37] Beckett NS, Peters R, Fletcher AE, et al. Treatment of hypertension in patients 80 years of age or older. New England Journal of Medicine. 2008; 358 (18):1887-1898.

[38] Iyer S, Naganathan V, McLachlan AJ, Le Couteur DG. Medication withdrawal trials in people aged 65 years and older: A systematic review. Drugs Aging. 2008;25(12): 1021-1031.

[39] Bain KT, Holmes HM, Beers MH, et al. Discontinuing medications: A novel approach for revising the prescribing stage of the medication-use process. Journal of the American Geriatrics Society. 2008;56(10): 1946-1952.

Chapter 11

Use of Primary Healthcare Facilities for Care and Support of Chronic Diseases: Hypertension

Maseabata Ramathebane, Maja Lineo and Sello Molungoa

Abstract

Hospitalisation of chronic diseases can be costly and time-consuming to patients with chronic diseases, and success of management of chronic diseases is in the primary care. This chapter gives a detailed description of primary health and its role in the management of chronic diseases. Hypertension as a chronic disease of interest and its management in the primary healthcare (PHC) context are also to be discussed in detail. However, to give this chapter clarity, a brief description of the country Lesotho will be given. The summary of the country will highlight major barriers to health care which mainly include poverty, difficult topography with no or poor infrastructure which hinder access to primary health care. Situational analysis is made with regard to current practice. The potential role of a pharmacist in the care and treatment of hypertension is explored. Best practices, need for policy change, guidelines and implementation plans will be highlighted. The aim of the chapter is to evaluate how chronic diseases are managed at the primary health care. The objectives include: a) to explore primary health care concept, b) to critically evaluate PHC concept in an African country and c) to describe human resource needs to meet the demands of PHC chronic diseases management.

Keywords: primary health care, hypertension, nursing, pharmacist

1. Introduction

The Lesotho Kingdom is a relatively small country, 30,360 km^2 divided into 10 administrative districts and further divided into four ecological zones, namely the lowlands, foothills and highlands (mountains) and the Senqu valley [1]. The mountainous terrain makes ground travel very difficult in Lesotho [2]. The mountainous topography and harsh winters make it difficult to access essential services, including healthcare services [1]. The Republic of South Africa surrounds Lesotho, with a population of slightly more than 2 million [1]. About 99% of Lesotho people are ethnic Basotho, with Christianity being the majority religion. The national languages are Sesotho and English [2]. Altitudes in Lesotho range from 4500 to over 13,000 feet, and 33% of Lesotho population resides in the urban areas leaving the majority of the population living in the mountain areas. High mountains cover about two-thirds of the country, and snow is expected in the winter months [3].

Lesotho, classified as a lower-middle-income country with a per capita income of US$1879, ranks 161 out of 187 countries on the UN Human Development ranking [4].

National poverty figures indicate that 57.1% of the population lives below the national poverty line [4]. Poverty is particularly acute in the mountainous areas, which are hard to reach [5]. Besides, Lesotho's economy is dependent on clothing and textiles; diamond extraction; exports of water to South Africa and workers' remittances from the Southern African Customs Union (SACU) [4]. The agricultural sector, which accounts for only 8.6% of Gross Domestic Product (GDP), is the primary source of income for the majority of the rural population [4].

The World Bank and UNICEF report indicates that the main priority for the Ministry of Health (MoH) should be to strengthen its control systems both for compliance which now appear extremely weak as well as performance at all levels (centre, district, facility level) [6]. The health system looks very fragmented, with several pools of resources from donors and government and different service providers operating according to different priorities and operating mechanisms and without any accountability for results.

The health outcomes for major indicators remain poor despite the increase in funding by the government [6]. Considering the fact that HIV prevalence and incidence are slowly improving, TB incidence, maternal and infant mortality rates remain among the highest in the world [6]. The Government of Lesotho (GoL) should strive to meet the objective of universal health coverage, the quality and cost-effectiveness of health care and increase access to underserved populations within a very tight budget [6]. Therefore, more quantifiable efforts have to be taken towards getting outputs worth the investment made on health system.

To clarify this further, the government of Lesotho has incurred increased expenditure in the District Health Management Teams (DHMTs) (135%) and Christian Health Association of Lesotho (CHAL) (121%). Another increased expenditure was seen in laboratories (126%), planning (163%) and pharmaceuticals (162%) [6]. Perhaps, the increase in DHMT expenditure may be understandable as it is the main implementer of decentralisation of health service delivery at the primary healthcare level [6]. However, looking at the topography of the country, it is believed that the community councils may play a similar role with better cost-effective health outcomes.

2. The concept of primary health care

In Lesotho, PHC is provided at health centres (HCs) and health posts and at community level [2]. Community health workers, also known as village health workers (VHWs), are patients' first formal contacts with the health system. The VHWs are trained community members who help patients in the community and form a link between communities and health centres [7]. Implementers at the health centres can, therefore, play an important role in decreasing the need for higher-level referral by providing integrated service delivery [8].

Lesotho adopted the Alma-Ata Declaration in 1979 [9]. The Lesotho National Health Policy, which has been used in draft form since 2004 [9], is largely based on the Alma-Ata Declaration on PHC and involves the establishment of 18 health service areas. The District Health Management Teams (DHMTs) are responsible for PHC activities in health centres at a district level. The staffing of health centres (HCs) is determined by whether the facility is rural and small in size or urban and larger in size. Rural HCs are manned by registered nurses while urban ones have registered nurses, doctors, pharmacists and laboratory technologists [9].

Primary health care (PHC) was conceptualised and agreed to be a global solution to the problem of providing comprehensive health services to all at the Alma-Ata Conference in 1978. The conference defined PHC as,

> *'essential health care based on practical, scientifically sound and socially acceptable methods and technology made universally accessible to individuals and families in the community, through their full participation and a cost that the community and country can afford to maintain, at every stage of their development in the spirit of self-reliance and self-determination' [10].*

Sadly, the implementation of comprehensive service delivery as determined by the Alma-Ata Declaration failed to be consistent and was fragmented based on financial, disease-specific and strategic reasons; therefore service provision of varying degree is continuously offered. However, the integration of essential services and strengthening of health services comprise quantifiable comprehensive service delivery [11, 12].

The low-and-middle income countries, including Lesotho, have selected and serious health problems that are given special attention, and this results in fragmented services. An overwhelming disease burden, donor-driven care and unclear frameworks, guidelines or indicators of PHC are responsible for the prevailing fragmentation of care [11]. The issues of a holistically, patient-centred approach can be met by adopting an integrated service delivery models. The integration of PHC services approach not only embraces the 'best practice' model, and can prevent duplication of services, reduce the risk of adverse events and consequently improve quality of care [11, 13].

The sustainability of health care can be maintained by paying attention to all diseases, not only to prioritised diseases as this creates gaps instead of strengthening the health system [11]. Consequently, the prevalence of preventable illnesses has increased. Conditions, such as hypertension and diabetes, are increasing yearly despite highly specialised care [14]. This results in increasing prevalence of these preventable conditions, patients who receive fragmented service delivery have to visit health centres to receive different specialised services on different days for different, but related, health needs [15]. The consequences of separate, specialised services undermine holistic individualised patient care, patients' adherence to medication, multiple clinic visits, each time enduring long waiting periods, with endless referrals between departments, resulting in high patient 'no-show rates' for appointments [11, 16].

The National Health Sector Strategic Plan 2012–2017 and the Lesotho PHC Revitalisation Plan 2011–2017 show how Lesotho recommitted itself to the original Alma-Ata Declaration for all health centres, including the health centres in Maseru district [7]. Also the Ministry of Health (MoH) undertook several health reforms [7, 8].

It is, however, indicated that lack of formal framework with documented strategies leads to haphazard implementation of integrated primary health care (IPHC), and the Lesotho national policy is also wanting in this regard [8, 17]. It is therefore indicated that when the registered nurses implement IPHC, they based themselves on their own understanding. According to Posholi, to date, PHC has had very few comprehensive implementation frameworks or guidelines [17]. Again, Valentijn et al. stipulate a serious need for standardised, tabulated, systematic procedures for implementation of IPHC [12]. In the absence of standardised protocols across settings, PHC implementation remains subjective and, sometimes, misguided [17, 18]. Even the WHO has cautioned that the absence of standard guidelines for implementation has the potential to derail the initial vision of PHC [19].

It was indicated that the MoH depends on registered nurses to implement IPHC. They are the key personnel who attend to the patients visiting health centres, then referred to a higher level of care, if needed, based on the patient's diagnosis [20]. The registered nurses employed at the health centres report to the registered nurse in charge of the health centre, who in turn report to the relevant DHMT [21].

As initially planned, PHC brings health promotion, disease prevention, cure and care together in a safe, effective and socially acceptable manner to the community [22]. The report by Stender et al. further discusses the skills that are acquired and the training that healthcare workers at the PHC level receive [22]. These included history taking, performing a physical examination and making a nursing diagnosis during a client consultation, problem-solving and decision-making skills especially in the absence of a doctor and completing patient records as well as an appreciating the importance of recordkeeping. Stender et al. point out one of the key elements of PHC which involves bringing health care closer to where people live by conducting home visits and facilitate community involvement in health care through community outreach [22].

3. Healthcare human resources

Health worker density is the most widely used indicator to determine available human resources [23]. The WHO has set a density indicator of 2.23 healthcare professionals per 1000 population as the minimum threshold for access to public healthcare services [24]. Within that benchmark, significant variance exists between regions regarding the particular skills-mix of doctors, nurses and midwives. In the Africa continent, there are on average five nurses/midwives per doctor [25]. Zimbabwe's health worker density at 1.45 per 1000 of the population is higher than those of Sierra Leone and South Sudan but is still less than the WHO's density benchmark [23]. In Botswana, according to Nkomazana et al., the health worker density is 3.4 doctors and 28.4 nurses per 10,000 of the population [25]. In Lesotho, however, health workforce is challenged to meet the needs of its population. The nursing and midwifery workforce is 6.0 per 10,000 compared with neighbouring South Africa's 41 per 10,000 and 11 per 10,000 for the Africa region [24].

The Lesotho government staff establishment has not been reviewed; therefore it does not take care of health cadres that are needed resulting from the use of modern health technologies, for example, equipment, devices and protocols [26]. Furthermore, there is an acute shortage of expertise within the health sector with many posts on the establishment list of the MoH remaining unfilled. The overall establishment list of the MoH was at the beginning of the year 2015 was 4610. Over half (54%) of nurse and midwife posts remain vacant in rural areas [27]. At the end of the 2015 financial year, only 23% of all vacancies were filled. Several factors have been associated with this, such as local circumstances that negatively impacted on training, pay, infrastructure and working conditions [26]. However, the country could consider changing some of the posts to cover other cadres in order to add diversity to the nursing cadres and leave nursing within the mandatory scope of work that is done well.

4. Community pharmacy as primary healthcare facilities

Stimulating a professional relationship between a pharmacist and patient begins at the community level because patients must perceive pharmacists as necessary experts within the healthcare system [28]. The role of a pharmacist in dealing with minor health problems is well established, and pharmacists are also viewed as professionals who are an accessible source of information and advice [24]. This, therefore, implies that the community's health is in the hands of the community pharmacists; hence their practice should be well regulated and monitored. **Figure 1** depicts the scope of pharmacy in Lesotho in terms of regulation, education practice and research.

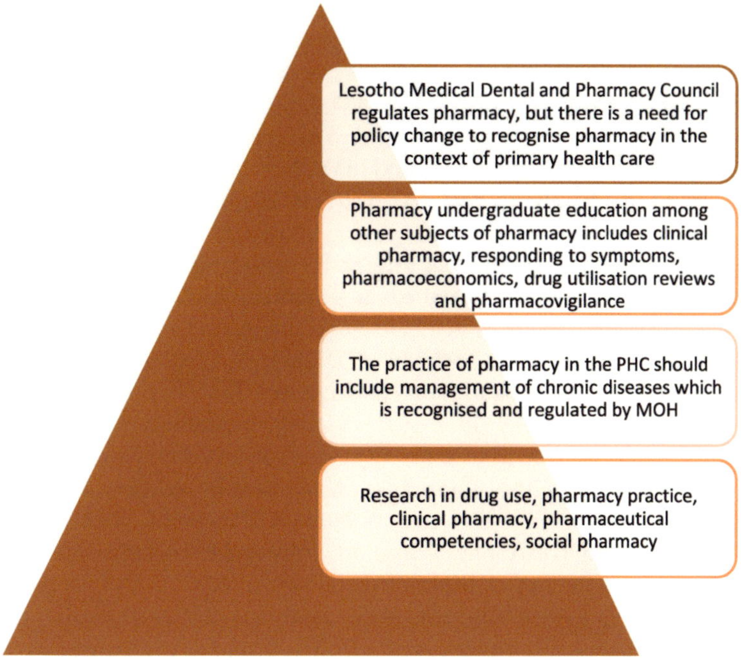

Figure 1.
The scope of pharmacy practice in Lesotho.

5. Disease burden

The country is faced with enormous health challenges; as nearly one-quarter of adults 15 – 49 years of age are living with HIV (22.9%) [29], and Lesotho is considered to have the world's second highest tuberculosis incidence rate at 916 cases per 100,000 population [30, 31]. Lesotho as a country also has one of the highest maternal mortality ratios in the world at 490 per 100,000 live births, with a lifetime risk of maternal death at 1 in 64 [32]. According Lesotho Demographic and Health Survey (LDHS), there were 19% of women and 13% of men aged 15–49 who have hypertension [26]. One in five women and one in seven men with hypertension (5% of all women and 2% of all men age 15–49) have their hypertension controlled with medication [26].

6. Hypertension as a chronic disease

Worldwide, the leading risk factor associated with morbidity and mortality from non-communicable diseases (NCDs) and the highest cause of premature deaths is reported to be of those of hypertension [33]. The global prevalence of hypertension in adults aged 18 years and over was around 24.1% for men and 20.1% for women in 2015 [33]. Based on the statistics of hypertension reports for the past years, the WHO predicts that, by the year 2025, almost 75% of the world's hypertension population will be found in developing countries [33]. However, the global action plan has a target of a 25% reduction of the global prevalence of hypertension [34].

Nonetheless, recent statistics on the prevalence of chronic diseases in Lesotho indicate that the presence of hypertension was reported to be at 41% in 2015 [35]. Inevitably, hypertension ranks among the top causes of morbidity and mortality and is the third-most common cause of hospital admissions in the country [2, 36].

An accurate measurement of blood pressure with a well-fitting calf remains an important part of diagnosis of primary hypertension [37]. In an adult, the normal blood pressure is said to be 120/80mmHg [38]. A definite diagnosis of hypertension is when their blood pressure reading is above 139/89 mmHg on three consecutive clinical visit within two days up to a maximum of 7 days in between [39, 40]. This definition is consistent with the one found in the Lesotho national guidelines on the management of diabetes and hypertension at PHC level. Regarding sign and symptoms of hypertension, the following are said to be associate and these are tiredness, headaches, confusion, vision changes, angina-like pain and the presence of blood in the urine, nosebleeds, irregular heartbeat as well as ear noise or buzzing sounds [41].

The WHO recommends that once a patient is diagnosed with hypertension, as based on the nation's guidelines, both pharmacological and non-pharmacological management measures must be initiated immediately [34]. In Lesotho, the treatment of increased blood pressure is guided by the national guidelines on the management of diabetes and hypertension at primary care level [39]. With regard to pharmacological management, the guidelines advise that diuretics, beta-blockers, calcium antagonists, converting enzyme inhibitors and angiotensin II receptor blockers are suitable for initial and follow-up treatment, as monotherapy and in combination [39].

Further advice on the prescription of the drugs, dosages and expected intervals for medication taking is included. However, treatment differs according to the individual's blood pressure and compliance to treatment at the time of check-up. Furthermore, the guidelines recommend psychosocial support in terms of the suggested lifestyle changes (exercise, reduced dietary salt intake, reduced alcohol and tobacco intake) [39]. Patients with uncontrolled blood pressure despite medication adherence and lifestyle changes are referred to the secondary level of care for further investigations and management [39].

The effectiveness of hypertension treatment and experiencing its benefits relies critically on strict compliance to treatment instructions [42]. Rao et al. mention compliance is to treatment as a primary determinant of the effectiveness of treatment, which intensifies optimum clinical benefit and promotes good health [43]. Additionally, it is a cost-saving measure for a larger society, because the incidence of complications is decreased leading to less need for additional medications [33].

Globally, in comparison with acute diseases, chronic diseases treatment compliance rates are typically low and continue dropping radically despite increased awareness of the effect of chronic conditions [44]. There is still a need for improvement even among populations with relatively high adherence rates. According to Ivarsson et al., good compliance is a requirement worldwide, as reported in a national population-based cohort study conducted in pulmonary arterial hypertension centres in Sweden [45].

Hacihasanoglu and Gozum report that in Turkey, 40% of hypertension patients did not take their medications as prescribed and 50% defaulted on their appointment dates [46]. In contrast, Mafutha and Wright argue that medication-taking behaviour is not affected by failure to comply with follow-up appointments to collect medications [47]. Their study at primary healthcare clinics in Tshwane, South Africa, reported that 81% of patients were compliant regarding medication-taking, yet 57% were non-adherent to follow-up appointments [47]. Perhaps appointment keeping should be viewed in a broader context as the patient may come to the PHC facility before or after the appointed date or pick medicines from other facilities.

Some of the factors that are associated with missed appointments include lack of hypertension knowledge, experience of medication side effects, forgetfulness, transportation challenges, a feeling that appointments are not helpful, lack of trust and health professionals' communication behaviour during consultations [48, 49]. Consequently, a particular factor associated with non-compliance of an individual hypertensive patient should guide interventions that improve appointment keeping compliance [49, 50].

There are few studies that address the compliance of patients suffering from non-communicable diseases in Lesotho. Most of the published research works on hypertension compare the knowledge of patients regarding antihypertensive treatment with treatment outcomes. Khothatso, et al. conducted an observational, descriptive cross-sectional study at a district hospital in Lesotho, the main findings are that there is low level of knowledge regarding their treatment and its adherence among hypertensive patients [51].

The study of Mugomeri, et al. reported that inadequate knowledge about anti-hypertensive treatment is significantly associated with uncontrolled high blood pressure and the associated complications [52]. A study conducted at Domicilliary Health Clinic in Maseru, Lesotho, reports that the prevalence of chronic, uncontrolled high blood pressure remains high in patients on treatment and claims an important intervention in this population would involve identifying factors that can help improve compliance to the hypertension treatment [36]. A report of a selective literature review study in various countries indicates, furthermore, that it is desirable to carry out studies on the promotion of compliance in Germany and countries facing the same national challenge of conditions prevailing in the healthcare system [53].

In their study, Wells et al. found that hypertension appeared to be one of the highest risk factors of heart failure [54]. Hypertensive patients have a higher risk of having heart attack, heart failure, stroke, kidney disease than normotensive people [55]. Saseen mentions that hypertension complications include atherosclerotic vascular disease which can be coronary artery disease, carotid artery disease, peripheral arterial disease and abdominal aortic aneurysm [56]. Other complications include cardiovascular diseases (CVDs) such as heart failure, chronic kidney disease and retinopathy.

Beaglehole et al. stated the need to distinguish approach between the management of chronic diseases and acute illnesses; they further mentioned the importance of the organisational or structural interventions in managing chronic disease [57]. It was highlighted that the PHC needed to be strengthened in order to undertake opportunistic case finding, for assessment of risk factors, early detection of disease and identification of high risk status for chronic disease can be carefully undertaken [57]. The development of management plans must take into account patients' needs and preferences as chronic patients are said to be their own primary carers [57]. According to Siantz et al., in order to minimise functional limitations and disability, effective management of chronic conditions requires behavioural and lifestyle adjustments [58]. Therefore, an appropriate theoretical framework fitting the health problem of interest to change behaviour needs to guide the planned organisational interventions [59].

Patient must take up an active role in knowing and managing their own health, by expressing their concerns, preferences and participating in medical decisions; this can be achieved through patient empowerment, patient involvement and shared decision-making [60]. It is believed that informed patients improve their decisions by collaborating with their healthcare providers [61]. This results in increased patient's involvement leading to a positive effect on the health outcomes.

On the other hand, Maimela et al. mentioned that PHC professionals often lack the resources such as quality equipment's and promotional materials which could be used to assist local community self-management support services such as education programmes [62]. More so, the lack of continuous availability of medicines has become another important barrier for chronic disease management (CDM) in practice, and this plays an essential part in the provision of health care for chronic conditions [63]. The study of Wagner et al. suggested the need to transform a health system from responding mainly when a person is sick which is being reactive, but, rather be proactive and focused on keeping a person as healthy as possible which eventually improves the health of people with chronic illnesses [64].

7. Interventions models

It is noteworthy that Nyangu and Nkosi mentioned that registered nurse midwives and nurse clinicians manage the majority of PHC facilities, and their professional titles did not affect service provision [65]. However, it was suggested that there is a need to provide more staffing to address staff shortages and reduce patients waiting times at facilities [65]. Ideally, Uys and Klopper recommended that at least one specialist nurse, five registered nurse midwives and four enrolled nurses were needed for the effective running of PHC settings [66]. Additionally, the finding of Rampamba et al. revealed that encouragingly, the pharmacist intervention highly satisfied patients in PHC facilities in South Africa, and this laid a strong foundation for improving collaboration in the future [67]. Consequently, the study recommended that this intervention model be further developed and tested, with a greater focus on lifestyle changes and clinical outcomes. Pharmacists can further improve future control of blood pressure (BP) by routinely investigating and reviewing patient diaries [67].

Similarly, in Ghana, pharmacy curriculum for training pharmacists includes health promotion and health education, making it possible to undertake health promotion and disease preventative activities [68]. However, the national policy on prevention and control of chronic NCDs acknowledges the role of primary community facilities with no mention of community pharmacies [69].

Additionally, Afia et al. state that due to the increasing level of hypertension in low-income countries, community pharmacies could participate more in hypertension management interventions [70]. Nevertheless, the requirements for meaningful participation should be considered and realised which include the relevant staffing compliment, health promotion skill, pharmacy setting and referral systems [70]. Moreover, this service requires the constant presence of a pharmacist, screening space with privacy for counselling, staff training and referral linkages with the nearest health centre/clinic/hospital for referrals [70].

Furthermore, Omboni evaluated blood pressure telemonitoring (BPT) programmes involving a pharmacist; it was stated that this may require investment in laboratory monitoring and technologies [71]. Again, larger use of medications and more contacts with patients than standard care occur, there was a significantly improved BP control at relatively low cost or with an only minimal increase in healthcare costs compared with usual care. This would consequently lead to the reduced cost for future cardiovascular events. Interestingly, the economic analyses suggested that pharmacist case management provided the clinical gains as the current evidence to high-risk patients with stroke, evaluating the longer-term impact and cost-effectiveness of BPT with suggested by [72]. More so, the future analysis must consider cost savings from a reduction in cardiac events and long-term complications, as well as indirect or intangible costs such as travel time to clinic or time missed from work that would be relevant to an economic analysis from the societal perspective, particularly over several years [71].

8. Clinical management pathways

It is noted that the investment in predisposing factors awareness and health promotion with full participation of patients holds manifestation of the disease.

Similarly, the key elements of management of chronic disease such as hypertension are in maintaining normal blood pressure, which leads to prevention of progression of disease and consequently its complications. Therefore, service provision takes into consideration prevention of disease, treatment of the disease, compliance to treatment, periodic reviews and close disease outcome monitoring. Is it possible to cover all this in the primary health care that has competing interest such as those imposed by communicable and acute illnesses? Is primary health care not burdened with mother and child health services, such as antenatal clinics and post-natal service?

Eventually, what remains unclear is, are the general nursing skills sufficient to carry the disease burden to desired treatment outcomes, for all the diseases in Lesotho? Is it time to look at how other countries manage hypertension using other professionals whose aim is to achieve desired treatment outcome? Is a pharmacist viewed in the context of medicines chain supply and dispensing or his/her clinical role in the management of diseases recognised? Is the pharmacist in a good position to play a role in the management of chronic diseases either in community pharmacy or primary healthcare setting? Is the pharmacist exposed to clinical pharmacy throughout the training, covering clinical management of diseases and pharmacy practice clarifying the role of a pharmacist in disease management, not only covering drug supply chain but also covers responding to symptoms in the pharmacy, pharmacoepidemiology, pharmacovigilance, pharmacoeconomics and drug utilisation reviews? Will these in due course benefit treatment outcomes of hypertension, improve treatment adherence, manage medication adverse drug reaction and based on treatment outcome in order to select the best treatment for the patient and carry out appropriate referral where needed?

Accordingly, study of Hallit et al. clarified that the PHC strategy of the Ministry of Public Health (MOPH) includes several programmes: communicable diseases, immunisation, mother and child health, nutrition, environmental health, non-communicable diseases, health awareness and essential medication [73]. Based on the above scenarios, in order to prevent disease progression, hospitalisation and poor prognosis of patients with hypertension, the following are proposed:

1. Retail pharmacists can be viewed as primary healthcare facilities, as patients who do not want long queues in the public sector sort services for their ill health. Currently, services include management of minor illnesses through over-the-counter (OTC) medicines and referrals where necessary. Also chronic diseases screening, prescription refills, monitoring and follow-up. Sale of gargets for blood pressure monitoring and education on how to use them to monitor their response to treatment at home.

Consequently, collaboration or community pharmacy with the public sector in terms of referral and further management is necessary. What is proposed as new is a service agreement with the public sector whereby patients who would otherwise be seen at the PHC clinic come to the retail pharmacy to receive care and treatment at the cost of public sector. This is already being done through contracted service in many countries; it just needs to extend to the resource-limited countries. For example, in England, the study of Albasri et al. showed that there is strong trial evidence for the involvement of community pharmacy in the long-term management of hypertension [74]. Systematic reviews and meta-analyses of these trials demonstrate that when compared with usual care, the results consistently show a 6–7 mmHg reduction in systolic blood pressure [74].

2. The PHC facilities that are run by nurses could also include the services of pharmacists, who have competencies to run pharmacy-led chronic disease clinics. This addition will complement the skills of nurses and give them time to

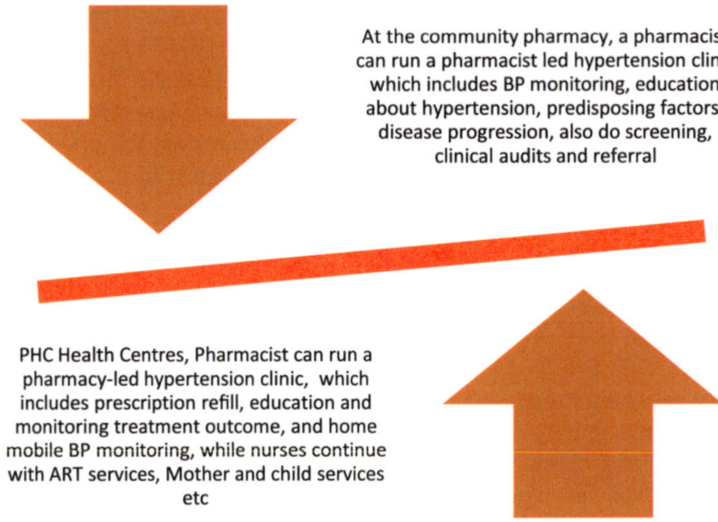

Figure 2.
Summary of the role of a pharmacist in the management of hypertension in the community pharmacy and primary health care clinic.

manage other programmes in the PHC facilities such as mother and child services immunisations. If Lesotho has high disease burden, doing similar activities have to be avoided because poor results in maternal mortality rates, infant mortality rates and failure in other programmes will prevail. It is suggested that pharmacist-led chronic disease management be included in the policy and treatment guidelines.

The study of Buis et al. considered primary care patients with uncontrolled hypertension whose blood pressure was effectively reduced by a pharmacist-led mobile health (mHealth) intervention which was intended to promote the home blood pressure monitoring and clinical pharmacist management of hypertension [75]. The data in this study also support the feasibility and acceptability of these types of interventions for patients and providers [75].

In Sweden, when collaboration between community pharmacy and primary health care was reflected, it was viewed as a golden opportunity [76]. The primary health care has strategic plans and national policy documents which do not include community pharmacy as a partner, and this is considered as a major challenge [76]. This was a similar case to Ghana community pharmacy and primary health care [69]. **Figure 2** summarises what the pharmacist will be doing at the community pharmacy and at the PHC clinic if he/she works for the facility. This has to be done through government policies and be properly regulated through relevant laws.

9. Conclusion

Primary health care is a good place to manage preventable diseases. Treatment outcome can be monitored at the PHC level and lifestyle modification can be instituted according to patients' needs. There is evidence that involvement of pharmacist at the community pharmacy and at the primary healthcare facility can improve treatment outcome of hypertension.

Therefore, it is recommended that there should be policy change that allows for involvement of pharmacy in the management of hypertension.

Acknowledgements

I would like to thank the Department of Pharmacy National University of Lesotho and Senkatana Project administrator for her assistance. I would also like to thank my daughter and sons who are always there and making my life worth living.

Conflict of interest

The authors declare no conflict of interest.

Acronyms and abbreviations

BP	Blood pressure
BPT	Blood pressure telemonitoring
CDM	Chronic disease management
CHAL	Christian Health Association of Lesotho
CVDs	Cardio Vascular Diseases
DHMTs	District Health Management Teams
GDP	Gross Domestic Product
GoL	Government of Lesotho
IPHC	Integrated primary health care
mmHg	Millimetres of Mercury
MoH	Ministry of Health
MOPH	Ministry of Public Health
NCDs	Non communicable diseases
OTC	Over the counter
PHC	Primary health care
SACU	Southern African Customs Union
UN	United Nations
UNICEF	United Nations International Children's Emergency Fund
VHW	Village health workers
WHO	World Health Organisation

Author details

Maseabata Ramathebane*, Maja Lineo and Sello Molungoa
National University of Lesotho, Maseru, Lesotho

*Address all correspondence to: mvramathebane@gmail.com; mv.ramathebane@nul.ls

References

[1] Lesotho, Ministry of Planning. Bureau of Statistics Census results 2016. Maseru, Government Printers; 2016

[2] Lesotho, Ministry of Health. Annual Joint Review Report (2009/2010). Maseru: Government Printers; 2010

[3] UNICEF (United Nations International Children Emergency Fund). Lesotho National Budget Brief-Fiscal Year 2018/19. 2018. Available from: https://wwwuniceforg/esaro/UNICEF-Lesotho-2018-National_Budget_Briefpdf [Accessed Date: 27 September 2021]

[4] Lesotho, Ministry of Health. Standard Treatment Guidelines for Lesotho. 2nd ed. Maseru: Government Printers; 2017

[5] Bertelsmann, S. BTI 2014 - Lesotho Country Report. 2014. Available from: http://wwwbti-projectorg [Accessed Date: 27 September 2021]

[6] World Bank and UNICEF. Lesotho Public Health Sector Expenditure Review. Washington: 2017. Available from: http://www.worldbank.org. [Accessed: 26, November 2021]

[7] Lesotho, Ministry of Health and Social Welfare. PHC revitalization plan 2011-2017. Maseru: Government Printers; 2011

[8] Lesotho government. National Strategic Plan 2012-2017. Maseru: Government Printers; 2012

[9] Lesotho MoH (Ministry of Health). Lesotho National Health Policy. Maseru: Government Printers; 2011a

[10] WHO (World Health Organisation). Primary health care: Report of the international conference of primary health care Alma-Ata, USSR, 6-12 September 1978. Geneva: WHO; 1978

[11] Collins C, Hewson DL, Munger R, Wade T. Evolving models of behavioural integration in primary care. New York: Milbank Memorial Fund; 2010

[12] Valentijn PP, Schepman SM, Opheij W, Bruijnzeels MA. Mint: Understanding integrated care: A comprehensive conceptual framework based on the integrative functions of primary care. International Journal of Integrated Care. 2013;**13**(1):1-12

[13] Acharya B, Maru D, Schwarz R, Citrin D, Tenpa J, Hirachan S, et al. Mint: Partnerships in mental healthcare service delivery in low-resource settings: developing an innovative network in rural Nepal. Globalization and Health. 2017;**13**(1):2

[14] Zhang XH, Lisheng L, Campbell NR, Niebylski ML, Nilsson P, Lackland DT. Mint: World hypertension league implementation of world health organisation package of essential non-communicable disease interventions (WHO PEN) for primary health care in low-resource settings: A policy statement from the world hypertension league. The Journal of Clinical Hypertension. 2016;**18**(1):5-6

[15] Chen AH, Murphy EJ and Yee Jr HF. Mint: eReferral—a new model for integrated care New England Journal of Medicine, 2013;**368**(26):2450-2453

[16] Nicholson C, Jackson C, Marley L. Mint: A governance model for integrated primary and secondary care for the health-reforming first world results of a systematic review BCM. Health Services Research 2013;**12**(528):1-12

[17] Posholi M, Wilke M. Strategies Registered Nurses use to Implement Integrated Primary Health Care in Maseru District, LESOTHO [thesis]. South Africa: University of the Free State; 2019

[18] Goodwin N. Mint: Understanding integrated care. International Journal of Integrated Care. 2016;**16**(4):1-4

[19] WHO (World Health Organisation). The World Health Report: Primary Health Care Now More Than Ever. Geneva: WHO; 2008a

[20] Lesotho MOH (Ministry of Health). Rapid Assessment of the Status of HIV and Sexual and Reproductive Health Linkages and Integration in. Lesotho Maseru: Government Printers; 2011a

[21] Lesotho MOH (Ministry of Health) 2011a Lesotho national health policy Maseru: Government Printers, 2011b.

[22] Stender S, Phafoli S, Christensen A, Skolnik L, Nyangu I, et al. Lesotho Nursing and Midwifery Primary Health Care Clinical Placement. World Health & Population; December 2015;**16**(2):46-53. DOI: 10.12927/whp.2016.24493

[23] MacKinnon J, MacLaren B. Human Resources for Health Challenges in Fragile States: Evidence from Sierra Leone. South Sudan and Zimbabwe Ontario: The North-South Institute; 2012. Available from: wwwnsi-insca//2012-Human-Resources-for-Health-Challenges-in-Fragile-Statespdf [Accessed Date: 27 September 2021]

[24] WHO (World Health Organisation). Assessment of Medicines Procurement and Supply Management System in the Health Sector A Country Report Ghana. Geneva: WHO Press; 2009

[25] Nkomazana O, Peersman W, Willcox M, Mash R, Phaladze N. Mint: Human resources for health in Botswana: The results of in-country database and reports analysis. African Journal of Primary Health Care and Family Medicine. 2014;**6**(1);Art. #716, 8 pages. DOI: 10.4102/phcfm.v6i1.716

[26] Lesotho Ministry of Health and ICF International. Lesotho Demographic and Health Survey. 2014. Maseru, Lesotho: Ministry of Health and ICF International; 2016

[27] Ntlale ME, Duma SE. Mint: The costs and benefits of nurse migration on families: A Lesotho Experience. Curationis. 2012;**13**:1. DOI: 104102/Curationis34i113

[28] McPherson T , Fontane P. Mint: Pharmacists' social authority to transform community pharmacy practice Idea Paper, 2011; **2**(2): 42. Available from: https://pubslibumnedu/indexphp/innovations/article/download/225/219/ [Accessed Date: 27 September 2021]

[29] UNAIDS Lesotho. Follow-Up to the 2011 Political Declaration on HIV/AIDS: Intensifying Efforts to Eliminate HIV/AIDS. 2014. [Accessed Date: 27 September 2021]

[30] World Health Organization (WHO). WHO Global Tuberculosis Report. Geneva: WHO Press; 2014

[31] World Health Organization (WHO). Global Tuberculosis Report 2014 Key Indicators for the WHO African Region. 2014b. Available from: http://wwwwhoint/tb/publications/global_report/indicators_african_regionpdf?ua=1 [Accessed Date: 27 September 2021]

[32] World Health Organization (WHO). Trends in Maternal Mortality 1990 - 2013: Estimates by WHO, UNICEF, UNFPA, the World Bank and the United Nations Population Division. Geneva: World Health Organization; 2014c. [Accessed Date: 27 September 2021]

[33] World Health Organization (WHO). Epidemiology of Hypertension. Geneva: WHO; 2012a

[34] World Health Organization (WHO). Global Action Plan for Prevention and Control of Non-Communicable Diseases 2013-2020. Geneva: WHO; 2013

[35] Bosu W K, Aheto J M K, Zucchelli E Reilly S. Mint: Mint: Prevalence, Awareness, and Associated Risk Factors

of Hypertension in Older Adults in Africa: A Systematic Review and Meta-Analysis Protocol BioMed Central, 2017;**6**:192-200

[36] Thinyane KH, Mothebe T, Sooro M, Namole LD, Cooper V. Mint: An observational study of hypertension treatment and patient outcomes in a primary Health Care Setting. Pan Africa Medical Journal. 2015;**20**(1):424-432

[37] Uys L. Integrated Fundamental Nursing. 2nd ed. South Africa: Pearson; 2017

[38] World Health Organization (WHO). New Data Highlight Increases in Hypertension, Diabetes Incidence. Geneva: WHO; 2012b

[39] Lesotho Ministry of Health and Social Welfare. National Guidelines on Management of Diabetes and Hyper-tension at Primary Care Guidelines. Maseru: Government Printers; 2009

[40] Lesotho Ministry of Health. Standard Treatment Guidelines and Essential Medicines List for Lesotho Maseru Government Printers. 2017

[41] WHO (World Health Organisation). Factsheet: Hypertension. Geneva: WHO Press; 2021

[42] Vrijens B, Antoniou S, Burnier M, De la Sierra A, Volpe M. Mint: Current situation of medication adherence in hypertension. Frontiers in Pharmacology. 2017;**100**(8):1-8

[43] Rao CR, Kamath VG, Kamath A. Mint: Treatment compliance among patients with hypertension and type 2 diabetes mellitus in a coastal population of Southern India. International Journal of Preventive Medicine. 2014;**5**(8): 992-998

[44] Njuguna B, Vedanthan R. Mint: Find and plug the leak: Improving adherence to anti-hypertensive medicines. Cardiovascular Drugs Therapy. 2017;**31**(5-6):485-487

[45] Ivarsson B, Hesselstrand R, Rådegran G, Kjellström B. Mint: Adherence and medication belief in patients with pulmonary arterial hypertension or chronic thromboembolic pulmonary hypertension: A national population-based cohort survey. The Clinical Respiratory Journal. 2018;**2**(2): 692-703

[46] Hacihasanoglu R, Gozum S. Mint: The effect of patient education and home monitoring on medication compliance, hypertension management, healthy lifestyle behaviours and BMI in a primary health care setting. Journal of Clinical Nursing. 2011;**20**:692-705

[47] Mafutha GN, Wright SCD. Mint: Compliance or non-compliance of hypertensive adults to hypertension management at three Primary healthcare day clinics in Tshwane. Curations. 2013;**36**(1):1-6

[48] Martin KD, Roter DL, Beach MC, Carson KC, Cooper LA. Mint: Physician communication behaviours and trust among black and white patients with hypertension. Medical Care. 2013;**51**(2): 151-157

[49] Nwabuo CC, Morss Dy S, Weeks K, Young JH. Mint: Factors associated with appointment non-adherence among African-Americans with severe. Poorly Controlled Hypertension. Journal Pone. 2014;**9**(8):1-7

[50] Himmelfarb CRD, Commodore-Mensah Y. Mint: Expanding the role of nurses to improve hypertension care and control globally. Annals of Global Health. 2016;**82**(2):243-253

[51] Khothatso T, Moshoeshoe T, Saroni Z, Ross A. Mint: Knowledge of hypertensive patients about treatment in the Seboche Hospital, 2013. South African Family Medicine. 2015;**58**(1):27-38

[52] Mugomeri E, Ramathebane MV, Maja L, Chatanga P, Moletsane L. Mint: Knowledge of disease condition and medications among hypertension patients in Lesotho. Journal of the American Society of Hypertension. 2016;**10**(1):41-46

[53] Matthes J, Albus C. Mint: Improving Adherence with Medication– a Selective Literature Review based on the Example of Hypertension Treatment. Deutsches Arzteblatt International. 2014;**111**(4): 41-47

[54] Wells BG, DiPiro JT, Schwinghammer TL, Schwinghammer CV. Pharmacotherapy Handbook. 7th ed. New York: McGraw-Hill; 2009

[55] Chobanian AV, Bakris GL, Black HR, Cushman WC, Green LA, Izzo JL. The Seventh Report of the Joint National Committee on Prevention, Detection, Evaluation, and Treatment of High Blood Pressure (JNC7) Bethesda: National Heart, Lung, and Blood Institute. 2004. Available from: https://wwwncbinlmnihgov/books/NBK9630/pdf/Bookshelf_NBK9630pdf [Accessed Date: 27 September 2021]

[56] Saseen J. Essential hypertension. In: Koda-Kimble MA, Young LY, Alldredge BK, Corelli RL, Guglielmo BJ, Kradjan WA, Williams BR, editors. Applied Therapeutics; The Clinical Use of Drugs. 9th ed. Philadelphia: Lippincott Williams & Wilkins; 2009. pp. 1-42

[57] Beaglehole R, Epping-Jordan J, Patel V, Chopra M, Ebrahim S, Kidd M, et al. Mint: Improving the prevention and management of chronic disease in low income and middle-income countries: a priority for primary health care. Lancet. 2008;**372**:940-949

[58] Siantz E, Aranda MP. Mint: Chronic disease self-management interventions for adults with serious mental illness: a systematic review of the literature. General Hospital Psychiatry. 2014;**36**: 233-244

[59] Leidy NK, Kimel M, Ajagbe L, Kim K, Hamilton. Mint: A Designing trials of behavioural interventions to increase physical activity in patients with COPD: Insights from the chronic disease literature. Respiratory Medicine. 2014;**108**:472-481

[60] Bastiaens H, van Royen P, Pavlic DR, Raposo V, Baker R. Mint: Older people's preferences for involvement in their own care: A qualitative study in primary health care in 11 European countries. Patient Education and Counseling. 2007;**68**:33-42

[61] Lorig KR, Hurwicz M, Sobel D, Hobbs M, Ritter PL. Mint: A national dissemination of an evidence-based self-management program: a process evaluation study. Patient Education and Counseling. 2005;**59**:69-79

[62] Maimela E, Van Geertruyden J, Alberts M, Modjadji S, Meulemans H, Fraeyman J, et al. Mint: The perceptions and perspectives of patients and health care providers on chronic diseases management in rural South Africa: A qualitative study. BMC Health Services Research. 2015;**15**:143. DOI: 101186/s12913-015-0812-5

[63] Beran D, Yudkin JS. Mint: Diabetes care in sub-Saharan Africa. Lancet. 2006;**368**:1689-1695

[64] Wagner EH, Austin BT, Von Korff M. Mint: Improving outcomes in chronic illness. Managed Care Quarterly. 1996;**4**(2):12-25

[65] Nyangu I, Nkosi ZZ. Mint: Antiretroviral therapy program accessibility across Lesotho districts' primary health care centres. Journal of Public Health and Diseases. 2019;**2**(2): 32-40

[66] Uys LR, Klopper HC. Mint: What is the ideal ratio of categories of nurses for

the South African public health system? South African Journal of Science. 2013;**109**(5-6):1-4

[67] Rampamba EM, Meyer JC, Helberg EA. Mint: Godman B Empowering hypertensive patients in South Africa to improve their disease management: A pharmacist-led intervention. J Res Pharm Pract. 2019;**8**:208-213

[68] Parliament of Ghana. Health Professions Regulatory Bodies Act 857 Part four Establishment of the Pharmacy Council. Accra. 2014

[69] Ministry of Health Ghana. National Policy for the Prevention and Control of Chronic Non-Communicable Diseases in Ghana Ministry of Health Ghana. 2012. Available from: http:// wwwiccp-portalorg/sites/default/files /plans/ national_policy_for_the_prevention_ and_control_of_chronic_- non-communicable_diseases_in_- ghana (1)pdf

[70] Afia FA, Marfoa F, Owusu-Daakua T. Mint: Evaluation of a pharmacist-led hypertension preventative and detection service in the Ghanaian community pharmacy: an exploratory study. International Journal of Pharmacy Practice. 2016;**24**:341-348. DOI: 10.1111/ ijpp.12263

[71] Omboni S. Mint: Pharmacist-led hypertension management combined with blood pressure telemonitoring in a primary care setting may be cost-effective in high-risk patients. Journal of Clinical Hypertension (Greenwich). Feb 2019;**21**(2):169-172. DOI: 10.1111/ jch.13467. Epub 2018 Dec 20. PMID: 30570221.

[72] Padwal RS, So H, Wood PW, Mcalister FA, et al. Mint: Cost-effectiveness of home blood pressure telemonitoring and case management in the secondary prevention of cerebrovascular disease in Canada. J Clin Hypertens (Greenwich). Feb 2019;**21**(2):159-168. DOI: 10.1111/ jch.13459. [Epub: 2018 Dec 2020]. PMID: 30570200

[73] Hallit S, Abou Selwan C, Salameh P. Mint: Primary health care policy and vision for community pharmacy and pharmacists in Lebanon. Pharmacy Practice. 2020;**18**(2):2003

[74] Albasri A, Clark CE, Omboni S, McDonagh STJ, McManus RJ, Sheppard JP. Mint: Effective detection and management of hypertension through community pharmacy in England. The Pharmaceutical Journal. 2020;**304**:7935. DOI: 10.1211/ PJ.2020.20207532

[75] Buis LR, Roberson DN, Kadri R, Rockey NG, Plegue MA, Danak SU, et al. Mint: Understanding the feasibility, acceptability, and efficacy of a clinical pharmacist-led mobile approach (BPTrack) to hypertension management: Mixed methods pilot study. Journal of Medical Internet Research. 2020;**22**(8): e19882. https://www.jmir.org/2020/8/ e19882. DOI: 10.2196/19882

[76] Westerlund T, Marklund B. Mint: Community pharmacy and primary health care in Sweden - at a crossroads. Pharmacy Practice. 2020;**18**(2):1927

Chapter 12

Impact of Cardiovascular Diseases on the Outcome of Patients with COVID-19

Seeta Devi Akyana and Dipali Dumbre

Abstract

The prevalence of COVID 19 disease cases in India stands too high; this disease is caused by the coronavirus called SARS-CoV-2. Noval coronavirus virus was firstly detected in a group of people suffering from Pneumonia in Wuhan, China. Several studies are conducted to understand the different aspects of novel coronavirus SARS-CoV-2 in causing severe respiratory infections. However, the impact of risk factors on the severity of the symptoms and outcome of COVID 19 is not clearly understood. Similarly, most studies reported that patients who suffer from comorbidities with COVID 19 had a poor prognosis. Most COVID 19 patients who had preexisting medical conditions such as hypertension, diabetes, obesity, smoking habit, etc., required ICU admission and mechanical ventilation. On the other hand, studies reported that COVID 19 infection is responsible for causing the predominant cardiovascular diseases due to myocardial damage, thromboembolism arrhythmias, and ACS.

Keywords: Cardiovascular risk factors, Diabetes, Hypertension, outcome patients, COVID- 19

1. Introduction

Coronaviruses belong to a large family of viruses that causes various illnesses in humans and animals, ranging from the common cold to severe acute respiratory syndrome. COVID 19 is the most recently discovered virus of the coronavirus family. The prominent significant symptoms of coronavirus are cold, cough, fever, headache, and sometimes even diarrhea [1]. It is transmitted from one person to another by tiny droplets from the nose or mouth, expelled by a person with COVID-19 coughs, sneezes, or speaks. These droplets are moderately thick, do not travel far, and quickly sink to the ground [2]. People can also be infected by touching the objects or surfaces with coronavirus and then touching their eyes, nose, or mouth. The person who has contacted a COVID 19 positive and has cold, cough, and fever symptoms needs to be self-quarantined for 14 days to prevent the spread of infection to others within the community. The duration between exposure to COVID 19 and the beginning of symptoms is around five to six days, but it ranges from 2 to 14 days. It is one of the main reasons why the person is quarantined for 14 days after exposure. A research study showed that children and adolescents are as likely to be infected as any other age group and can spread the disease. The severity of the symptoms is equally noticed in all age groups [3].

The effect of COVID 19 among patients with cardiovascular disease conditions and diabetes was found to be high. Similarly, the prevalence of cardiovascular disease conditions was also found to be high among the patients who were infected with COVID 19. The hypothetical reasons are myocardial damage, myocarditis, and cardiomyopathy caused by stress due to COVID 19. The other important causes of cardiovascular problems in COVID 19 are pneumonia, increased cardiac output, electrolyte imbalance, side effects of drugs used to treat the COVID 19 [4].

The infection occurs in myocardial muscles due to damage or injury to the major organs. The inflammation chances will increase, which induces the cytokine storm and vascular hyper-permeability, leading to multi-organ failure and death. The occurrence of cytokines storm is high in patients with diabetes [4].

The thromboembolic action is intense in diabetic patients as it has a significant association with prothrombotic events, which are responsible for causing fibrinolysis and clotting factors. The coagulation activity is likely to be increased further among the patients with COVID 19 diseases. Due to endothelial dysfunction, hypoxia occurs, which can cause intra-vessel coagulation problems [5].

The following are the main cardiovascular risk factors;

1. Diabetes

2. High blood pressure (hypertension)

3. Obesity

4. Family history of CVD

5. Smoking

2. Impact of diabetes on COVID-19 virus

2.1 Pathogenesis of COVID-19 virus

SARS- CoV – 2 is an RNA virus that is the zoonotic source in origin. The transmission of the coronavirus is possible from person to person by respiratory droplets. The symptoms of COVID -19 are range from no signs to mild to moderate. The transmission of coronavirus is possible by specific procedures such as bronchoscopy, endotracheal intubation, and tracheostomy [6].

It enters the human body with S- glycoprotein receptors and binds with the host's ACE2 (Angiotensin-converting enzyme2) receptors, located on the cell membrane. S- Glycoprotein consisting of subunits of S1 and S2 that are found on spikes of the virus [7].

The volume of Furin is more in diabetic patients, which is believed to enhance the viral entry into the human body. The enrichment of the viral entry occurs by the S1 and S2 subunits of spike proteins. Other factors include an acidic environment, and the presence of proteases in diabetic patients increases the replication of the virus [8].

The entry of coronavirus in the body occurs via the pulmonary system. However, it spreads to the other organs comprised of lungs, kidneys, heart, and intestines [9]. Severe acute respiratory syndrome coronavirus (SARS-CoV) and Middle East respiratory syndrome coronavirus (MERS-CoV) cause dangerous respiratory symptoms while other coronaviruses cause the common cold (**Figure 1**) [10].

After entry of the coronavirus into the human body, inflammation begins with the development of cytokines and chemokines. The presence of leukocytosis and

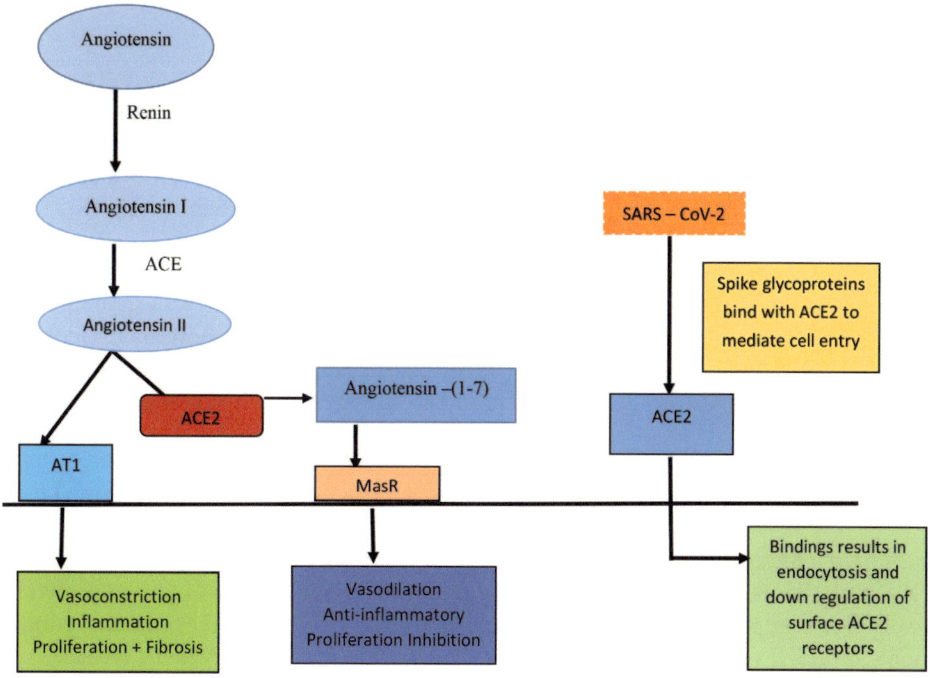

Figure 1.
The role of ACE2 in the regulation of angiotensin system and SARS-CoV-2 infection.

elevated ESR, C- reactive protein levels is commonly observed in laboratory investigation, indicating coronavirus progression in the body [11].

2.2 Pathogenesis of diabetes mellitus

A lack of insulin causes type 1 diabetes, and type 2 diabetes is caused by insulin resistance. The long-term rise of blood glucose levels causes glucotoxicity in body tissues. This mechanism causes chronic complications to include diabetic ketoacidosis (DKA). The treatment of insulin and sulfonylurea cause hypoglycemia [12].

The infection is the primary responsible factor in causing diabetic ketoacidosis and hyperglycemia; thus, it increases the requirement of insulin, leading to cause uncontrolled hyperglycemia. The presence of C-reactive proteins, plasminogen activator inhibitor-1 in laboratory investigations indicate the association of inflammation and diabetes [13].

3. Relationship between diabetes and COVID 19

3.1 Dipeptidyl peptidase-4

Typically incretins, including the Glucagon peptide and gastric inhibitory peptide, are essential to increase insulin secretion. Nonetheless, these incretin values in type 2 diabetes are reduced due to degraded levels of dipeptidyl peptidase-4 in the small intestinal gut. The dipeptidyl peptidase-4 is a transmembrane glycoprotein that exists in the body as a dimer. The primary function of D dimer is to block the degrading enzyme and enhance the activity of incretins in insulin secretion [14].

This enzyme has been indicated as one of the components responsible for the entry receptors of the coronavirus. The place of the enzyme is at the entry of the bronchial tree.

3.2 ACE2 receptors

These receptors play a crucial role in facilitating the entry of SARS-CoV-2 into the human body cells. ACE2 receptors are mainly located on the cell membranes of the lungs, intestine, kidney, and vessels. ACE2 levels are known to be increased in diabetic patients, which is also associated with non-communicable diseases such as diabetes, hypertension, stroke predisposing to develop the SARS-CoV 2 infection [15, 16].

3.3 ACEi and ARBs

ACEi and ARBs are commonly used antihypertensive medications by patients with diabetes and hypertension. These medications are believed to increase the ACE2 levels within the body. However, clinical evidence is yet to be proved [17].

4. Potentials of spreading COVID-19 infection to diabetes individuals

There is adequate evidence to say that people with diabetes at high risk get COVID – 19 infection than the general population. Diabetic patients are more likely to develop complications if they are infected with COVID 19 infection. Their condition worsens if they have other comorbidities, including coronary heart disease, above 60 years old.

Diabetic patients with COVID 19 are at high for the development of serious complications. They are most likely to suffer from moderate to severe symptoms and other complications. These symptoms and complications are less in the patients who have controlled and managed their blood glucose levels well. COVID 19 infection can cause inflammation and endothelial damage; this inflammation is responsible for generating complications in people with diabetes.

The differences in the complications results depend on viral load, host immunity, patient's age, and other long-term diseases. The mortality and morbidity rate are similar in diabetic patients with the corona infection of SARS and MERS.

Diabetic Patients with COVID 19 are at high risk for uncontrollable inflammation due to hypercoagulable response [18]. In Type 2 Diabetes, inflammation induces poor regulation in the homeostatic glucose levels and peripheral insulin sensitivity [19]. Many other factors are also responsibly increasing the severity of SARS-CoV-2 disease in diabetic patients.

5. Effect of diabetes on COVID-19

Patients with diabetes are at high risk for the acquired infection of viruses and bacteria, which affect the respiratory system. The main responsible factor for this increased risk is less function of leukocytes in DM patients. Further, it increases the risk of SARS-CoV-2 inclinations in patients. The lung's deference in terms of gaseous exchange will be impaired due to microangiopathy. This mechanism causes the proliferation of the microorganism in the airway, especially SARS-CoV-2. These changes in the respiratory tract will petrogenetically affect the lung capacity and diffusing capacity of the pulmonary system [20].

Muniyappa and Gubbi concluded that the following mechanisms are responsible for causing the mortality and morbidity of SARS-CoV-2 among patients with diabetes [21].

a. Cellular binding capacity raises the entry of the virus.

b. Reduced leukocyte and the function of T- cells.

c. Vulnerability increased to high inflammation.

Studies conducted in Italy proved that ischemic heart disease and hypertension are commonly observed among patients with comorbidities. A survey conducted in Wuhan regarding the feature of COVID 19 results revealed that the prevalence of COVID 19 about 2–20% is high among the patient's DM and created the requirement of ICU admission about 7.1%. The study results on the clinical features on COVID 19 patients with diabetes reported that approximately 20% of cases reported with COVID 19 positive, and 7% of the cases required the ICU admission. In another study also similar results were observed that 17% and 12.1% accordingly [22].

Hyperglycemia plays a vital role in damaging the endothelial function, causing the cytokine storm and injuries to multiple organs. Patients with COVID 19 and hyperglycemia cause a reduced expiratory volume of the lungs. Phillips et al. [22] results revealed that high blood glucose levels in blood on the respiratory system would reduce its distinctive immune capacity. The cardiovascular mortality rate is also increased due to hyperglycemia by enhancing the inflammatory process in the endothelial system and platelet aggregation [23], in case-controlled blood glucose levels worsen the mortality rate [24].

6. Effect of COVID-19 on diabetes

COVID 19 infection in patients multiplexes the glucocorticoids and catecholamines in the circulation. These are two factors causing uncontrolled glucose levels in the blood, damage the majority of vital organs, and worsen the outcome of the disease.

6.1 Effect of corticosteroids

In case of severe infection, to suppress the inflammatory progress, corticosteroids include hydrocortisone. However, the complications due to administration of these drugs found high comprise as raising 80% of blood glucose levels among diabetic patients and lesser in non-diabetic patients. The mortality rate was higher among diabetic patients with CIVID 19 infection after administration of corticosteroids due to uncontrolled blood glucose levels, necrosis, and psychosis [25, 26]. Glucose monitoring is essential for the patients who all are on the corticosteroids [27].

7. Relationship between hypertension and COVID 19

Hypertension is characterized by increased blood pressure (BP) to the extent of 140/90 mmHg. The essential modifiable factors are associated with the development of cardiovascular illnesses with high BP. Hypertension is one of the primary diseases causing worldwide non-communicable infections [28].

Coronavirus infection mainly influences respiratory tract disease. The spreading of infection is extreme in patients who are at risk of cardiovascular diseases. Hypertension causes massive pathophysiological changes in the cardiovascular system includes left ventricular hypertrophy and fibrosis, which makes parson more susceptible to SARS-CoV-2 [28].

8. Regulation of blood pressure by RAAS

Angiotensin-converting enzyme 2 is a biochemical pathway of the Renin-Angiotensin-Aldosterone System (RAAS), which plays an essential role in regulating blood pressure.

In reaction to stimulation of the sympathetic nervous system, the blood flow to the kidneys and serum sodium levels are reduced. Renin is emitted from the juxtaglomerular apparatus in the kidney.

Renin is an enzyme that converts the angiotensinogen to angiotensin I. Angiotensin-converting enzyme (ACE) converts angiotensin I into angiotensin II (A-II), a potent vasoconstrictor that increases vascular resistance; thus, it increases blood pressure levels.

Angiotensin-II increases blood pressure by stimulating the adrenal cortex to produce aldosterone, which causes sodium and water preservation by the kidneys, bringing about expanded blood volume and expanded cardiac output.

Due to vasoconstriction in blood vessels, blood pressure values that cause atherosclerosis, renal illness, heart hypertrophy) [29].

9. Link between coronavirus and RAAS

RAAS is the neurohormonal pathway that controls blood pressure and fluid balance. The mechanism of the rennin angiotensin is the formation of angiotensin 2, a vasoactive hormone attached to the receptor of the type I angiotensin, which is present in the renal, cardiac, and respiratory systems. It has a vital role in causing the hypertrophy of the myocardium and fibrosis. Further, it causes inflammation, remodeling of vascular endothelium, and formation of atherosclerosis plaque. The Angiotensin-converting enzyme 2 is present in human body tissues, and it affects the mechanism of angiotensin II and the reducing of vasoconstriction effect [29].

SARS-CoV-2 connected to the ACE2 receptor by releasing the spikes protein into host cells causes the regulation of ACE2 and bringing about the local aggregation of angiotensin II. Respiratory severe illness is a sign of COVID-19 and an essential reason for morbidity and mortality; RAAS is proposed to cause an extreme lung injury. Angiotensin-converting enzyme II is considered as the entry for SARS-CoV-2.

The entry of COVID-19 infection in the human body occurs if the virus comes in contact with the angiotensin-converting enzyme II cell surface. This enzyme acts with SARS-CoV-2 by restricting the receptor binding space of the viral spike protein. In the human lung, type II alveolar epithelial cells, ACE2 and transmembrane protease serine III are viewed as fundamentally liable for virus entry in COVID-19 [29].

10. The possible impact of RAS inhibitors on COVID-19

At the start of the COVID 19 episode, the patients with hypertension utilizing angiotensin-converting enzyme inhibitors might provide unfavorable results. The studies mentioned that mineral corticoid receptor antagonists (MRAs) increase the movement of angiotensin-converting enzyme II in the heart and kidney. The antihypertensive medications initiate the ACE2 increase the chances of the portal of entry for the COVID infection [30].

11. Key comorbidities of hypertension comparable to COVID-19

Many research studies have shown that the death rate in COVID 19 was more in patients aged above 50–60 years with hypertension [31].

Obesity with hypertension is also the determinant factor in increasing the seriousness of the disease, which deteriorates the patient's outcome by affecting the expansion of the diaphragm, decreasing the expiratory reserve volume, compromising the ventilation. Obesity increases the release of increased cytokines, causes atherosclerosis, and leads to cardiac problems, which reduces the recovery of the patients with COVID - 19 [31].

12. Coronavirus and thromboembolic problems

The patients with COVID 19 have shown a higher risk of forming arterial and venous thrombus and embolic complications. The patient with severe clinical infection shows the neurological components and the increment level of the D – dimer values, indicating that thromboembolic complications increase mortality among the COVID 19 patients. Among thromboembolic difficulties, VTE (Venous Thromboembolic complication) was a common problem in hospitalized patients [32].

13. Potential mechanisms of SARS-CoV-2-instigated endothelial injury

The organ damage from the coronavirus was mainly related to the inflammatory response; the stimulation of the inflammatory mediator such as cytokine leads to endothelial injury. The virus damages the endothelial cell, directly and indirectly, leading to the endothelial cell's dysfunction and the formation of the clots. Endothelial cell damage increases the permeability of the cell membrane, leading to complications such as acute respiratory distress syndrome and pulmonary fibrosis and pulmonary edema, which is not related to the cardiac problem but due to the increase in vascular permeability. Thus, endothelial injury due to the COVID virus can affect the patient's respiratory function and impacts the patient's recovery [33].

14. Myocardial injury related with COVID-19

There are different types of cardiovascular problems observed in the patient of COVID-19. The issues include congestive cardiac heart failure, dysrhythmia, cardiogenic shock, myocardial infarction, and myocarditis. The studies also stated that the diagnostic studies related to cardiac system problems such as cardiac injury in COVDI-19 patients indicated a positive test of Troponin T, changes in the ECG, and 2d echo. The pathogenesis of the myocardial injury is indescribable in the situation of COVID 19. Due to the viral infection, the inflammatory mediator triggers the inflammatory process, leading to the rupture of the plaque and development of the thrombus and ending in atherosclerotic diseases. The production of the inflammatory mediator comprises of cytokine causes instability in the plaque results in atherosclerosis, and myocardial dysfunction shows clinical conditions like inflammation of myocardium and cardiomyopathy [33].

Apart from this, essential risk factors such as smoking, obesity, hypertension, diabetes, etc., cause atherosclerosis. It increases the viral load in circulation causes hypoxemia and unusual hemodynamic changes in patients with COVID-19. This mechanism probably acts in corresponding to cause the damage to the cardiovascular system, leads myocardial infarction, ventricular arrhythmias, and congestive cardiovascular failure. Viral infection also affects the respiratory system, which reduces the oxygen levels in the blood. This process alters the hemodynamic parameters, including saturation level, blood pressure changes, leading to cardiovascular complications and atherosclerosis plaque formation. This process of pathogenesis causes significant cardiac damage and significant complications such as myocardial infarction, dysrhythmias, and the cardiac failure [34].

15. Impact of obesity on COVID 19

People with obesity are at high risk for the contraction of COVID – 19 infection. Adipose tissue is increased in ACE2 receptors, which facilitates the SARS-CoV-2 to enter the human cells quickly [35]. The viral load is significantly increased along with the prolonged viremia due to the massive number of adipocytes in obese people. Visceral adiposity causes cytokine proliferation, which causes the low-grade inflammation to advance the cytokines storm in COVID- 19 [36]. Obesity is responsible for reducing individuals' immunity and susceptibility to infection due to various pathogenic organisms. Because increased cytokines in the circulatory system reduce adiponectin levels, thus the immune response to infection is reduced. This mechanism causes damage to the lymphoid tissue and decreasing the B and T cells in the immune system, susceptible to viral infection [37]. Obesity and procoagulant factors are interlinked together that play a vital role in causing thromboembolic complications in patients with COVID-19. Obesity also reduces pulmonary function, reducing reserve volume and respiratory system compliance, at high risk for COVID 19 complications. Obesity with dysfunctional adipose tissue is associated with type 2 diabetes, hypertension, and CVD, which impair individuals' health during COVID 19 infection [38].

16. Impact of family history on COVID 19

There are certain non-modifiable risk factors involved in the pathogenesis of hypertension; one of the essential factors is family history. Various family grounds the inherited character of hypertension examines, exhibiting the relationship of circulatory strain among kin and guardians and youngsters [39].

Hereditary attributes identified with hypertension, for example,

- Counter-Transport in High Level of Sodium and Lithium L,
- Reduced Exertion Of The Urinary Kallikrein,
- Increased Level Of Blood Uric Acid,
- High Blood Sugar Level,
- Changes In The High-Density Lipoprotein And Low-Density Lipoprotein,
- Changes In The Glycemic Index,
- Body Mass Index

- The Environmental Factors Like More Intake Of Sodium In The Diet [40].

The prevalence of CVD and family history are interlinked. The patient with hypertension with a family history is double in value than the patient with no family history [15]. Various types of research indicate that the person having a family history of hypertension leads to premature changes in the cardiac system, including ventricular wall thickness and differences in vascular permeability and stress responses [41, 42].

17. Impact of smoking on COVID 19

The side effect of smoking is prominent, and it causes mortality in all the body system linked with cardiovascular, respiratory systems, and diabetes. Smoking is a significant risk factor for all kinds of cardiovascular infections. It has expanded the risk of getting coronary heart disease. The rate of mortality has increased by 70% from coronary heart disease because of smoking.

It impacts the myocardium, obstructs the blood supply, and increases the chances of atherosclerosis, which directs myocardial infarction and different infections from cardiovascular problems, including cardiomyopathy. The tobacco content incorporated the nicotine and carbon monoxide directly impacts vascular endothelium, which causes inflammation and thrombosis. The majority of individuals with smoking are in danger of developing atherosclerosis.

Smoking has equally been troubled in the progression of corpulmonale. However, a close relationship with congestive cardiovascular breakdown has not been set up.

The proportion of myocardial oxygen supply and demand is influenced by nicotine and carbon monoxide, resulting in vascular endothelial injury, prompting the atherosclerosis plaque's progression [43].

18. Effect of smoking on coronary heart disease

Cigarette smoking is a significant modifiable factor for developing coronary illness. Due to cigarette smoking, the patients breathe tar; this substance contains 4,000 synthetics and cancer-causing agents, including cyanide, formaldehyde, and smelling salts. The nicotine is delivered by smoking which stimulates the sympathetic nervous system, causes peripheral vasoconstriction, and displays tachycardia, hypertension, and increased cardiac workload. Smoking affects the respiratory tract by causing hyperplasia that enhances the abnormal production of mucus. Hyperplasia obstructs the airway due to excessive secretion. Smoking causes the enlargement of the distal air spaces with obliteration of the alveolar walls. Thickening and narrowing of the airway wall cause the inflammatory exudates in the airway lumen.

Carbon monoxide (CO) is a part of tobacco smoke, which absorbs the increased hemoglobin and reduces the O2-carrying capacity to blood. Smoking causes inflammation, vasoconstriction, clot formation, and hypoxia in the endothelial system. Individuals who smoke are at high risk for the development of atherosclerosis. Endothelial injury causes thrombosis [44]. Coronary thrombosis can cause cataclysmic heart damage that leads to sudden death. Nicotine acts on the sympathetic nervous system and decreases myocardial oxygen, causing angina [45]. Tobacco smokers are bound to encounter intense cardiovascular occasions at an early age and prior illness. It has been proved that smoking can adversely affect the lungs, destructing the immune system and making it prone to developing infections.

Smokers are prone to develop pulmonary infections and reduce pulmonary immune function. World Health Organization (WHO) expressed that individual who smokes, carries the fingers to the lips, and that expands the chances of hand to mouth infection transmission, which is generally seen in COVID patients [46].

19. Preventive measures to be followed by patients

- People with diabetes to be careful in preventing the contraction of COVID 19 disease. The recommendations made available for the general public are doubly important for people with diabetes.
- A thorough and regular hand washing is essential.
- Do not touch the face beforehand, washing and drying of the hands.
- The objects or materials are frequently touched to be disinfected thoroughly.
- The food items, clothes, vessels, tools, etc., should not be shared with others.
- The mouth and nose should be closed with tissue when there is coughing and sneezing.
- Avoid exposure with people with symptoms of COVID – 19, such as respiratory infections.
- Try to avoid contact with anyone showing symptoms of respiratory illness such as coughing.
- Unnecessary gatherings and traveling's use of public transportation should be avoided.
- Patients with diabetes to be prepared if they are infected.
- Diabetic patients need to be more cautious in controlling their glucose levels. To prevent diabetic complications, their blood glucose levels to be monitored daily.
- If patients suffer from flu-like symptoms, such as increased temperature, cough, and breathing difficulties, they need to consult health care professionals. If cough consists of phlegm, suspected of infection, they need to get medical advice and treatment urgently.
- Patients need to be ensured for the sufficient supply of diabetic medication; this would help if he has to be quarantined.
- Patients should have enough provisions to correct the hypoglycemia if their blood sugar levels drop down suddenly.
- Diabetic patients need to be advised to adequate sleep and to avoid excessive workout [47].

20. Conclusion

The amount of the Furin is more in the diabetic patients that promote the entry of virus in the human body.

The enhancement of the viral entry occurs by the S1 and S2 subunits of spike proteins of the virus. ACE2 inhibitors play a crucial role in enriching the entry of SARS-CoV-2 into the human body. They are usually located on the vital organs' cell membranes, including the lungs, intestine, kidney, and vessels. They are known to be more in diabetic and hypertensive patients. ACE2 values are high in the patients using antihypertensive and antidiabetic medications.

Similarly, diabetic patients are at increased risk of acquiring viral infections due to the decreased function of the leukocytes. Further, it enhances the multiplication of SARS-CoV-2. Many studies revealed that diabetes and hypertensive patients infected with COVID 19 causes endothelial destruction and lead to venous thrombus and embolic complications. That leads to an increase in the D – dimer values, which indicates the thromboembolic complications increase mortality among the COVID 19 patients with diabetes and hypertension. The spreading of COVID 19 disease is high in the obesity population, as increased levels of fatty tissues consist of ACE2 receptors that easily facilitate the SARS-CoV-2 entry into the human system. Smoking is also one of the crucial modifiable risk factors in contacting the COVID 19 infection as it destructs the endothelial system and damages the respiratory system. Therefore, through this chapter, we understand an association between cardiovascular risk factors and the outcome of the patients with COVID 19.

Author details

Seeta Devi Akyana* and Dipali Dumbre
Symbiosis College of Nursing, Symbiosis International Deemed University, Pune, Maharashtra, India

*Address all correspondence to: sitadevi@scon.edu.in

References

[1] WHO Director-General's opening remarks at the media briefing on COVID-19 - 11 March 2020: World Health Organisation; 2020.

[2] Li BO, Yang J, Zhao F, et al. prevalence and impact of cardiovascular metabolic diseases on COVID-19 in China. Clin Res Cardiol. 2020; 109(5): 531- 538.

[3] Diabetes atlas: international diabetes federation 2019, 9th. https://www.diabetesatlas.org/en/

[4] Shereen MA, Khan S, Kazmi A, Bashir N, Siddique R. COVID-19 infection: origin, transmission, and characteristics of human coronaviruses. J Adv Res. 2020; 24: 91- 98.

[5] Wilson N, Corbett S, Tovey E. Airborne transmission of covid-19. BMJ. 2020; 370: m3206.

[6] Standards of Medical care in diabetes-2019. Diabetes Care. 2019;2(Suppl 1).

[7] Management of patients with confirmed 2019-nCoV [Online]. Available from: https://www.cdc.gov.

[8] Mode of transmission of virus causing COVID 19: implications for IPC precaution recommendations. Scientific brief [Online]. Available from: who.int/news-room/commentaries [Accessed 2020 May 26].

[9] Wan Y, Shang J, Graham R, Baric RS, Li F. Receptor recognition by novel Coronavirus from Wuhan: an analysis based on decade-long structural studies of SARS. J Virol. 2020;94(7): e00127–e00120.

[10] Hulswit RJ, de Haan CA, Bosch BJ. Coronavirus spike protein and tropism changes. Adv Virus Res. 2016; 96:29-57.

[11] Fernandez C, Rysä J, Almgren P, Nilsson J, Engström G, Orho-Melander M, et al. Plasma levels of the proprotein convertase furin and incidence of diabetes and mortality. J Intern Med. 2018;284(4):377-387.

[12] Yang P, Feng J, Peng Q, Liu X, Fan Z. Advanced glycation end products: potential mechanism and therapeutic target in cardiovascular complications under diabetes. Oxid Med Cell Longev. 2019 Dec 6;2019:9570616.

[13] Gosmanov AR, Gosmanova EO, Kitabchi AE. Hyperglycemic crises: diabetic ketoacidosis (DKA), and hyperglycemic hyperosmolar state (HHS) [updated 2018]. In: Feingold KR, Anawalt B, et al., editors. Endotext [Internet]. South Dartmouth, MA: MD Text.com, Inc.; 2000

[14] FDA Drug safety communication: FDA warns that DPP-4 inhibitors for type 2 diabetes may cause joint pain [Online]. Accessed 2020 May 20.

[15] European Societies of Cardiology. Position statement of ESC Council on Hypertension on ACE-inhibitors and angiotensin receptor blockers. March 13, 2020 [Online]. Accessed 2020 May 16.

[16] Liu C, Li Y, Guan T, Lai Y, Shen Y, Zeyaweiding A, et al. ACE2 polymorphisms associated with cardiovascular risk in Uygurs with type 2 diabetes mellitus. Cardiovasc Diabetol. 2018;17(1):127.

[17] Castelnuovo AD, Iacoviello L. ACE inhibitors, angiotensin II type I receptor blockers and severity of COVID 19.

[18] Guo W, Li M, Dong Y, Zhou H, Zhang Z, Tian C, et al. diabetes is a risk actor for the progression and prognosis of COVID19. Diabetes/metabolism Res Rev (2020) e3319.

[19] Yang JK, Feng Y, Yuan MY, Yuan SY, Fu HJ, Wu BY, et al. Plasma glucose levels and diabetes are independent predictors for mortality and morbidity in patients with SARS. Diabetic Med (2006) 23(6):623-628.

[20] Chen Y, Gong X, Wang L, Guo J. Effects of hypertension, diabetes and coronary heart disease on COVID-19 diseases severity: a systematic review and meta-analysis. medRxiv (2020) 14(4):303-10.

[21] Zhou F, Yu T, Du R, Fan G, Liu Y, Liu Z, et al. Clinical course and risk factors for mortality of adult inpatients with COVID-19 in Wuhan, China: a retrospective cohort study. Lancet (2020) 395(10229):1054-1062.

[22] Li F. Receptor recognition mechanisms of coronaviruses: a decade of structural studies. J Virol (2015) 89(4):1954-1964.

[23] Hoffmann M, Kleine-Weber H, Schroeder S, Krüger N, Herrler T, Erichsen S, et al. SARS-CoV-2 Cell Entry Depends on ACE2 and TMPRSS2 and Is Blocked by a Clinically Proven Protease Inhibitor. Cell (2020) 181(2):271-80.e8.

[24] Brufsky A. Hyperglycemia, hydroxychloroquine, and the COVID-19 pandemic. J Med Virol (2020) 92(7):770-775.

[25] Yang JK, Lin SS, Ji XJ, Guo LM. Binding of SARS coronavirus to its receptor damages islets and causes acute diabetes. Acta Diabetol (2010) 47(3):193-199. doi: 10.1007/s00592-009-0109-4

[26] Philips BJ, Meguer JX, Redman J, Baker EH. Factors determining the appearance of glucose in upper and lower respiratory tract secretions. Intensive Care Med (2003) 29(12):2204-10. 65.

[27] Rao S, Lau A, So H-C. Exploring diseases/traits and blood proteins causally related to expression of ACE2, the putative receptor of SARS-CoV-2: A Mendelian Randomization analysis highlights tentative relevance of diabetes-related traits. medRxiv (2020) 43(7):1416-26.

[28] Arnett DK, Blumenthal RS, Albert MA, et al. 2019 ACC/AHA Guideline on the Primary Prevention of Cardiovascular Disease. J Am Coll Cardiol 2019;74:e177–e232.

[29] Fryar CD, Ostchega Y, Hales CM, Zhang G, Kruszon-Moran D. Hypertension prevalence and control among adults: United States, 2015-2016. NCHS Data Brief 2017;289:1-8.

[30] Shah SJ, Stafford RS. Current trends of hypertension treatment in the United States. Am J Hypertens 2017;30: 1008-1014.

[31] Chen N, Zhou M, Dong X, et al. Epidemiological and clinical characteristics of 99 cases of 2019 novel coronavirus pneumonia in Wuhan, China: a descriptive study. Lancet 2020;395:507-513.

[32] Onder G, Rezza G, Brusaferro S. Case-fatality rate and characteristics of patients dying in relation to COVID-19 in Italy. JAMA 2020 March [Epub ahead of print].

[33] Grasselli G, Zangrillo A, Zanella A, et al. Baseline characteristics and outcomes of 1591 patients infected with SARS-CoV-2 admitted to ICUs of the Lombardy Region, Italy. JAMA 2020 April

[34] Bunyavanich S, Do A, Vicencio A. Nasal gene expression of angiotensin-converting enzyme 2 in children and adults. JAMA 2020 May

[35] Frühbeck G, Baker JL, Busetto L, Dicker D, Goossens GH, Halford JC, et al. European Association for the Study of Obesity Position Statement on the Global COVID-19 Pandemic. Obes Facts. 2020;13(2):292-296.

[36] Honce R, Schultz-Cherry S. Impact of obesity on influenza A virus pathogenesis, immune response, and evolution. Front Immunol. 2019 May;10:1071.

[37] Kanneganti TD, Dixit VD. Immunological complications of obesity. Nat Immunol. 2012 Jul;13(8):707-712.

[38] Simonnet A, Chetboun M, Poissy J, Raverdy V, Noulette J, Duhamel A, et al.; LICORN and the Lille COVID-19 and Obesity study group. High prevalence of obesity in severe acute respiratory syndrome coronavirus-2 (SARS-CoV-2) requiring invasive mechanical ventilation. Obesity (Silver Spring). 2020 Jul;28(7):1195-9.

[39] Zhou F, Yu T, Du R, Fan G, Liu Y, Liu Z, et al. Clinical course and risk factors for mortality of adult inpatients with COVID-19 in Wuhan, China: a retrospective cohort study. Lancet. 2020;395:1054-1062.

[40] Tocci G, Nati G, Cricelli C, Parretti D, Lapi F, Ferrucci A, et al. prevalence and control of hypertension in the general practice in Italy: updated analysis of a large database. J Hum Hypertens. 2017;31:258-62.

[41] Shi Y, Yu X, Zhao H, Wang H, Zhao R, Sheng J. Host susceptibility to severe COVID-19 and establishment of a host risk score: findings of 487 cases outside Wuhan. Crit Care. 2020;24:108

[42] Li X, Xu S, Yu M, Wang K, Tao Y, Zhou Y, et al. Risk factors for severity and mortality in adult COVID-19 inpatients in Wuhan. J Allergy Clin Immunol. 2020.

[43] Åberg A, Bergstrand R, Johansson S, Ulvenstam G, Vedin A, Wedel H, Wilhelmsson C, Wilhelmsen L. Cessation of smoking after myocardial infarction: effects on mortality after 10 years. British Heart Journal. 1983; 49(5):416-422.

[44] Abu-Hayyeh S, Sian M, Jones KG, Manuel A, Powell JT. Cadmium accumulation in aortas of smokers. Arteriosclerosis, Thrombosis, and Vascular Biology. 2001;21(5):863.

[45] Adler AI, Stevens RJ, Neil A, Stratton IM, Boulton AJM, Holman RR. UKPDS 59: hyperglycemia and other potentially modifiable risk factors for peripheral vascular disease in type 2 diabetes. Diabetes Care. 2002;25(5): 894-899.

[46] Aicher A, Heeschen C, Mohaupt M, Cooke JP, Zeiher AM, Dimmeler S. Nicotine strongly activates dendritic cell-mediated adaptive immunity: potential role for progression of atherosclerotic lesions. Circulation. 2003;107(4):604-611

[47] WHO Director-General's opening remarks at the media briefing on COVID-19 - 11 March 2020: World Health Organisation; 2020.

Chapter 13

Aplication Arterial Oscilography to Study the Adaptive Capacity of Subject with COVID-19 in Primary Care

Dmytro Vakulenko, Liudmyla Vakulenko, Leonid Hryshchuk and Lesya Sas

Abstract

The aim of study is finding complex pathological process markers occurred in COVID-19. Adaptive capacity, cardiovascular features, autonomic, central nervous systems in 67 patients with severe COVID-19 were studied and evaluated using (suggested by authors) temporal, spectral, correlation analysis of arterial oscillograms (AOG). The method is based on mathematical analysis adaptation of electrocardiographic signal heart rate variability to arterial pulsation variability analysis recorded during blood pressure measurement using an electronic tonometer VAT 41–2. Received results were compared with AOG 480 healthy (including 68 people after exercising) and 26 patients in a closed ward at psychoneurological hospital. Study results showed patients with severe COVID-19 have disorders at (four) cardiovascular system (CVS) regulation levels. It's confirmed by lack of adequate sympathetic-adrenal response to a stressful situation due to severe COVID-19; higher than in healthy, parasympathetic part activity of autonomic nervous system. AOG spectral analysis revealed violation of management centralization, communication and coordination between CVS regulation levels. This leads to functional reserves decrease, low stress resistance of body and finally to a disease severe course and recovery processes. Arterial oscillography can be used to search markers of complex pathological processes occurred in COVID-19 and to improve methods of diagnosis, treatment, control of long-term results in clinical and family medicine.

Keywords: Arterial oscilography, adaptive capacity of the body, heart rate variability, COVID-19, primary care

1. Introduction

The urgency of the work is associated with pandemic COVID-19 [1, 2]. Due to a large-scale pandemic, the SARSCoV-2 virus has become the focus of researchers around the world [3]. To date, the pathogenetic mechanisms of development of COVID-19 are insufficiently studied [4]. Changes in the mental status of patients complicate the course of the disease [5–7]. The search for markers of complex pathological processes that occur in COVID-19 to improve methods of diagnosis, treatment, control of long-term results of this dangerous disease, which course largely depends on the adaptive capacity of the body is continued [3].

The level of adaptability of the body is one of the important health criteria [8]. The circulatory system with its neurohumoral control apparatus and self-regulation is a universal indicator of the adaptive activity of the whole body [9].

An available method for assessing global hemodynamic processes is blood pressure (BP) monitoring [8–16]. The response of blood vessels to compression indicates: the state of coordination between local self-regulatory mechanisms and the central, neurohumoral regulation of the cardiovascular system (CVS) [13–16]; the level of the autonomic nervous system (ANS) [11, 12]; functional ability of the heart, reflex reaction of CVS [14, 15]; the state of the peripheral vascular bed (tone, elasticity, resilience, patency) [15, 16], the activity of the mechanisms of the urgent reaction to compression (baroreceptors, chemoreceptors, ischemia reflex), etc [14–16].

Various invasive and non-invasive devices are used to record the arterial signal [17–22]. The introduction of information technology for its analysis makes it possible to significantly expand the informativeness of blood pressure measurement results [23–28]. The methods used in the mathematical analysis of heart rate variability (HRV) are promising for assessing arterial pulsations [19, 20, 22].

HRV is an integral indicator of the functional state of the body, reflecting the activity of the main physiological systems. It makes it possible to obtain information from 4 levels of CVS regulation activity: peripheral, autonomic, hypothalamic–pituitary, central nervous system [8, 9, 24–26]. A minimum number of levels of the system is involved with optimal regulation to ensure the adaptation of the body. The inclusion of higher levels of regulation is due to the inability of the previous ones to cope with their functions and, if necessary, to coordinate the activities of several subsystems. The higher the body's adaptive capacity, the more reliable the protection, the lower the risk of disease [8, 9, 12, 13, 28–30].

How do adaptation processes occur in patients with COVID-19? To date, the pathogenetic mechanisms of development of COVID-19 are insufficiently studied [4]. Our study is devoted to the determination of the adaptive capacity of the body and the mechanisms of their violation in the severe course of COVID-19 using arterial oscillography AOG.

2. Methods

The studies are based on the results of temporal, spectral, correlation analysis of AOG, registered during the measurement of BP. 67 patients with severe COVID-19 who were treated at the Ternopil Regional Phthisio-Pulmonology Center (main group) were examined. The control group (573 patients) included students of I. Horbachevsky Ternopil National Medical University and Volodymyr Hnatiuk Ternopil National Pedagogical University, as well as 28 patients who were treated in a Closed Department of Ternopil Regional Psychoneurological Hospital.

The main group included 67 patients with COVID-19, who were prescribed intensive care at the Ternopil Regional Phthisio-Pulmonology Center. Among them – 34 (50.7%) men and 33 (49.3%) women. By age – up to 20 years – 1 (1.5%), 21–40 – 19 (28.4%), 41–46 – 29 (43.3%), over 60 years – 18 (26.8%). The most typical complaints of patients on admission: fever and cough (100%), shortness of breath (79.1%), general weakness (71.6%), sore throat (47.8%), loss of smell (38.8%) and taste (23.9%), chest pain (31.3%), hyperhidrosis (28.4%). Complaints of depression or euphoria, insomnia, mood swings with aggression, sometimes psychomotor agitation were observed in 26.8% of patients. The study was conducted from March to September 2020.

The diagnosis was made on the basis of anamnesis, complaints, contact with other patients, laboratory tests, in particular the detection of genetic material (RNA) SARS-CoV-2 by polymerase chain reaction. A positive result of the polymerase chain reaction was observed in 57 (85.1%). Saturation is less than 95% – in 26 (38.8%), changes in the lungs on the radiograph – in 65 (97.0%) patients. Among laboratory indicators lymphopenia (34.3%) and accelerated ESR (41.8%) were noted. Nonspecific flora was found in the sputum of 19 people (28.4%). Among comorbidities, cardiovascular diseaes (46.3%). After performed treatment, patients in satisfactory condition were discharged to continue outpatient treatment.

AOG was recorded during BP measurement when patient's admission and during treatment. 282 AOGs were registered. The article presents an analysis of 68 of them (registered on admission).

The control group included 548 people aged 18–22 without health complaints (CG-1), selected by random, voluntarily, by oral consent. CG-2 included 28 patients treated in a closed department of a psychoneurological hospital. AOG was recorded in them during the BP measurement in the process of treatment. The research results were used for comparative assessment of the adaptive capacity of the cardiovascular, autonomic, central nervous systems of the experimental and control groups.

CG-1 consitsed of 3 groups. CG 1-a – the largest one, included 548 people aged 18–22 without health complaints. AOG was registered in them at rest. The obtained results were used for their general assessment as a standard of indicators of AOG of healthy and comparison with patients with COVID -19 [19].

CG 1-b included 54 persons of the control group, electrocardiogram (ECG) synchronously with AOG was recorded, who were also subjected to temporal and spectral analysis [9, 10, 20, 21]. The obtained results were used for comparative analysis of the correspondence of individual indicators of HRV electrocardiographic signal [8–10, 25] and AOG [19–22].

CG 1-c included 68 members of the control group (45 males and 23 females) aged 18–22 without health complaints. AOG was recorded at rest, immediately after the Ruffier test (30 squats in 45 second, [9, 27] and after 2 minutes of rest). Used to study the dynamics of AOG under the influence of stress (physiological) factors, assessment of adaptation mechanisms at the same time and comparison with indicators of patients with severe COVID-19.

CG-2 included 28 patients (aged 32–65) who were treated at the Ternopil Regional Clinical Psychoneurological Hospital (TRCPH), in a Closed Department for patients with mental disorders. The choice for monitoring CG-2 is due to the appearance in the information sources of indications for the presence of patients with COVID-19 mental disorders in the form of depression, euphoria, insomnia, mood swings with aggression, sometimes psychomotor agitation on the background of severe hypoxia [3, 5–7]. Complaints and indicators of temporal and correlation analysis of AOG in patients of the closed department were closest to AOG in patients with COVID-19 [21].

The CG-2 examination program included clinical and psychological studies (clinical and psychological interview, collection of psychological history). The main range of diagnoses: paranoid schizophrenia, bipolar disorder and severe depressive disorders with psychotic inclusions, requiring systematic and long-term, usually lifelong use of antipsychotropic drugs.

Arterial oscillography. The information technologies of temporal, spectral, correlation analysis of AOG registered at BP measurement (in shoulder compression growth) by means of the electronic tonometer VAT 41–2, ICS Techno [19–21] are developed in the work. For their analysis, the methods, indicators, terminology used in the study and evaluation of the results of mathematical analysis of HRV electrocardiographic signal were used [8, 9, 14, 24–34]. We analyzed both the indicators obtained during the compression of the shoulder, and in its individual (five) periods [19–22] to study and evaluate the process of adaptation of the body to shoulder compression.

Temporal analysis of oscillograms was performed by statistical analysis of the variability of the pulsation duration [19–21]. The values of indicators were studied: SDSD, RMSSD, pNN50, Mo, AMo, BP; IVR, VPR, IN, HVR index. Temporal analysis makes it possible to assess the state of the cardiovascular, autonomic nervous systems and the level of centralization management of their activities [8, 9, 14, 24–34].

Spectral (frequency) analysis of oscillograms. Realization of rhythmic activity of heart is possible only in certain phase relations between oscillating brain and cardiac processes. The control system of these rhythms is functionally and morphologically part of a single adaptive vertical, ensuring the adaptation of the body to conditions of external and internal environment [8, 9, 14, 24–34].

Spectral analysis of AOG was performed by determining the power of the spectrum in the range from 0 to 0.4 Hz: HF – high frequencies, LF, VLF, ULF (low, very low and ultra-low frequencies). Fast, slow, very slow and ultra-slow regulation is controlled by all links (parasympathetic, sympathetic, humoral, thermoregulatory, etc.). The influence of PSL is greater in fast, sympathetic - in slow and very slow, and humoral - in very slow and ultra-slow regulation [8, 9, 14, 24–34]. Due to indicators in the ranges: 0–4 Hz (Delta), 4–8 Hz (Theta), 8–13 Hz (Alpha), 13–25 Hz, 25 Hz and more Hz (Beta) were able to determine the level of brain activity. For this purpose, Fourier and Hilbert-Huang transform methods were used, which reflect the general and instantaneous adaptive response to shoulder compression [24, 34].

Correlation analysis. In the correlation analysis of the arterial oscillogram, the values of the Pearson correlation coefficient from 0.9 to 1 and – 0.9 to –1 were taken into account. The selected correlation values were subject to Cluster analysis (k-means clustering) [35–38], where the calculated correlation values were grouped separately in the middle of one experiment in 12 clusters.

2.1 Statistical methods

Statistical analysis of the data was conducted using the software package "OscEcgReoPuls", which was developed in "Matlab". The statistical significance of differences between the arithmetic average and relative values was estimated by Student's t-test (t) for the normally distributed data set. For samples that differed from the normal distribution, the Wilcoxon method was used. During the comparison of all variants of indicators within the limits of one experiment, we conducted a liaison analysis of the correlation coefficient (r) by the Pearson method [37, 38]. Statistical calculation was additionally processed in Statistica 10 software.

The urgency of the work is associated with the pandemic COVID-19. The obtained results will help doctors to pay attention to possible variants of mechanisms of pathogenetic processes at COVID-19, to plan preventive, diagnostic, medical, rehabilitation process [4].

The obtained results will help doctors to pay attention to possible variants of mechanisms of development of pathogenetic processes at COVID-19, to plan preventive, diagnostic, medical, rehabilitation process.

3. Results

The results of the temporal analysis of AOG in the main and control groups.

Temporal analysis of oscillograms (by analogy with HRV) reflects the state of the ANS and the level of management centralization of the cardiovascular system.

Healthy persons of CG 1-b. To confirm the reliability of AOG in healthy, the representatives of CG 1-b underwent a temporal analysis of AOG and ECG, recorded synchronously at rest in 54 people aged 18–22 (**Figure 1**).

Cases of strong correlation between Mo, heart rate are obtained. RMSSD (0.97 ± 0.02, $p < 0.05$) on synchronously recorded ECG and AOG make it possible to conclude that the noted indicators characterize not only the level of control of the cardiac activity, but also blood vessels "peripheral heart" [8, 9, 14, 24–34] and confirm the high informativeness of the selected research methods. Similar results were obtained in the analysis of ECG time indicators from literature sources. So, according to I. V. Babunts [25], the Mo index is (0.8 ± 0.03) s, RMSSD – (0.43 ± 0.19) s, which coincides with our results and confirms the reliability of the indicators obtained in the analysis of AOG registered by us.

The results of the temporal analysis of AOG of healthy, patients with COVID-19 and patients undergoing treatment in a closed department of a psychoneurological hospital (PPNH) separately and in comparison with each other are presented in **Table 1**.

Patients with COVID-19 (main group). As can be seen from **Table 1**, in patients with COVID-19 (compared to healthy) there was an increase in SDSD, pHN50, BP ($P < 0.05$) and Mo ($P > 0.05$), a decrease in IVR, IN ($P < 0.05$) and AMo ($p > 0.05$). The results obtained (by analogy with the HRV ECG [8, 9, 14, 25, 26]) indicate a slight increase in the activity of the parasympathetic link of the ANS, the lack of sympathetic-adrenal response and management centralization of the body defenses of patients with COVID-19. Homeostasis can be maintained by increasing the activity of the sympathetic division of the ANS [8, 9]. The abovementioned is a vegetative correlator of anxiety and leads to a decrease in functional reserves and stress resilience.

Healthy persons of CG 1-c (Ruffier test). To study the reaction of healthy people to an extreme situation, we used a physiological stress situation – physical activity (30 squats in 45 seconds, Ruffier test). Normally, physical activity promotes the activation

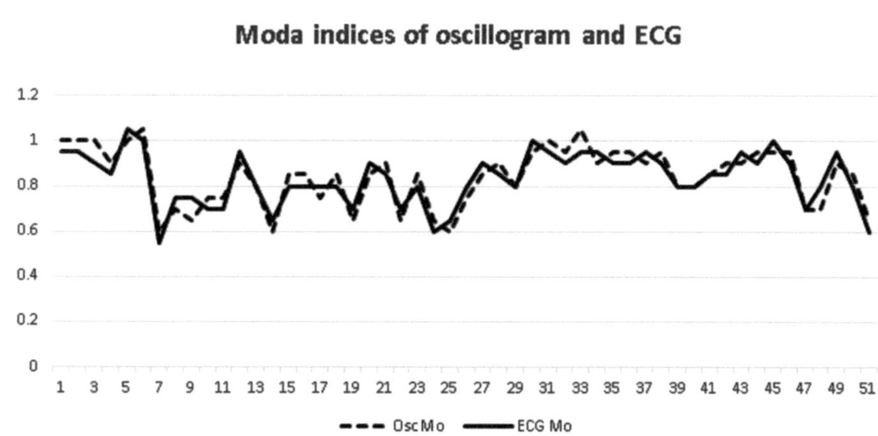

Figure 1.
Mode indicators (Mo), obtained by analysis of AOG and ECG. Note. On the X axis – A representative sample of 30 people, on the Y axis – On the left the duration of R-R intervals (s).

The studied indicator	The impact of growth on the stateANS**	COVID-19	Healthy	COVID-19 - healthy		PPNH			COVID-19 – PPNH	
		M±m	M±m	%	P	M±m	PPNH -3d		%	P
							%	P		
Mo, (s)	L-PS	0.848 ± 0.003	0.7945 ± 0.002	6.37	>0.05	0.7134+ 0.008	−10.15	>0.05	−15.87	>0.05
pNN50, (%)	L-PS	22.503 ± 0.094	14.894 ± 0.084	33.81	<0.05	26.10+ 0.247	75.24	<0,01	−1.39	>0.05
SDSD, (s)	L-PS	0.381 ± 0.002	0.16966 ± 0.001	55.64	<0.01	0.335+ 0.004	98.22	<0,01	−18.52	>0.05
AMo, (%)	L-S	31.68 ± 0.049	33.49 ± 0.143	−5.88	>0.05	31.19+ 0.407	−6.87	>0,05	−1.39	>0.05
IN, (y.o)	L-S	12.53 ± 0.037	22.80 ± 0.139	−32.04	<0.05	14.07+ 0.167	−38.0	<0,05	−18.52	>0.05
BP, (s)	L-S	0.89 ± 0.001	0.58 ± 0.003	25.64	<0.05	0.857+ 0.006	47.76	<0,01	9.87	>0.05
RMSSD, (s)	L-PS	0.38 ± 0.001	0.40 ± 0.002	−5.26	>0.05	0.335+ 0.004	−16.2	>0,05	−11.84	>0.05

*Note: * - informative value of the studied indicators: Mo (mode) - the range of oscillation duration values, which are most common (s); pHN50 - the percentage of consecutive intervals (separately highs and lows), the difference between which exceeds 50 ms; SDSD - standard deviation of differences between adjacent normal extremes (s); AMo (mode amplitude) - the number of intervals that correspond to the value of the mode (%); IN-voltage index of regulatory systems), BP (variation range) - the difference between the maximum and minimum values of the duration of the intervals between adjacent oscillations (s); RMSSD - the square root of the mean squares of the difference between adjacent extremes (s);*
***- value of increase (B) of indicators concerning activity of sympathetic (S) and parasympathetic (PS) links of ANS. More details are in the following text.*

Table 1.
Indicators of temporal analysis of AOG of healthy, patients with COVID-19 and persons undergoing treatment in a closed department of a psychoneurological hospital and their ratio.

of the central control circuit, accompanied by increased sympathetic activity and manifested by stabilization of the rhythm, reducing the scatter of the duration of cardio intervals, increasing the number of similar intervals [8, 9, 14, 25, 26, 34]. This is confirmed by the results of our research. A significant decrease in SDSD, pHN50 (**Figures 2-1a**), Mo ($P < 0.001$) (**Figures 2-2a**) and an increase in AMo ($P < 0, 01$), IVR, IN and HVR-index, standard deviation of oscillation amplitudes ($P < 0.001$) was registered on AOG in patients of group CG 1-c immediately after exercise. After 2 minutes of rest in most of the examined these indicators returned (or approached) to the initial ones (**Figure 2-b**).

For example, we demonstrate the dynamics of pNN50 and Mo registered in 30 members of group CG 1-c before, after exercise and in 2 minutes of rest (**Figure 2**).

As can be seen from **Figure 2**, after the Ruffier test, an increase in pNN50 (1) and Mo (2) and a return (approach) to the initial data after 2 minutes of rest is recorded. The observed dynamics of the studied indicators (by analogy with HRV on the ECG) indicates an increase in the tone of the sympathetic link of the ANS and increase the level of centralization of circulatory system management [8, 9, 14, 24–26, 34]. Return to the initial level of the studied indicators after 2 minutes of rest indicates a high level of regenerative capacity of the body after stress [27].

In patients with COVID-19, despite the extremely stressful situation, no similar dynamics of the studied parameters was observed. They were even lower than in healthy people at rest [9, 14, 24, 27, 34].

Patients of CG-2 (patients of psychoneurological hospital). As can be seen from **Table 1**, the results obtained of the temporal analysis of AOG in patients of the closed department in most cases had indicators similar to COVID-19, the difference between them was insignificant, had no reliability. This may indicate the same direction of pathological processes in patients with severe COVID-19 and in patients with mental disorders who are taking neuroleptics and are in a closed stay.

Spectral analysis of AOG indicators of the main and control groups.

The results of spectral analysis of AOG of healthy, patients with COVID-19 and PPNH are presented in **Table 2**.

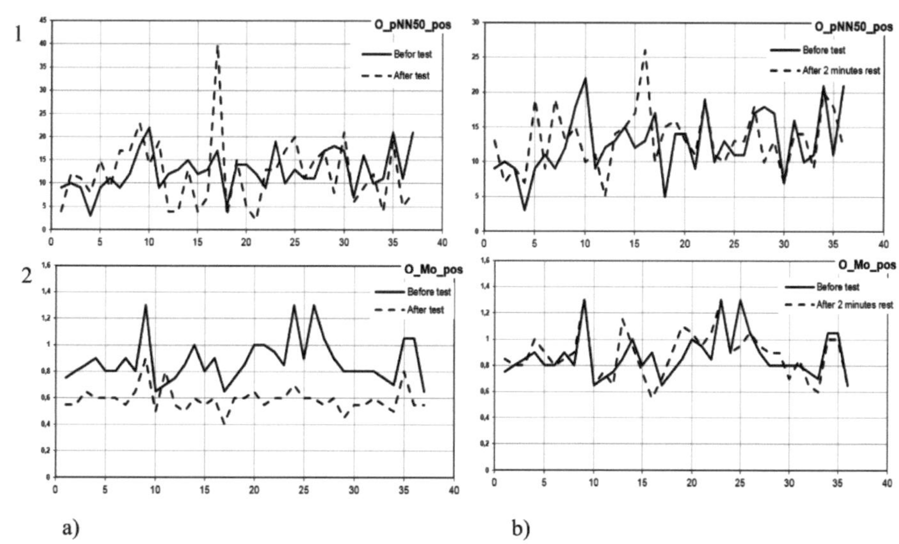

Figure 2.
Dynamics of pNN50 (1) and Mo (2): a) before and after the Ruffier test; b) before the Ruffier test and after 2 minutes of rest. Note. On the X axis – A representative sample of 30 patients; along the Y axis: in figure 2.1– pNN50 (%); figure 2.2. – Mo (s) in each of the patient. The dash line is before the exercise, the solid line is after it.

	Patients with COVID-19 (Co-19)	Healthy			Patients of psychoneurological hospital (PPNH)				
		Index M±m	Co-19- healthy	Co-19- healthy	PPNH				
					Index M±m	PPNH –healthy	PPNH –healthy	Co-19- PPNH	Co-19- PPNH
			%	P		%	P	(%)	P
%ULF	1.15 + 0.019	0.85 + 0.012	+26.1	<0.05	1.443 + 0.030	41.1	<0.01	−25.5	<0.05
%VLF	19.788 + 0.277	20.244 + 0.189	−7.36	>0.05	31/582 + 0.917	48.66	<0.01	−59.60	<0.01
%LF	9.27 + 0.065	10.24 + 0.064	−10.51	>0.05	8.543 + 0.169	−16.57	>0.05	+7.80	>0.05
%HF	69.814 + 0.418	67.64 + 0.349	+3.15	>0.05	57.718 + 1.373	−21.0	>0.05	+17.3	>0.05

*Note. * - informative value of the studied indicators:% HF - measure of high-frequency power,% LF - measure of low-frequency power,% VLF - measure of very low-frequency power,% ULF - measure of power of low-frequency domain in the general frequency spectrum. The influence of parasympathetic activity is greater in fast, sympathetic - in slow and very slow, and humoral - in very slow and ultra-slow regulation [8, 9, 14, 24–34]. These are described in more detail below.*

Table 2.
Indicators of spectral analysis of AOG of healthy, patients with COVID-19, patients of psychoneurological hospital (PPNH) and their ratios.

Patients with COVID-19 (main group). As can be seen from **Table 2**, there is a specific adaptive pattern in patients with COVID-19. A slight increase in the percentage of high-frequency domain power (% HF) in the total frequency spectrum (compared to healthy ones) is noteworthy. This (as well as the results of temporal analysis) indicates a shift in the autonomic balance in the direction of increasing the activity of the parasympathetic division of the ANS. While the degree of its inhibition (not the growth) is an indicator of increase of the tone of the sympathetic link of the ANS, necessary to maintain homeostasis [8, 9].

This was confirmed by the fact that the percentage of power of the LF spectrum was 10% lower than in healthy people. The LF spectrum is an indicator of the activity of the vasomotor center, reflects the sympathetic and parasympathetic effects from the level above the peripheral and to the centers of autonomic innervation in the medulla oblongata [9, 14, 24–26, 34]. They are regulated by the subcortical nodes and the cerebral cortex [8, 9].

% VLF was lower than in healthy. It reflects the influence of higher autonomic centers on the cardiovascular subcortical center. It can be used as a marker of the degree of connection of autonomous (segmental) levels of blood circulation regulation with suprasegmental, including pituitary–hypothalamic (with its nervous and humoral regulation) and cortical level [9, 24, 34].

It should be noted that according to the literature (according to HRV on the ECG) normally the power of % VLF in the total frequency range is 15–30% [9], that also corresponds to the indicators of our studies. The lack of dynamics of %VLF in patients with severe COVID-19 compared to healthy may indicate a violation of the above connections and functions of the corresponding levels of regulation.

At the same time, the %ULF in the total frequency spectrum is higher than in healthy (26%). The latter integrates and adapts the restructuring of the functional state of the body under the influence of external factors [9, 14, 24–26, 34]. The absence of a significant difference in %HF, %LF, %VLF in patients with COVID-19 and healthy may be due to the inability of the central control loop to integrate and adapt the restructuring of functional activity in severe disease. This can be attributed to the lack of necessary connections and coordination between the levels of regulation of the circulatory system in patients with COVID-19.

Since in this vertical the %VLF is already lower than in healthy ones (−3%), it is possible at this level the connection and coordination between the cortex and the lower levels of regulation of the circulatory system are suppressed.

It should be noted that recently there has been an assumption that patients with SARS-CoV-2 the cause of respiratory failure may be not only "damage to the lungs, but the brain stem, where the command center is located, which provides breathing even in unconsciousness" [36]. Probably, the information noted by us is a direction of markers search of the difficult pathological processes arising at COVID-19. Research is ongoing.

Healthy CG 1-c (Ruffier test). Spectral analysis of oscillograms (**Table 2**) showed that fast (HF) waves (indicator of the state of the parasympathetic link of the ANS) also dominated at rest in the general frequency spectrum.

Exercise helped to increase the percentage of spectrum power of low (%LF – $P < 0.01$) and ultra-low (%VLF – $P < 0.01$) frequencies, power of the Theta rhythm spectrum ($P < 0.01$) and reduce the level of high (%HF, $P < 0.01$) frequencies in the total frequency spectrum (**Figure 3**) At the same time, the synchronicity of changes in the %VLF and Theta spectra is noteworthy. This indicates an increase in the activity of the sympathetic division of the ANS after exercise, an increase in the centralization of the impact on the activity of the CVS and high stress resistance of the body in the examined patients [8, 9, 14, 24–26, 34]. After rest (**Figure 3**), the studied indicators returned (or approached) to the initial, which confirm the high

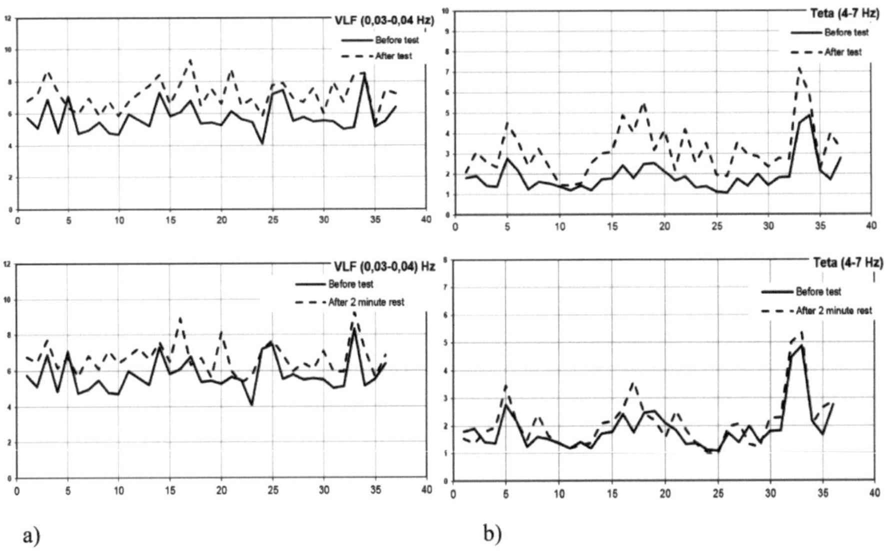

Figure 3.
Dynamics of VLF (left column) and Theta spectrum (right column) before, after the Ruffier test and after 2 minutes of rest. Note. On the X axis – A representative sample of 30 people, on the Y axis – The power of the spectrum (ms²); top line – Before and after exercise. Bottom line – Before exercise and after 2 minutes of rest. Before exercise – A dash line, after exercise – A solid line.

adaptability of the body of the patients [8, 9, 14, 24–26, 34]. Its slowing down is about the decrease of functional reserves and low stress resistance of the organism, which is a vegetative marker of anxiety [9, 10, 19, 24, 34].

It was noteworthy that (despite the difficult stressful situation due to the severe course of the disease) in patients with COVID-19 the marked direction of the adaptive response of the healthy body was not observed. This confirms the violation of function, coordination and communication in the hierarchical regulation of the circulatory system, which leads to a decrease in functional reserves and low stress resistance of the body.

Patients of CG-2 (PPNH). Frequent analysis of AOG of PPNH (**Table 2**) revealed a slight decrease in the percentage of weight of the spectrum of high (HF), low (LF) and a significant increase in the percentage of VLF (49%) and ULF (41%) frequencies compared to healthy. The last two reflect the activity of the central control circuit by the functional capacity of the cardiovascular system [12, 13, 28–30]. Their activities are closely related to psycho-emotional tensions [9]. It should be noted that in the norm, the power of the central control circuits occurs as a result of the reaction to a stressful situations and disappears in their absence [12, 13, 28–30], confirmed by the results of our (Ruffier test) studies. It is possible to predict that long tension of activity of the central contour of regulation integrating and adapting reorganization of functional activity of the body, can cause mental disorders of the presented group of patients.

When comparing the spectral analysis of patients with COVID-19 and PPNH, the long-term tension of %ULF in the total frequency spectrum was common, which can be associated with the presence of mental disorders.

3.1 Correlation analysis of AOG of the examined patients in main and control groups

Patients with COVID-19 (main group). Analysis of correlations in COVID-19 showed a limitation in their number. If in healthy people (group CG 1-c) 28 pairs of correlates were registered, in patients with COVID-19 – only 10. There were no temporal analysis indicators in the correlation pairs. Waves LF, VLF, HF occurred, respectively, in 15, 15, 5 percent of cases. Among the indicators of brain activity in pairs of correlates Theta rhythm was most common, Alpha, Beta, Gamma (20%, 15%, 10%, 5% – respectively) – less common. The highest aspect that connects the waves of brain activity with human health is the ability to change these states according to the requirements of the situation [24, 34, 39, 40]. In patients with COVID-19, only maximal compression provoked a slight inclusion in the correlations of brain activity, indicating a profound violation of the ability to adapt to external factors.

Healthy, CG 1-c (Ruffier test). Before exersice, correlations were recorded in 28 pairs of correlates, mainly between the temporal parameters of the oscillogram: Mo, AMo, NN50, IVR. In addition, between the waves of high (HF) and the slowest (VLF) frequency of spectral analysis and with temporal parameters in different numerical and percentage values and periods of compression.

Immediately after the Ruffier test, 19 pairs of correlates were recorded. The correlations of rest mostly disappeared. Participation in HF correlates also decreased from 16 to 8 cases. New ones appeared – most often between the absolute and percentage content of Theta, Alpha, Beta, Delta brain rhythms. They occurred (respectively) in 16%, 13%, 8%, 8% of cases and were registered during the entire shoulder compression. Gamma waves were not met.

The obtained results indicate an increase in the rhythms of brain and cardiac activity in healthy people after exercise of coordinated wave activity. Two minutes after the squats, the restoration of the vast majority of correlations inherent in the indicators before exercise was registered in the examined patients.

If we compare the results of the correlation analysis of AOG of healthy people after physiological stress (exercise) and patients with COVID-19, the main differences are that the number of correlates in healthy people is greater, they include indicators of temporal, spectral analysis and brain activity. The reaction in healthy people was manifested from the beginning to the end of compression, in patients – only in its last phases, with maximum compression of the shoulder.

Patients of CG-2 (PPNH). Surveys showed that among the 4 departments of the psycho-neurological hospital on AOG, the fewest correlations were registered in patients treated in a closed department. Actually, they were subject to study. The most common components of 12 correlation pairs were: Beta (20%), Gamma (14%), Delta (11%) rhythms of brain activity. In correlation pairs, Beta and Gamma, VLF and LF were combined. Ultra-low frequencies (VLF) occurred in 20%, %LF and %HF – once. The correlations is noticeable only in the last phases of shoulder compression.

If we compare the correlation portraits of patients with COVID-19 and the closed department, the Theta waves predominate in the first and Beta and the appearance of Gamma waves – in the second. The limited number of correlations between the rhythms of brain and heart activity in both groups was noteworthy. At the same time, they appeared only in the last phases of shoulder compression, which indicates a deep violation of the adaptive capacity to the influence of external factors. According to the results of research, we can predict the common pathogenetic mechanisms of mental disorders in patients with COVID-19 and PPNH [5–7].

4. Discussion

The research is aimed at finding markers of complex pathological processes that occur in COVID-19 and lead to a significant reduction in functional reserves, low stress resistance of the body and as a result - to severe disease and recovery processes in COVID-19. For this purpose (proposed by the authors), the temporal, spectral, correlation analysis of AOG [19–21] was used. The method is based on the adaptation of the mathematical analysis of heart rate variability (HRV) of the electrocardiographic signal [8, 9, 14, 24–34]. to the analysis of variability of the arterial pulsations registered during measurement of arterial pressure by means of the electronic tonometer of BAT 41–2.

The AOG method was developed by the authors for the first time. It is based on the personal experience of scientific researches on morphological, temporal, spectral, correlation analysis of 3500 AOG people of different ages and health conditions. In healthy people AOG was registered at rest and after exposure to various (mechanical, thermal, physical, psychological, etc.) factors. Patients with diseases of the cardiovascular, respiratory and nervous systems were submitted to oscillographic examination [19].

To substantiate the reliability of the results of arterial oscillography, a comparative analysis of the results of mathematical analysis of ECG and AOG synchronously registered at rest (54 people). Cases of strong correlation between Mo, heart rate are obtained. RMSSD (0.97 ± 0.02, $p < 0.05$) on synchronously recorded ECG and AOG make it possible to conclude that the observed indicators characterize not only the level of control of the heart, but also blood vessels "peripheral heart" [8, 9, 14, 24–34] and confirms the high informativeness of the selected research methods which ECG does not register [19–21].

For this study, we used temporal, spectral, correlation analysis of AOG, conducted and evaluated in 67 patients with severe COVID-19. The results compared with AOG of 28 patients at the closed ward of the psychoneurological hospital and 548 healthy (including 68 people after exercise and after 2 minutes of rest).

In patients with COVID-19, dysfunction, coordination and communication at all (four) levels of regulation of CVS activity, which is a universal indicator of adaptive activity of the whole organism [9]. There was a significant decrease in functional reserves and low stress resistance of the body due to the lack of sympathetic-adrenal response and centralization of body defense control, disruption of communication and coordination at all levels of the adaptive vertical. This is confirmed by the following research results.

1. An increase in SDSD, pHN50, BP ($P < 0.05$) and Mo ($P > 0.05$), decrease in IVR, IN ($P < 0.05$) and AMo ($p > 0.05$) compared to healthy people. The results obtained (by analogy with the HRV ECG) [8, 9, 14, 25, 26, 34] indicate the absence of sympathetic-adrenal response and centralization of the defense in patients' bodies with severe COVID-19. For comparison, the analysis of AOG was performed in 68 people without health complaints before and after exercise (Ruffier Test). After exercise (physiological stress), the statistically significant opposite dynamics of the above indicators was registered. This indicates an increase in the activity of the sympathetic ANS and the centralization of the impact on the CVS after exercise [9] and their recovery after 2 minutes of rest.

2. Examined patients with severe COVID-19 in terms of time and spectral parameters of AOG had the activity of the parasympathetic division of the ANS even higher than in healthy people at rest. While homeostasis can be maintained by increasing the activity of the sympathetic division of the ANS, which can be assessed by the degree of inhibition of its parasympathetic division [8, 9]. And the state of the autonomic response to external influences is the most accurate marker of reactivity and resistance of the organism [9, 14, 24, 27, 34, 39].

3. There was a decrease (compared to healthy) power % VLF, very low-frequency domain in the general frequency spectrum, a marker of the degree of connection of autonomous (segmental) levels of blood circulation regulation with suprasegmental, including pituitary–hypothalamic and cortical levels [9, 34]. Its decrease (compared to healthy) in severe COVID-19 may indicate a violation of the above links and functions of the relevant levels of regulation.

4. The growth of power % ULF, ultra-low-frequency domain in the total frequency spectrum, which integrates and adapts the restructuring of functional activity of the organism under the influence of external factors [9, 14, 24–26, 34] against the background of decreasing% VLF levels suppress the relationship between the cerebral cortex and the lower levels of regulation of CVS activity.

5. Analysis of correlations [35–38] in COVID-19 showed a limitation of their number both separately in the segments of time and spectral indicators, and between them. If 28 pairs of correlates were registered in healthy people (group KG 1-s), then only 10 in patients with COVID-19 were noted. At the same time, they appeared mainly in the last (maximum) phases of shoulder compression. This confirms a significant reduction in the adaptive capacity of the body, when only the maximum compression of the shoulder had the ability to bring them out of this state.

6. The appearance of mental disorders in patients with COVID-19 [5–7]. provoked us to compare the adaptation model which their body builds under the influence of the disease and in patients of a closed ward of a psychoneurological hospital who are constantly taking neuroleptics. At the last ones, it was found most similar to other members of psychiatric wards. There was no significant difference in the results of temporal, correlation analysis of AOG and a significant increase in both cases% ULF in the total frequency spectrum (whose activity is closely related to psycho-emotional stress). This may indicate the same direction of pathological processes in both groups of subjects and justify the presence of mental disorders in patients with COVID-19.

7. The conducted researches gave the chance to reach the set purpose and to inform readers about the following.

    A. At patients with COVID-19 mechanisms of decrease in adaptive ability of an organism, disturbance of a functional condition of cardiovascular, autonomic, central nervous systems, mental frustration are revealed and proved. The obtained results will help doctors to pay attention to possible variants of mechanisms of development of pathogenetic processes at COVID-19 and to consider them at a choice of means of correction of the noted disturbances and to include in the protocol of diagnosis, treatment and rehabilitation of patients with COVID-19 at inpatient and outpatient stages of treatment.

    B. Informative and effective application of arterial oscillography (according to D.V. Vakulenko, L.O. Vakulenko), which can be a mean of finding markers of complex pathological processes that occur in COVID-19. It can be used to improve methods of diagnosis, treatment, rehabilitation, control of long-term results of this dangerous disease in clinical and family medicine.

    C. For implementation in practice new models of electronic blood pressure monitors it is necessary to provide the possibility of using the AOG method (D. Vakulenko, L. Vakulenko). The device has the ability to record the values of cuff pressure during compression and export the values for further analysis. AOG includes: measurement of blood pressure, sending data to the personal account of VEP-service Oranta-AO, obtaining the results of the analysis in the form of values of indicators and recommendations of the expert system for further decision-making by the doctor.

8. The authors continue research in various fields, collaborate with physiologists, cardiologists, neurologists and other specialists for further substantiate AOG methods.

9. Prospects for research on this problem: morphological analysis of AOG, comprehensive analysis of the dynamics of AOG patients with COVID-19, testing of the expert system to support decision-making at the stages of inpatient treatment and rehabilitation after the disease in outpatient treatment, under the supervision of a family doctor.

5. Conclusion bioethics commission

Protocol No. 7, Meeting of the Bioethics Commission of I. Horbachevsky Ternopil National Medical University of the Ministry of Health of Ukraine of January 25, 2021.

Resolved: Materials of the article by D.V. Vakulenko L.O. Vakulenko L.A. Hryshchuk I.M. Sas On topic: "The use of arterial oscillography to study the adaptive capacity of the body of patients with COVID-19", on examination of patients, performing laboratory, scientific researches meets requirements of norms and principles of bioethics.

Funding

The study did not receive a specific grant from any funding agency in the public, commercial, or nonprofit sectors.

Conflict of interest figures and tables

The authors declare no conflict of interest.

Authors' contributions

Vakulenko D. V. developed the concept and design of the work. Registered AOG downloaded to a PC and subjected to temporal, spectral, correlation analysis using the OscEcgReoPuls program, developed by the authors of the study; conducted statistical processing, analysis, interpretation of the results; participated in the design of the article.

Vakulenko L. O. – co-author of the methods of temporal, spectral, correlation analysis of AOG; made a significant contribution to the concept and design of work; conducted analysis and interpretation of AOG data; participated in the design of the article.

Hryshchuk L. A. conducted examination, treatment, registration of AOG in patients with COVID-19; participated in the analysis and interpretation of AOG data.

Sas L. M. conducted examination, treatment, registration of AOG in patients of the closed department of the psychoneurological hospital; participated in the analysis and interpretation of AOG data.

Author details

Dmytro Vakulenko[1*], Liudmyla Vakulenko[2], Leonid Hryshchuk[1] and Lesya Sas[1]

1 I. Horbachevsky Ternopil National Medical University, Ternopil, Ukraine

2 V. Hnatiuk Ternopil National Pedagogical University, Ternopil, Ukraine

*Address all correspondence to: dmitro_v@ukr.net

References

[1] Zhu, N., Zhang, D., Wang, W., Li, X., Yang, B., Song, J., Zhao, X., Huang, B., Shi, W., Lu, R., et al. 2020. A novel coronavirus from patients with pneumonia in China, 2019. New England Journal of Medicine. 382:727-733. https://doi.org/10.1056/NEJMoa 2001017.

[2] World Health Organization. 2020. Q&A on coronaviruses (COVID-19). Retrieved on May 1, 2020 from https:// www.who.int/news-room/q-a-detail/ q-a-coronaviruses.

[3] Komisarenko, S. World COVID-19 crisis. Kyiv: LAT & K, 2020. 120 p. ISBN 978-617-7824-26-7 https://files.nas.gov. ua/PublicMessages/.../0/.../2009241523 50305-1709.pdf. Ukrainian. https:// medikom.ua/koronavirus-simptomy-i-profilaktika/.

[4] Singh R, Sarsaiya S, Singh TA, Singh T, Pandey LK, Pandey PK, Khare N, Sobin F, Sikarwar R, Gupta MK. Corona Virus (COVID-19) Symptoms Prevention and Treatment: A Short Review. JDDT [Internet]. 15Apr.2021 [cited 25May2021];11(2-S): 118-20. Available from: http:// jddtonline.info/index.php/jddt/article/ view/4644

[5] Carod-Artal F.J. Neurological complications of coronavirus and COVID-19. Revista de Neurologia. 2020. 70(9): 311– 322. DOI: https://doi. org/10.33588/rn.7009.2020179

[6] Brooks M. COVID-19 Tied to Wide Range of Neuropsychiatric Complications. Medscape. June 29, 2020. https:// www.medscape.com/ viewarticle/933136

[7] Cormier Z. How Covid-19 can damage the brain. BBC News. 23 June 2020. https://www.bbc.com/future/ article/ 20200622-the-long-term-effects-of-covid-19-infection

[8] Heart rate variability. Standards of measurement, physiological interpretation, and clinical use Task Force of The European Society of Cardiology and The North American Society of Pacing and Electrophysiology (Membership of the Task Force listed in the Appendix. Heart Journal, Mar. 1996, vol. 17, p. 354-381

[9] Baevsky, R.M., Berseneva, A.P. Estimation of adaptive possibilities of an organism and risk of development of diseases. Moscow: Meditsina. 1997. 265 p. Russian.

[10] Nirmalan M, Dark PM. Broader applications of arterial pressure wave form analysis. Continuing Education in Anaesthesia Critical Care & Pain 2014; 14(6): 285-290.

[11] Moxham IM. Understanding arterial pressure waveform. Southern African Journal of Anaesthesia and Analgesia 2003; 9(1): 40-42, doi: 10.1080/22201173.2003.10872991.

[12] Caro CG, Pedley TJ, Schroter RC, et al. The mechanics of the circulation. 2nd ed. London: Cambridge University Press; 2012.

[13] Tartiere JM, Tabet JY, Logeart D, et al. Noninvasively determined radial dP/ dt is a predictor of mortality in patients with heart failure. Am Heart J 2008; 155(4): 758-763.

[14] Goldberger AL, Stein PK. Evaluation of heart rate variability. UpToDate [cited 02.09.2018]. Available from URL: https://www.uptodate. com/ contents/evaluation-of-heart-rate-variability.

[15] Pokrovsky, A.V. Clinical angiology. Moscow: Meditsina; 1979. Russian.

[16] Warner HR, Swan SH, Connolly DC, et al. Quantitation of beat-to-beat changes in stroke volume from the aortic pulse contour in man. J Appl Physiology 1953; 5: 495-507.

[17] Langewouters GJ, Wesseling KH, Goedhard WJ. The static elastic properties of 45 human thoracic and 20 abdominal aortas in vitro and the parameters of a new model. J Biomech 1984; 17(6): 425-435.

[18] Chamos C, Vele L, Hamilton M, et al. Less invasive methods of advanced hemodynamic monitoring: principles, devices, and their role in the perioperative hemodynamic optimization. Perioper Med (Lond) 2013; 2(1): 19, doi: 10.1186/2047-0525-2-19.

[19] Vakulenko, D.V. Information system of morphological, temporal, frequency and correlation analysis of arterial oscillograms in physical rehabilitation: monograph. Ternopil: TSMU; 2015. Ukrainian.

[20] Vakulenko DV, Martseniuk VP, Vakulenko LO, Selskyy PR, Kutakova OV, Gevko OV, Kadobnyj TB. Cardiovascular system adaptability to exercise according to morphological, temporal, spectral and correlation analysis of oscillograms. Fam Med Prim Care Rev 2019; 21(3): 253-263, doi: https://doi.org/10.5114/fmpcr.2019.88385.

[21] Vakulenko, D.V., Vakulenko, L.O., Kutakova OV. Application of spectral and correlation methods of analysis of biosignals in psychophysiology. Psychophysiological and visceral functions in normal and pathology": VIII International Scientific Conference dedicated to the 175th anniversary of the Department of Physiology and Anatomy of Man and Animals of Kyiv Taras Shevchenko National University. October 17-20, 2017. Kyiv Taras Shevchenko National University. Kyiv, RA AMT LLC. Ukrainian.

[22] Martsenyuk V, Vakulenko D, Vakulenko L, Kłos-Witkowska A, Kutakova O. Information System of Arterial Oscillography for Primary Diagnostics of Cardiovascular Diseases. Lecture Notes in Computer Science (including subseries Lecture Notes in Artificial Intelligence and Lecture Notes in Bioinformatics), 17th International Conference, CISIM 2018; 2018 Sep 27-29; Olomouc, Czech Republic. Berlin: Springer; 2018: P. 46-56.

[23] Shachak A, Borycki E, Shmuel P. ReisHealth Professionals' Education in the Age of clinical information systems, mobile computing and social networks. Academic Press; 2017.

[24] "Dynamics" computer complex for assessing the functional state of the human body: user documentation. St. Petersburg: Dynamics, 2011. 59 p. Russian.

[25] Babunts, I.V., Miridzhanyan, Z.M., Mashaekh, Yu.A. Heart rate variability ABC [E-book]. Stavropol; 2002. Russian.

[26] Yabluchanskyy, N.I., Martynenko, A.V. Heart rate variability to aid the practitioner. For real doctors. Kharkiv: [b. v.]. Russian.

[27] Amosov, N.M., Bendet, Y.A. Physical activity and heart. 3rd ed. Kyiv: Zdorovia; 1989. Russian.

[28] Lombardi F, Stein PK. Origin of heart rate variability and turbulence: an appraisal of autonomic modulation of cardiovascular function. Front Physiol 2011; 2: 95, doi: 10.3389/fphys.2011.00095.

[29] Sassi R, Cerutti S, Lombardi F, et al. Advances in heart rate variability signal analysis: joint position statement by the e-Cardiology ESC Working Group and

the European Heart Rhythm Association co-endorsed by the Asia Pacific Heart Rhythm Society. Europace 2015; 17(9): 1341-1353, doi: 10.1093/europace/euv015.

[30] Klaus Forstner, inventor. Microlife Intellectual Property Gmbh, assignee. System and method for processing and presentation of arrhythmia information in the detection and treatment of arrhythmias. US 7907996 B2 (Patent) 2011 March. Available from URL: https:// patents.justia.com/inventor/klaus-forstner.

[31] Goss CF, Miller EB. Dynamic Metrics of Heart Rate Variability 2013; 1-4. arXiv:1308.6018. Bibcode:2013arXiv 1308.6018G. Available from URL: https://arxiv.org/abs/1308.6018.

[32] Takahashi N, Kuriyama A, Kanazawa H, et al. Validity of spectral analysis based on heart rate variability from 1-minute or less ECG recordings. Pacing Clin Electrophysiol 2017; 40(9): 1004-1009, doi: 10.1111/pace.13138.

[33] Chantler PD, Lakatta EG, Najjar SS. Arterial-ventricular coupling: mechanistic insights into cardiovascular performance at rest and during exercise. J Appl Physiol 2008; 105: 1342-1351

[34] Smirnov K.Yu., Development and research of methods of mathematical modeling and analysis of bioelectric signals / K.Yu. Smirnov, Yu.A. Smirnov. - St. Petersburg: Dynamics, 2001. 60 p.

[35] E.M. Mirkes, K-means and K-medoids applet.\ MirkesE.M. University of Leicester, 2011

[36] Winters R, Winters A, Amedee RG. Statistics: a brief overview. Ochsner J 2010; 10: 213-216.

[37] Lee Rodgers J, Nicewander WA, Thirteen ways to look at the correlation coefficient. Am Stat 1988; 42(1): 59-66.

[38] Coates A, Ng AY. Learning Feature Representations with K-means. Stanford University, 2012. Available from URL: https://www-cs.stanford.edu/~acoates/papers/coatesng_nntot2012.pdf. COVID-1938

[39] Mintser O., Martsenyuk V., Vakulenko D. (2020) On Data Mining Technique for Differential Diagnostics Based on Data of Arterial Oscillography. In: Zawiślak S., Rysiński J. (eds) Engineer of the XXI Century. Mechanisms and Machine Science, vol 70. Springer, Cham, https://doi.org/10.1007/978-3-030-13321-4_23

[40] Siver David. Mind machines. Rediscovering ABC Technology, 2000. Available from: http://www.mindmachine.ru/book/. Russian.

Section 5

Mental Health Prevention in Primary Care

Chapter 14

The Need to Strengthen Primary Health Care Services to Improve Mental Health Care Services in South Africa

Kebogile Elizabeth Mokwena and Velaphi Anthony Mokwena

Abstract

Despite the reported increase in the prevalence of mental disorders, including substance abuse disorders, required services in South Africa have not been improved to meet the demands for these challenges. Although South Africa has invested in a process to conduct a re-engineering of primary health care services to address a range of common health challenges in communities, this process has not demonstrated adequate policy and practice changes toaddress emerging challenges in providing services for mental health disorders at primary health care level. In particular, primary health care services do not include routine screening for common mental disorders, which include depression, anxiety, postnatal depression and substance abuse, although there are easy to use tools for such screening. This has resulted in a failure for early detection of these mental health challenges by the health system. The chapter argues that making moderate changes to the current offerings of primary health care can result in major achievements in offering mental health services, which in turn will benefit the patients and assist health services to address the increasing scourge of mental disorders, which include substance abuse.

Keywords: Primary health care re-engineering, South Africa, mental health, substance abuse, screening

1. Introduction

The increase in the prevalence of non-communicable diseases has been widely reported, and among these is the category of mental disorders. Recent literature has reported that mental disorders have been on the rise exponentially, and account for an estimated 25% of all health-related disability worldwide [1], which highlights the need to prioritize treatment for this group of disorders. Although some health systems in some world regions and countries have acknowledged and have started to respond to this need, others lag behind. Health care systems are generally ideally organized to treat more people at lower levels of care, and decrease the proportion as the level of care increases. This is feasible because the less severity of illness can be easier managed at lower levels of care, where the illness requires less specialization and treatment costs are less because at this level

 IntechOpen

most illnesses have not yet complicated. This approach has resulted in the globally accepted and promoted approach of placing Primary Health Care (PHC) services to offer optimal health services to the majority of citizens of a country. Primary healthcare (PHC) is thus acknowledged to be the foundation of well-functioning healthcare systems, and is the success indicator of attempts to improve health provision services. In fact, the 1978 Alma Ata declaration confirmed this view, by establishing and promoting PHC as a cornerstone of global health services provision [2]. The significance of the position of PHC services applies despite differences in regional and country wealth, and if well resourced and well run, PHC services can improve the offering of health services for the poor, and so decrease the differences in health outcomes across wealth bands. The South African government envisages the provision of primary health care as a service that should be provided to the whole population, which includes communities of low socio-economic status. During the Millennium Development Goals (MDG) era, and transcending to the Sustainable Development Goals (SDG) era, countries that were able to make strides towards achieving their goals, such as Brazil and Thailand, are those that prioritized the improvement of their PHC systems [3]. It is for that reason that PHC should be the focus of service provision for the increasing scourge of mental illness.

1.1 Substance abuse within mental disorders

The use of psychoactive substances affects mental function at both the short and long- term basis, hence the treatment of substance abuse disorders by mental health professionals. Moreover, literature also shows a bilateral association between the use of psychoactive substances and mental disorders [4], which implies that not only is mental illness a risk factor for later substance abuse [5], but substance abuse is also a risk factor for the development of mental illness [6]. This makes interventions for the prevention of substance dependence an important secondary outcome of interventions for early-onset mental disorders. For purposes of this chapter, reference to mental disorders includes substance abuse.

2. Cues and guidelines from the National Development Plan 2030

The South African National Development Plan (NDP) is the blueprint of how the South African government plans to improve the quality of services to achieve transformation that will improve the lives of the majority of people who were previously marginalized [7]. The NDP further identifies the need for a functional monitoring process as the basis of offering and improving the envisaged outcomes because without monitoring, it is not possible to determine the progress made towards any one goal. Chapter 10 of the National Development Plan acknowledges the promotion of health as a key to speed up transformation. The NDP further proposes to address a variety of social determinants of health, including mental health and substance abuse trends. The NDP further acknowledges the importance of considering the needs of the community, as well as embracing and elevating the role of society in addressing community needs. The scourge of mental disorders fits the category of community needs, and addressing them is an example of using the NDP to guide government responses to service delivery. The NDP further promotes the systematic use of data incorporating community health, prevention and environmental concerns, which is a focus area of the Primary health Care programme.

DOI: http://dx.doi.org/10.5772/intechopen.99781

3. The scourge of mental disorders

As the prevalence on non-communicable diseases increase, mental health and wellbeing have been identified as central to reducing the global burden of this group of diseases [8]. The World Health Organization's mental health action plan for 2013-2020 advocates for this integration because of the significant associations between common mental health disorders and other cardio cardiovascular diseases and common mental disorders, as well as the two groups sharing risk factors. The integration of mental health services seems to be so natural that their separation is regarded as a false divide [1]. Primary health care services present opportunities to offer universal health care to Africa [9]. However, this can be achieved if such services are well planned and adequately resourced with the right quantity of the right categories of staff [10].

3.1 Substance abuse in schools as a mental health issue

There are reports of an increasing prevalence of substance abuse in schools in South Africa [11], both in rural [12], as well as urban areas [13, 14], which calls for prevention as well as treatment interventions to address the challenges of substance abuse in schools. However, the focus of schools is mainly on academic development and outcomes. This often leaves both short and long-term impacts of other behaviors such as substance abuse, not receiving adequate attention.

On their own, schools are not equipped to deal with substance abuse, which identified a gap, which can and should be met by primary health care services. The inability of the school system to address the challenges related to substance abuse is demonstrated by the existence of the National Policy on Drug Abuse Management in Schools of 2002, which was meant to counteract the use of substances by learners. However, a study to assess the extent to which this policy was being implemented by schools found that the policy is not even known, let alone used by schools [15]. For most communities and schools, there is nothing that has been put in place for the prevention, screening or treatment of substance abuse, and upgrading primary health care services to provide these services will be a highly beneficial asset.

4. The urgency of addressing mental disorders

As the prevalence of mental disorders increase, related mental health services remain chronically under-resourced. The impact of mental illness is not limited to the patient, but also extends to the family, as mental distress has been identified among family members of psychiatric patients [16]. Additionally, those family members also need health care services, thus a continuous addition of people who need mental health services. On the other hand, the high prevalence of substance abuse in South Africa increases demands for mental health services [17]. Mental health services remain chronically under-resourced [18], which implies major unmet needs for mental health care. The lack of adequate resources has been interpreted as apathy by governments and funders to mitigate this human, social and economic costs of mental illness [19].

As in other countries, and in the absence of a well developed primary health care system to address mental illness, the current system of relying on mental hospitals as a mode of service provision is dominant in South Africa. Not only is this mode unrealistic for resource-constrained countries, but it limits the extent to which mental illness needs are met, as these hospitals are too few and expensive to meet the needs of the people who need such services. Moreover, the dependence on this mode contributes to non-prioritization of development of community-based resources and infrastructure.

Primary care delivery platform has been identified as ideal to address behavioral health, including substance abuse and mental disorders, as this level can be enhanced to effectively address these conditions [20]. Due to inadequate access to specialty substance use disorders, it is estimated that only 10% of people with substance use disorders (SUD) actually receive treatment [21], and this could be improved if such disorders were treated at primary health care levels, which is, by design, able to treat a greater proportion of the population. Delays in treating such patients contributes to major poor prognosis.

5. Qualities of a responsive health care system

Optimal health systems are those that respond to the needs of the people who rely on such services, which explains the regional and country variations of availability of services. As an example, when the global number of HIV infections were rising, HIV related services at primary health care levels were strengthened, which enabled an increased number of patients to access treatment nearer their homes and communities. Primary health care services were also improved to offer comprehensive HIV related services, which were not limited to the contracting the virus, but included services such as prevention of HIV, promotion of positive behavior change and health literacy about HIV [22]. The development of extensive community health services were also trained at this level, which further increased access to PHC services and cater for community health needs [23]. This approach was effective because it utilized local community workers who were able to identify relevant community needs [24], and the model can be duplicated for the promotion of mental health and prevention of mental disorders.

6. The appropriateness of primary health care services for mental health services

The advantages of the PHC as appropriate for the delivery of health services are many, including that most of such facilities are in communities and many clients are within walking distance to the nearest clinic. However, the availability of a structure does not necessarily guarantee optimal health services, as some of the clinics fall short of providing intended basic services. This implies that there is a need to continuously assess the functionality of primary health care services, to determine their relevance and effectiveness in providing services that are determined by community needs and priorities. An example of this gap is the increase in substance abuse and mental health challenges that have been prevalent in the last few years, and the failure of the health system to respond to the needs in the context of related services. As with other African countries, the South African Primary health care (PHC) nurse led [25], which is confirmed by the proportion of nurses compared to other health professionals, and the services rendered at PHC levels. It is for that reason that government can afford to offer services at no cost to the client as the State bears such costs [26].

What substance abuse and mental health have in common is that both are significantly impacted upon by social issues, which means that failure to respond appropriately may subject more members of the affected communities to similar

DOI: http://dx.doi.org/10.5772/intechopen.99781

challenges, which just increases the community burden of substance abuse and mental disorders. The increasing prevalence in both substance abuse and mental disorders has been well documented, but there is silence on how the PHC system has been prepared to respond in the appropriate manner. On the contrary, there is inequitable access to substance abuse treatment services in South Africa, and that, even among those that have access, the quality of services is often not ascertained. This is demonstrated by the action of government limiting itself to ensuring access but not putting adequate efforts to ensure quality that will improve treatment outcomes [27, 28]. The strengthening of PHC services in the area of mental health will thus increase access to the benefit of those that lacked such access. The monitoring of substance abuse services at PHC level, which is essential for making decisions, is not optimal [29].

7. The importance of the 1978 Alma Ata declaration in health service provision

The 1978 Alma Ata declaration envisaged primary health care to be the vehicle to achieve health for all. However, this outcome can only be achieved if the key principles of the Alma Ata are implemented, which include the requirement that services be driven by community needs and priorities, which will encourage and enable community participation, and the strengthening of the capacity of the district management system [30]. Because the cost of care increases with the level of care, primary health care services are at the most cost effective level for offering health care, which is ideal for a resource-constrained country like South Africa. However, failing to offer such services increases health care costs because of additional complications which needs to be addressed at a higher level of care, and which comes with higher costs and requires longer treatment periods.

8. Re-engineering of primary health care

Although the health budget of South Africa is on the upper end if compared to some of its neighbors, its health outcomes do not reflect that. This discordant has been attributed to a weak primary health care system [31]. The purpose of the re-engineering of Primary Health Care (PHC) is to improve both access and quality of health services to the general public. The need for the re-engineering was identified when the South African government acknowledged that although PHC services have been in existence for many years, they did not meet acceptable levels of both access and quality of services. The re-engineering of PHC was based on the three pillars as described below:

a. **Ward based PHC outreach teams,** which supports the provision of home and community based health services, which are linked to the fixed PHC facilities.

b. **School health services**, which supported health services in schools.

c. **District based specialist teams**, which supports the provision of district level specialists to improve health services at clinic level.

Evaluation of PHC services in South Africa have reported psycho-social support to be low [32], which can be improved by the integration of community health workers, who were specifically tasked with providing follow-up clinic and hospital care, as well as psychosocial support for patients and their family members [33]. Moreover, the re-engineering of primary health care purposed to, among others, to offer health promotion and prevention services at community level, which is needed for all disease categories offered at PHC level [34].

Primary healthcare is the first contact a person has with the health system for any health problem, and if well functional, the PHC re-engineering was expected to be a mechanism of relieving overburdened tertiary hospitals in South Africa [35] as most patients' problems will be resolved at that level. A well-functioning district health system is the intended outcome of the re-engineering of primary health care process, which will result in a greater emphasis on health promotion, disease prevention, and community participation and empowerment [36]. Mental health services should therefore benefit for these intended good.

9. Advocating for primary health care for mental disorders

Traditionally, substance use services have not been provided by South African primary health care facilities, which has led to chronic limiting of access to treatment for people who use such services. A lack of mental health workers has slowed plans to integrate these services into the primary health care system [37]. However, careful consideration of how service delivery for mental disorders can be obtained for the majority, confirms the PHC model as being ideal for the prevention and management of mental disorders. Moreover, the low cost and increased access are advantageous for services at this level.

9.1 The cost

Primary health care services are offered at a lower cost, which is important for resource- constrained country like South Africa. This low cost can therefore enable more people to access mental health services. Institutionalization model of mental health services is much more costly, even for well-resourced countries like the USA, compared to primary health [38].

9.2 Improved accessibility of services

By its nature, PHC services are designed to be accessed by the majority of citizens, and resourcing and integrating extending such services to mental health will contribute to the improvement in treatment outcomes for the patients who need such services. That is why the need for interdisciplinary models of primary healthcare is likely to improve accessibility and quality of care for the broader population [39].

10. Examples of success of treating mental health disorders at PHC level

A number of countries have successfully integrated mental health services to mainstream primary health care services, with tremendous gains for both the country health system and the patients who receive such care. In Zimbabwe, the primary health care services for mental disorders include the use of lay health workers, which is advantageous for resource-constrained countries. The services they offer include screening for mental health disorders and administering primary care-based problem solving therapy with education and support for the clients [40].

In India, a similar program has been used for several years, and it has been found to be not only cost-effective, but also cost-saving [41]. The use of a lower cadre of health workers require task-shifting which, if properly utilized with effective training of the workers, can substantially reduce the number of high level health professionals, and thus close the mental health service gaps at primary health care level in South Africa at a minimal cost [42, 43].

10.1 Status of PHC services for mental health

Despite the high prevalence of mental health disorders in South Africa, mental health services at primary health care level are not prioritized. With the high level of stigmatization of mental illness, the health-seeking behaviors are compromised, despite the high prevalence of such disorders. This low prioritization also contributes to poor capacity planning and implementation of mental health care plans, scarcity of trained generalists in mental health care, poor integration of mental health into integrated care, and lack of dedicated mental health budget [44]. Specifically, the resource limitations need to be addressed, by allocation of more funding for PHC services and to upgrade mental health legislation and policies [45].

In order for primary care providers to diagnose substance abuse and mental illness among clinic attendees, they need to receive specific training, specifically in the use of self-reported screening tools which are easy to administer and efficient to make a substance abuse diagnosis in primary care settings. Early diagnosis and a brief behavioral change counseling are effective in managing substance abuse before it develops into dependency.

The acknowledgement of increasing prevalence of mental disorders which include substance abuse in South Africa, renders them to be a priority in the offering of primary health care services, and literature has reported that mental health care can be effectively integrated into primary health care [46]. However, in order to do this, governance should be improved [44]. This improved governance is what this chapter regards as a major intervention to improve PHC services and to set them to adequately address mental health matters.

10.2 Integrating mental health into mainstream primary health care services

Integration of mental health services into mainstream services has been recommended globally [47], and this has been found to be both effective for intended treatment outcomes, as well as economically cost-effective [21, 48]. While treatment effectiveness benefits the patients, cost-effectiveness has a direct benefit on the health system and an indirect benefit to the patients as the quality of treatment can be improved as more resources are available. Although compared to other African countries, South Africa is reported to be doing better in offering mental health services [49], a lot still needs to be done to implement integration of mental health services to reap envisaged health system benefits. With the high prevalence of mental disorders, which are ranked third as contributors to disability-adjusted life-years [50], integration of mental health into primary health care remains incomplete, which contributes to inconsistent care and difficulties such as unidentified symptoms, defaulting treatment and the revolving-door phenomenon [47, 51].

The integration of mental health services requires a vision contained in the South African Mental Health Policy and Strategy Plan, whose implementation can make a difference to the quality of services required by mental health care users [52]. Additionally, strong political will can assist in providing the resources required.

11. Recommended primary health care mental health services

A functional primary health care system should provide adequate services for most patients, so that only a selected few of these need referrals to higher levels of care. For that reason, primary healthcare services should be able to provide the following comprehensive mental health services:

11.1 Screening

The purpose of screening is for early detection, which is essential for both substance abuse and mental disorders, because if left unattended, these conditions tend to worsen and complicate, with poor treatment outcomes. Screening is therefore essential as it can assist with the early identification of both substance-related problems and mental illness, and guide the provision of appropriate services [53].

One of the key examples of failure to screen for pregnant mothers is the Fetal Alcohol Spectrum Disorders, which are often only detected after the child is born [54]. Specifically, the continuous neglect of screening for maternal depression has major negative implications for the children of such mothers, to the extent that the children's constitutional rights are violated [55].

11.2 Prevention of mental illness and promotion of mental health

Both the prevention of mental illness and active promotion of mental health interventions are public health interventions for holistic approach for positive health outcomes [56]. This requires the identification of associated risk factors, and act on them. Because key contributors to mental illness are mostly socially derived, the negative social factors operational in communities need to be considered as points of attention. Prevention of mental illness and promotion of mental health has an economic value [57], hence the need to put efforts for their promotion.

11.3 Treatment

Although a few PHC clinics offer some mental services, the quality of treatment received does not meet the recommended mental health guidelines, and is therefore compromised [58]. In particular, promotion of mental health is often missing. Within the re-engineered primary health care package, which includes the utilization of a well-resourced district-based specialist teams, primary health care services will be enhanced to offer quality and effective treatment. However, not all clinics have functional district-based specialist teams, which needs to be improved.

With political commitment and following the spirit of the National Development plan and the core principles of Primary Health care, PHC services in South Africa can be an effective strategy in achieving the goal of health for all, including mental health services. This also applies to other African countries, which can use this strategy to coordinated efforts to achieve the health care components of the SDGs [9].

11.4 Ongoing support

A key success indicator for the treatment of chronic mental illness is the ability of the health system to provide ongoing support. This is necessitated to counteract possible relapse, which is common as the patients often experience treatment fatigue. Patients with chronic mental illness also often move residence, due to various social problems, which exposes them to discontinuity of treatment [59].

In the absence of any efforts for ongoing support, they are often lost to follow-up, with negative outcomes. In the South African setting, the existence of the Ward based PHC outreach teams can be effectively utilized for this service.

12. Conclusion

The chapter acknowledges the major problem of high prevalence of mental disorders in South Africa, as well as inadequate resources to address the problem. However, moderate changes to the primary health care model currently used in South Africa can result in major achievements in offering mental health services, which in turn will benefit the patients and assist health services to address the increasing scourge of mental disorders. This can be achieved by utilizing community health workers (CHWs), who are able to work effectively with marginalized communities, where the need for services is greatest [60]. With proper training, these community health workers can change the landscape of provision of mental health services, with resultant positive health outcomes for affected communities [61].

It is recommended that primary health care services be strengthened to provide comprehensive mental health and mental health services that include screening, brief interventions, referral to treatment and ongoing support [62], which will go a long way in addressing mental health and substance abuse needs for South Africa. Such services are likely to improve the mental disorder treatment needs across the spectrum, and provide the much needed continuity of care across levels [3]. With the integration of community health workers in primary health care service provision, the broader community participation is enabled, which is likely to result in an increased number of mental health activists, and better treatment outcomes for patients.

Acknowledgements

This chapter was jointly-funded by the National Research Foundation, through the NRF Chair in Substance Abuse and Population Mental Health grant, as well as the South African Medical Research Council, through the Substance Abuse and Adolescent Mental Health grant.

Author details

Kebogile Elizabeth Mokwena* and Velaphi Anthony Mokwena
Sefako Makgatho Health Sciences University, South Africa

*Address all correspondence to: kebogile.mokwena@smu.ac.za

References

[1] Kroenke K, Unutzer J. Closing the false divide: sustainable approaches to integrating mental health services into primary care. Journal of general internal medicine. 2017 Apr;32(4):404-410.

[2] World Health Organization. Report of the Global conference on primary health care: from Alma-Ata towards universal health coverage and the Sustainable Development Goals. World Health Organization; 2019.

[3] Lahariya C, Sundararaman T, Ved RR, Adithyan GS, De Graeve H, Jhalani M, Bekedam H. What makes primary healthcare facilities functional, and increases the utilization? Learnings from 12 case studies. Journal of family medicine and primary care. 2020 Feb;9(2):539.

[4] Saban A, Flisher AJ, Grimsrud A, Morojele N, London L, Williams DR, Stein DJ. The association between substance use and common mental disorders in young adults: results from the South African Stress and Health (SASH) Survey. The Pan African Medical Journal. 2014;17(Suppl 1).

[5] Groenman AP, Janssen TW, Oosterlaan J. Childhood psychiatric disorders as risk factor for subsequent substance abuse: a meta-analysis. Journal of the American Academy of Child & Adolescent Psychiatry. 2017 Jul 1;56(7):556-569.

[6] Choi NG, DiNitto DM, Marti CN, Choi BY. Association of adverse childhood experiences with lifetime mental and substance use disorders among men and women aged 50+ years. International psychogeriatrics. 2017 Mar;29(3):359-372.

[7] National Development Plan 2030, accessed from https://www.gov.za/issues/national-development-plan-2030

[8] Stein DJ, Benjet C, Gureje O, Lund C, Scott KM, Poznyak V, Van Ommeren M. Integrating mental health with other non-communicable diseases. Bmj. 2019 Jan 28;364.

[9] Onokerhoraye AG. Achieving universal access to health care in Africa: The role of primary health care. African journal of reproductive health. 2016 Nov 15;20(3):29-31.

[10] Daviaud E, Subedar H. Staffing norms for primary health care in the context of PHC re-engineering. Cape Town: Medical Research Council. 2012 Oct.

[11] Mokwena K, Sindane P. Cigarette smoking and alcohol intake among high school learners in Pretoria, South Africa. Psychology and Education Journal. 2020 Dec 23;57(7):531-536.

[12] Tshitangano TG, Tosin OH. Substance use amongst secondary school students in a rural setting in South Africa: Prevalence and possible contributing factors. African Journal of Primary Health Care and Family Medicine. 2016 Jan 1;8(2):1-6.

[13] Moodley SV, Matjila MJ, Moosa MY. Epidemiology of substance use among secondary school learners in Atteridgeville, Gauteng. South African Journal of Psychiatry. 2012;18(1):2-7.

[14] Mohale D, Mokwena KE. Substance use amongst high school learners in the south of Johannesburg: Is this the new norm?. South African Family Practice. 2020 Jan 1;62(1):NA-.

[15] Mokwena AV, Mokwena K, Van Der Heever H, Mokgatle M. The National Policy of Drug Abuse Management in Schools in South Africa: Unknown and Unimplemented. Journal of Drug and Alcohol Research. 2020 Sep 17;9(5):1-5.

[16] Zauszniewski JA, Bekhet AK, Suresky MJ. Indicators of resilience in family members of adults with serious mental illness. Psychiatric Clinics. 2015 Mar 1;38(1):131-146.

[17] Mokwena KE. The novel psychoactive substance 'Nyaope'brings unique challenges to mental health services in South Africa. International Journal of Emergency Mental Health and Human Resilience. 2015 Mar;17(1):251-252.

[18] Lund C, Kleintjes S, Kakuma R, Flisher AJ. Public sector mental health systems in South Africa: inter-provincial comparisons and policy implications. Social psychiatry and psychiatric epidemiology. 2010 Mar;45(3):393-404.

[19] Vigo D, Thornicroft G, Atun R. Estimating the true global burden of mental illness. The Lancet Psychiatry. 2016 Feb 1;3(2):171-178.

[20] Crowley RA, Kirschner N. The integration of care for mental health, substance abuse, and other behavioral health conditions into primary care: executive summary of an American College of Physicians position paper. Annals of Internal Medicine. 2015 Aug 18;163(4):298-299.

[21] Jack HE, Oller D, Kelly J, Magidson JF, Wakeman SE. Addressing substance use disorder in primary care: The role, integration, and impact of recovery coaches. Substance Abuse. 2018 Jul 3;39(3):307-314.

[22] Thomas C. Health risk behaviours of high school learners and their perceptions of preventive services offered by general practitioners. South African Family Practice. 2009 May 1;51(3):216-223.

[23] Khuzwayo LS, Moshabela M. The perceived role of ward-based primary healthcare outreach teams in rural KwaZulu-Natal, South Africa. African Journal of Primary Health Care and Family Medicine. 2017 Feb 22;9(1):1-5.

[24] Labonté R, Sanders D, Packer C, Schaay N. Is the Alma Ata vision of comprehensive primary health care viable? Findings from an international project. Global health action. 2014 Dec 1;7(1):24997.

[25] Michel JE, D Tediosi F, D Egger MB, T McIntyre DR. Lest we forget, primary health care in Sub-Saharan Africa is nurse led. Is this reflected in the current health systems strengthening undertakings and initiatives?. Journal of Global Health Reports. 2018;2:e2018009.

[26] Nteta TP, Mokgatle-Nthabu M, Oguntibeju OO. Utilization of the primary health care services in the Tshwane Region of Gauteng Province, South Africa. PloS one. 2010 Nov 9;5(11):e13909.

[27] Myers BJ, Louw J, Pasche SC. Inequitable access to substance abuse treatment services in Cape Town, South Africa. Substance Abuse Treatment, Prevention, and Policy. 2010 Dec;5(1):1-1.

[28] Myers B, Petersen Z, Kader R, Parry CD. Moving beyond access: Towards a quality-orientated substance abuse treatment system in South Africa. SAMJ: South African Medical Journal. 2012 Aug;102(8):667-668.

[29] Myers B, Petersen Z, Kader R, Koch JR, Manderscheid R, Govender R, Parry CD. Identifying perceived barriers to monitoring service quality among substance abuse treatment providers in South Africa. BMC psychiatry. 2014 Dec;14(1):1-0.

[30] Sherr K, Cuembelo F, Michel C, Gimbel S, Micek M, Kariaganis M, Pio A, Manuel JL, Pfeiffer J, Gloyd S. Strengthening integrated primary health care in Sofala, Mozambique. BMC Health Services Research. 2013 May;13(2):1-2.

[31] Naledi T, Barron P, Schneider H. Primary health care in SA since 1994 and implications of the new vision for PHC re-engineering. South African health review. 2011 Jan 1;2011(1):17-28.

[32] James S, Pisa PT, Imrie J, Beery MP, Martin C, Skosana C, Delany-Moretlwe S. Assessment of adolescent and youth friendly services in primary healthcare facilities in two provinces in South Africa. BMC health services research. 2018 Dec;18(1):1-0.

[33] Le Roux K, Le Roux IM, Mbewu N, Davis E. The role of community health workers in the re-engineering of primary health care in rural Eastern Cape. South African Family Practice. 2015 Mar 1;57(2):1-5.

[34] Bheekie A, Bradley H. Re-engineering of South Africa's primary health care system: where is the pharmacist?. South African Family Practice. 2016 Nov 18;58(6):242-248.

[35] Mohapi MC, Basu D. PHC re-engineering may relieve overburdened tertiary hospitals in South Africa. SAMJ: South African Medical Journal. 2012 Feb;102(2):79-80.

[36] Dookie S, Singh S. Primary health services at district level in South Africa: a critique of the primary health care approach. BMC family practice. 2012 Dec;13(1):1-4.

[37] Myers B, Sorsdahl K. Addressing substance use within primary health care settings in South Africa: Opportunities and challenges.2014

[38] Roehrig C. Mental disorders top the list of the most costly conditions in the United States: $201 billion. Health Affairs. 2016 Jun 1;35(6):1130-1135.

[39] Ross LE, Vigod S, Wishart J, Waese M, Spence JD, Oliver J, Chambers J, Anderson S, Shields R. Barriers and facilitators to primary care for people with mental health and/or substance use issues: a qualitative study. BMC family practice. 2015 Dec;16(1):1-3.

[40] Chibanda D, Weiss HA, Verhey R, Simms V, Munjoma R, Rusakaniko S, Chingono A, Munetsi E, Bere T, Manda E, Abas M. Effect of a primary care–based psychological intervention on symptoms of common mental disorders in Zimbabwe: a randomized clinical trial. Jama. 2016 Dec 27;316(24):2618-2626.

[41] Buttorff C, Hock RS, Weiss HA, Naik S, Araya R, Kirkwood BR, Chisholm D, Patel V. Economic evaluation of a task-shifting intervention for common mental disorders in India. Bulletin of the World Health Organization. 2012;90:813-821

[42] Burns JK. The mental health gap in South Africa: A human rights issue. The Equal Rights Review. 2011 Jan;6(99):99-113.

[43] Petersen I, Lund C, Bhana A, Flisher AJ, Mental Health and Poverty Research Programme Consortium. A task shifting approach to primary mental health care for adults in South Africa: human resource requirements and costs for rural settings. Health policy and planning. 2012 Jan 1;27(1):42-51

[44] Marais DL, Petersen I. Health system governance to support integrated mental health care in South Africa: challenges and opportunities. International journal of mental health systems. 2015 Dec;9(1):1-21.

[45] Mugisha J, Abdulmalik J, Hanlon C, Petersen I, Lund C, Upadhaya N, Ahuja S, Shidhaye R, Mntambo N, Alem A, Gureje O. Health systems context (s) for integrating mental health into primary health care in six Emerald countries: a situation analysis. International Journal of Mental Health Systems. 2017 Dec;11(1):1-3.

[46] Petersen I, Fairall L, Bhana A, Kathree T, Selohilwe O, Brooke-Sumner C, Faris G, Breuer E, Sibanyoni N, Lund C, Patel V. Integrating mental health into chronic care in South Africa: the development of a district mental healthcare plan. The British journal of psychiatry. 2016 Jan;208(s56):s29-s39.

[47] Carey TS, Crotty KA, Morrissey JP, Jonas DE, Thaker S, Ellis AR, Woodell C, Wines RC, Viswanathan M. Future research needs for evaluating the integration of mental health and substance abuse treatment with primary care. Journal of Psychiatric Practice®. 2013 Sep 1;19(5):345-59.

[48] Cubillos L, Bartels SM, Torrey WC, Naslund J, Uribe-Restrepo JM, Gaviola C, Díaz SC, John DT, Williams MJ, Cepeda M, Gómez-Restrepo C. The effectiveness and cost-effectiveness of integrating mental health services in primary care in low-and middle-income countries: systematic review. BJPsych bulletin. 2021 Feb;45(1):40-52.

[49] Jack-Ide IO, Uys LR, Middleton LE. A comparative study of mental health services in two African countries: South Africa and Nigeria. International Journal of Nursing and Midwifery. 2012 May 30;4(4):50-57.

[50] Jacobs N, Coetzee D. Mental illness in the Western Cape Province, South Africa: A review of the burden of disease and healthcare interventions. South African Medical Journal. 2018;108(3):176-180.

[51] Gerber O. Practitioners' experience of the integration of mental health into primary health care in the West Rand District, South Africa. Journal of Mental Health. 2018 Mar 4;27(2):135-141.

[52] Schneider M, Baron E, Breuer E, Docrat S, Honikman S, Onah M, Sorsdahl K, Van der Westhuizen C, Lund C, Kagee A, Skeen S. Integrating mental health into South Africa's health system: current status and way forward. South African Health Review. 2016 Jan 1;2016(1):153-163.

[53] Carney T, Myers B, Louw J. Reliability of the GAIN-SS, CRAFTT and PESQ screening instruments for substance use among South African adolescents. South African Journal of Psychiatry. 2016 Aug 31;22(1).

[54] Williams JF, Smith VC, Committee on Substance Abuse. Fetal alcohol spectrum disorders. Pediatrics. 2015 Nov 1;136(5):e1395-406.

[55] Mokwena KE. Neglecting Maternal Depression Compromises Child Health and Development Outcomes, and Violates Children's Rights in South Africa. Children. 2021 Jul;8(7):609.

[56] Thieme A, Wallace J, Meyer TD, Olivier P. Designing for mental wellbeing: towards a more holistic approach in the treatment and prevention of mental illness. InProceedings of the 2015 British HCI Conference 2015 Jul 13 (pp. 1-10).

[57] McDaid D, Park AL, Wahlbeck K. The economic case for the prevention of mental illness. Annual Review of Public Health. 2019 Apr 1;40:373-389.

[58] Dube FN, Uys LR. Primary health care nurses' management practices of common mental health conditions in KwaZulu-Natal, South Africa. curationis. 2015;38(1):1-0.

[59] Mokwena KE, Ndlovu J. Why Do Patients with Mental Disorders Default Treatment? A Qualitative Enquiry in Rural Kwazulu-Natal, South Africa. InHealthcare 2021 Apr (Vol. 9, No. 4, p. 461). Multidisciplinary Digital Publishing Institute.

[60] Christopher JB, Le May A, Lewin S, Ross DA. Thirty years after Alma-Ata: a

systematic review of the impact of community health workers delivering curative interventions against malaria, pneumonia and diarrhoea on child mortality and morbidity in sub-Saharan Africa. Human resources for health. 2011 Dec;9(1):1-1.

[61] Rehm J, Anderson P, Manthey J, Shield KD, Struzzo P, Wojnar M, Gual A. Alcohol use disorders in primary health care: what do we know and where do we go?. Alcohol and alcoholism. 2016 Jul 1;51(4):422-427.

[62] Francis E, Bowers KS, Buchberger G, Ryan S, Milchak W, Kraschnewski J. Reducing alcohol and opioid use among youth in rural counties: an innovative training protocol for primary health care providers and school personnel. JMIR research protocols. 2020 Nov 6;9(11):e21015.

Section 6

Environmental Health and Infection Control in Primary Care

Chapter 15

Water, Sanitation, and Hygiene (WASH) and Infection Prevention and Control (IPC) in Primary Healthcare Facilities in Jordan in the Context of COVID-19

Yousef Khader, Mohamad Alyahya and Rami Saadeh

Abstract

Water, Sanitation, and Hygiene (WASH) and Infection prevention and control (IPC) are essential for preventing and containing outbreaks of disease. Nowadays, infection prevention is getting more attention due to the COVID-19 pandemic. The assessment of WASH/IPC indicators in the health sector is a major step in the preparation and management of such a pandemic. A facility-wide WASH and IPC assessment is the cornerstone for designing, developing, and implementing specific WASH and IPC activities at healthcare facilities. This type of assessment helps to identify and prioritize surveillance and prevention activities at the facility and provide healthcare policy makers at all levels with the evidence to strengthen WASH services and infection control policies, practices, and resources in health facilities. Moreover, this helps to motivate facilities to intensify efforts where needed to prevent, respond to, and control the spread of COVID-19. An assessment was conducted in primary healthcare facilities in Jordan to identify the strengths and gaps in the WASH and IPC practices, activities, and resources and to identify areas for quality improvement. This report demonstrates the results of a nationwide assessment of 33 healthcare centres. The assessment included eight domains (areas) pertaining to WASH/IPC with more than 150 indicators. The assessment tools were developed and adapted from the Water and Sanitation for Health Facility Improvement Tool (WASH FIT), the Infection Prevention and Control (IPC) Assessment Framework (IPCAF), Guide to Infection Prevention for Outpatient Settings: Minimum Expectations for Safe Care, the Systems for Improved Access to Pharmaceuticals and Services (SIAPS) tool, and COVID-19 Technical Guidance by WHO. The assessment revealed some deficiencies in basic WASH/IPC indicators such as lack of clear guidelines that support the management of health centres in planning and leadership, shortfalls in the budget needed to strengthen the infrastructure of WASH/IPC, inconsistent or under-provisioned training and education programmes for the development of staff skills to lead, plan, manage, and improve WASH/IPC at their facilities. Moreover, the report identified the unmet WASH/IPC needs at centres that should be addressed by policy makers and stakeholders as soon as possible for further steps of consideration in policy development. The report ends with specific recommendations to improve WASH/IPC services and practices.

Keywords: water, sanitation, hygiene, infection control

1. Introduction

1.1 Infection prevention and control (IPC)

Infection prevention and control (IPC) is a scientific approach and practical solution designed to prevent harm caused by infection to patients and health workers. In health facilities, IPC cannot be met without water, sanitation, and hygiene (WASH) services that provide the basis for adequate IPC. In the context of COVID-19, poor or inadequate WASH and IPC services and practices lead to transmission of the infection from healthcare facilities to communities and exacerbate the outbreak and spread of infections. The World Health Organization (WHO) in collaboration with the United Nations Children's Fund (UNICEF) 2015 Report underlined the importance of adequate WASH in healthcare facilities for the prevention of infections and spread of disease and for protecting staff and patients' health, dignity, and privacy [1]. WASH services strengthen the resilience of healthcare systems to prevent disease outbreaks, allowing effective responses to emergencies (including natural disasters and outbreaks), and bringing emergencies under control when they occur.

IPC has an immense role in reducing disease transmission generally and in healthcare facilities specifically; this fact has been well established in many studies. Madge et al. (1992) concluded that several IPC measures significantly reduced the incidence of nosocomial respiratory syncytial virus in the sample groups they observed [2]. According to Ershova et al. (2018), in middle-income countries, the employment of the IPC programme was highly effective in preventing nosocomial infection and in reducing antibiotic resistance [3]. Conducting evaluation studies for IPC in healthcare facilities helps find gaps and mistakes that should be corrected for the IPC programme to be more efficient and effective. In Jordan, this type of evaluation is seldom carried out. A survey of nosocomial IPC capacity among radiographers in Jordan reported moderate knowledge of IPC practices and that future training and improvement are needed [4]. Another study was conducted among nurses from 9 different hospitals in Jordan regarding safe injection handling. The study recommended focused and effective infection control educational programmes in Jordanian hospitals [5].

1.2 Water, sanitation, and hygiene (WASH)

WASH is the acronym of Water, Sanitation, and Hygiene. It has a major impact on public health and its importance is recognized globally. In 2015 members of the United Nations agreed on 17 Sustainable Development Goals; these goals require urgent actions from all countries [6]. The first two targets in SDG 6 (Ensure availability and sustainable management of water and sanitation for all) are focused on the availability of clean affordable water and proper conditions of sanitation and hygiene [7].

Proper WASH conditions are essential for the protection of human health during all types of disease outbreaks including the ongoing COVID-19 pandemic. According to WHO, routinely applied WASH and waste management in homes, communities, schools, marketplaces, and healthcare facilities help to prevent the viral transmission that causes COVID-19 [8]. Prüss et al. (2002) have estimated the global disease burden from water, sanitation, and hygiene to be 4.0 per cent of all deaths and 5.7 per cent of the total disease burden (in DALYs) [9].

According to Khader (2017), despite the major advancement Jordan has made in IPC by providing access to drinking water and improving sanitation and health waste management, several areas are yet to be improved in the Jordanian healthcare setting. Also, it is advisable to establish and implement a WASH monitoring system for the healthcare system [10].

1.3 Water

Water is essential to humans, not only for nourishment but also for better sanitation and hygiene. Each year, about 3,000 children under the age of 5 years old die from diarrhoeal disease resulting from lack of safe drinking water, hygiene, and sanitation; it also causes death to more than 829,000 humans each year [11]. The availability and quality of water are very strong factors in public health. According to the UNICEF, 663 million people do not have access to clean drinking water and nearly 60 million people use untreated water from unsafe sources like rivers [12, 13]. Jordan is ranked as the world's-second most-water scarce country with 100 m^3 per person, 400 m^3 less than the severe water scarcity threshold, and more than 50 per cent receive water once every week [12]. Regarding COVID-19, clean water is very crucial in controlling the pandemic as about 1.8 billion people globally use fecal contaminated water; this water can serve as an alternative route of infection [14]. The Hospital Water Supply as a Source of Nosocomial Infections study by Anaissie et al. (2002) mentioned that an estimated number of 1,400 annual deaths in the United States due to waterborne nosocomial lung infections caused by Pseudomonas aeruginosa alone [15]. A recently published article in Infection Control and Hospital Epidemiology by Stuckey et al. (2020) reviewed the National Health care Safety Network annual reports from 4929 hospitals in the United States. They reported that 1 in 10 hospitals did not have a water management programme and some hospitals did not include some basic practices like water temperature and disinfectant monitoring [16]. Hospitals in Low- and middle-income countries suffer from water shortage. Chawla et al. (2016) reported in their study, a systematic review that included 22 hospital in the LMICs area providing surgical services, that more than one-third of the hospital did not have a reliable water source. They recommended that both governments and non-governmental organizations should direct more effort to enhance the water infrastructure of hospitals [17].

1.4 Medical waste and sanitation facilities

Medical waste is a dangerous pollutant that may contain viruses, bacteria, chemical substances, and even radioactive waste. It must not be taken for granted as it can act as a source of infection and limit the efforts in controlling an outbreak, not to mention its environmental impact. Since the beginning of COVID-19 pandemic medical waste has increased significantly and managing it became more difficult [18]. It is important to evaluate waste management for an accurate infection prevention assessment. In Jordan, less than 78 per cent of sanitation systems are managed safely and one-third of schools have basic sanitation services [12]. Several studies found that viral materials of the SARS-COV2 virus (RNA) can be found in human waste like blood and stool [19–21]. A recent study by Chen et al. (2020) tested human waste for SARS-COV2 viral shedding and found that fecal samples of COVID-19 patients remained positive for the virus after the pharyngeal swaps turned negative; this means that a patient that tests negative might excrete the virus by fecal route. The study also suggests that the fecal-oral transmission may be another way for this virus to be transmitted. Wastewater epidemiology is a relatively new discipline and it was mainly used to detect drugs in wastewater to estimate drug use in a population. However, it is now applied to detect pathogens including SARS-COV2 as the first report of its detection in an Australian study by Ahmed et al. (2020) was followed by a number of studies that all recommended a safe wastewater management to help fighting the pandemic [22].

1.5 Hygiene

Hygiene is a term used to describe the behaviors performed to achieve a level of cleanliness that can lead to good health and provide a range of infection prevention. It includes practices like hands and face washing, douching with water and soap, and other personal hygiene etiquettes. Good hygiene practices have an immense effect on public health. A simple act like hand washing can reduce the risk of foodborne diseases that spread by hand, and can reduce the mortality of diarrhoeal associated diseases by 50 per cent [23]. Hand hygiene has a great impact in preventing nosocomial infections especially multidrug-resistant infections. Yet, studies estimated global compliance with hand hygiene in healthcare to be only around 40 per cent [24]. Przekwas and Chen (2020) have mentioned that, besides hand washing, washing the face is also recommended to prevent COVID-19 transmission as they stated that the virus may accumulate in some areas of the face and can then be inhaled [25]. Using the WHO methodology, a recent study in Tanzania compared hospitals that received WASH training and hospitals that did not receive it. It was shown that the compliance rate of hand hygiene was significantly higher among hospitals with the WASH training programme [26].

1.6 Assessment tools

Different studies have used different assessment tools. Recommendations on the suitability of different tools were made after the studies. A study was conducted by Tomczyk et al. (2020) to assess the WHO IPCAF at acute healthcare facilities in 46 counties. The study concluded that this is a necessary tool, and is effective for the improvement of IPC in health facilities [27]. Aghdassi et al. (2020) used the WHO IPCAF in their assessment and have stated in their paper that it was a useful tool that can detect shortfalls even in high-income settings at acute health facilities [28]. Maina et al. (2019) have reported in their paper, which examined WASH-FIT and WASH-FAST tools, that WASH-FIT is the tool of choice to assess WASH in smaller facilities. On the one hand, WASH-FAST is more suitable for hospitals at regional level [29]. On the other, a comprehensive study assessing different tools for WASH assessment has reported that none of the tools that they studied was comprehensive and concrete enough for assessing healthcare facility WASH activities [30].

2. Objectives

A facility-wide WASH and IPC assessment is the cornerstone for designing, developing, and implementing specific WASH and IPC activities at healthcare facilities. This type of assessment helps identify and prioritize surveillance and prevention activities at the facility, based on the risk of acquiring and transmitting infections in the facility [1, 23, 31]. This report will provide healthcare policy makers at the national, district, and facility levels with the evidence and the action plans needed to strengthen WASH services and infection control policies, practices, and resources in health facilities and to motivate facilities to intensify efforts where needed to prevent, respond to, and control the spread of COVID-19. This report identifies areas for quality improvement in primary healthcare facilities, including strengthening WASH and IPC policies and standards that will lead to lower infection rates, better health outcomes for patients and improved safety and morale. It also identifies the strengths and gaps in the WASH and IPC practices, activities, and resources in the primary healthcare facilities in Jordan in the context of COVID-19.

3. Methods

A national assessment of WASH and IPC in primary healthcare facilities, including primary health centres and comprehensive health centres, was conducted in Jordan during the period October–November 2020. A multistage cluster-sampling technique proportional to the size of the facility was used for the selection of health centres. A sampling frame of all MoH health centres was obtained from the MoH and stratified according to region (North, Middle, and South), facility type (primary health centres and comprehensive centres). A random sample of health centres was selected from each stratum. A total of 11 primary healthcare centres and 22 comprehensive centres were selected.

A comprehsnive assessment tool was developed for healthcare centres a based on the review and adaptation of several tools, mainly the Water and Sanitation for Health Facility Improvement Tool (WASH FIT) [32]. WASH FIT covers four broad domains and comprises 65 indicators, aiming to achieve minimum standards for maintaining a safe and clean environment. WASH FIT is primarily designed for use in primary healthcare facilities that provide outpatient services. The assessment tools developed included more indicators and standards from other tools such as: 'The Infection Prevention and Control Assessment Framework' (IPCAF) [33]; the Guide to Infection Prevention for Outpatient Settings: Minimum Expectations for Safe Care [34]; The Systems for Improved Access to Pharmaceuticals and Services (SIAPS) tool, and the coronavirus disease (COVID-19) technical guidance by WHO [8].

The health centre assessment tool covered eight broad areas (Domains): (1) Water, (2) Medical waste and sanitation facilities, (3) Hygiene, (4) Management, (5) Infection prevention and control programme, (6) Training and education, (7) Evaluation and feedback, and (8) COVID-19 precautionary measures. The Hygiene domain covered areas related to hand hygiene and facility environment, cleanliness and disinfection. The Infection prevention and control programme area was divided into subareas including (a) Basic indicators, (b) Guidelines in IPC unit, (c) Training and education for the Infection Prevention and Control Unit, (d) Healthcare associated infection monitoring, (e) Monitoring/auditing of infection control practices and outcomes, (f) Personal protective equipment, and (g) Availability of hygiene materials. Evaluation and feedback covered subareas including (a) Basic Indicators, (b) Respiratory safety, (c) Environmental cleaning, and (d) Sterilization of Reusable Devices.

Each area/subarea included indicators and targets for achieving minimum standards for maintaining a safe and clean environment. These standards are based on global standards as set out in the WHO Essential environmental health standards in health care [35] and the WHO Guidelines on core components of infection prevention and control programmes at the national and acute healthcare facility level [33]. The assessment tool included WASH-FIT indicators in addition to other indicators identified from available tools. Indicators were adapted to Jordan's needs and local priorities and/or national standards in order to meet quality improvement cycles and mechanisms implemented to improve quality of care. Indicators that are not relevant were removed. Additional indicators were added as necessary to represent levels of services.

A committed team with leadership skills and who are familiar with and trained on WASH and IPC was formed. The assessment team was composed of 12 assessors who were divided into three teams; one team for each region. The team had support from the MoH leadership and from facility's administration. A training workshop was held to train the assessment team on the assessment process, data collection, and use of assessment tools. During the workshop, the assessment team members were made aware of the assessment tools and their roles and responsibilities.

The assessment teams planed their visits to the health centres with the senior facility manager. During the facility visit, the assessment team worked the with facility team including those who have in-depth understanding and knowledge of WASH and IPC activities at the facility level to fill the assessment tool. If there were no professionals in charge of WASH and IPC or there was not yet an IPC programme established, the tool was completed by the team with the consultation with the senior facility manager. The IPC team consulted with other relevant teams in the facility to respond to questions accurately.

A comprehensive assessment of the facility was conducted using the agreed list of indicators and each indicator was recorded as whether it meets, partially meets, or does not meet, the minimum standards. The assessment forms were reviewed by supervisors to ensure all information is clear and correct and all members of the team agree on the findings of each assessment. As part of the assessment, hygiene promotion materials, WASH and IPC guidelines and budget were reviewed and observed.

The percentage of indicators, which meet or partially meet the standards, was calculated for each facility. The overall facility score (the percentage of all indicators meetings the standards) was calculated to make comparisons over time when future assessments are conducted. The mean percentages over all facilities were calculated. Data were described using means and percentages.

4. Results

4.1 Health centres' characteristics

A total of 33 healthcare centres were assessed using WASH and IPC assessment tools. One-third of these centres (n = 11, 33.3 per cent) were primary healthcare centres and 22 (66.7 per cent) were comprehensive health centres. Of all assessed health centres, 39.4 per cent were in the North of Jordan, 33.3 per cent in the Middle and 27.3 per cent in the South of the country.

Table 1 shows the characteristics and capacity of the 33 assessed health centres in Jordan. Primary healthcare centres were more consistent in the number of the medical staff they have than comprehensive healthcare centres; the median number of medical staff in each category was two for most specialties, while the median number of medical staff in the comprehensive healthcare centres ranged from two to six.

4.2 The WASH and IPC indicators

Table 2 shows the mean percentage of WASH and IPC indicators over health centres that met the targets for each assessed area in both the primary and comprehensive healthcare centres. Each assessed area has a different number of indicators. The mean percentages of indicators that met the targets considerably varied among various WASH/IPC areas and type of health centres.

Almost 61.7 per cent of water indicators in all health centres (64.9 per cent in comprehensive health centres and 55.2 per cent in primary centres) met the targets. However, only half of the medical waste and sanitation indicators (49.1 per cent) met the target. Almost two-thirds of hand hygiene indicators (64.2 per cent) and

	Primary healthcare centre			Comprehensive healthcare centre			Total		
Number	**Min.**	**Max.**	**Median**	**Min.**	**Max.**	**Median**	**Min.**	**Max.**	**Median**
Doctors	1	6	2	2	25	6	1	25	5
Nurses	0	8	2	1	8	3	0	8	3
Midwifes	0	6	2	1	6	2	0	6	2
Lab technicians	0	4	1	1	11	3	0	11	2
Radiology technicians	0	0	0	0	5	2	0	5	1
Pharmacists	1	6	2	1	9	3	1	9	3
Ambulance	0	0	0	0	1	0	0	1	0
MoH health technicians/inspectors	0	2	0	0	8	0.5	0	8	0

Table 1.
The characteristics and capacity of the 33 assessed health centres in Jordan.

environmental cleanliness and disinfection indicators (65.0 per cent) met the target. Only 41.8 per cent of management indicators (27.3 per cent in primary centres and 49.1 per cent in comprehensive centres) met the targets. While two-thirds of indicators pertaining to guidelines in IPC unit met the target, only 40.3 per cent of basic indicators of IPC programming, 38.4 per cent of indicators of the training and education for the Infection Prevention and Control Unit, and 43.4 per cent of the targets for healthcare-associated infection monitoring indicators were met. Moreover, 66.3 per cent of 'Monitoring/auditing of infection control practices and outcomes' indicators, 62.6 per cent of 'Personal protective equipment' indicators, 55.8 per cent of the 'Availability of hygiene materials' indicators, 44.7 per cent of the 'Training and education' indicators, 38.8 per cent of the 'Respiratory safety' indicators, and 48.5 per cent of the 'Environmental cleaning' indicators met the targets. The mean percentages of 'COVID-19 precautionary measures' indicators (49.7 per cent) that met the target were relatively low in both types of healthcare centres.

As expected, the mean percentages of indicators that had met the targets were higher for comprehensive healthcare centres than that for primary centres in all assessed WASH/IPC areas. For example, the mean percentage of 'respiratory safety' indicators in primary healthcare centres (14.5 per cent) was much lower than the mean percentage of 'respiratory safety' indicators in comprehensive healthcare centres (50.9 per cent).

4.3 Water indicators

The percentage of primary healthcare centres that met the target for most water indicators were lower than comprehensive care centres, except for a few indicators, as demonstrated in **Table 3**. The percentage of health centres that met water indicators varied between 21.2 per cent and 100 per cent. Improved drinking-water supply and the availability of hot water was weak in both primary and comprehensive healthcare centres. Less than two-thirds of centres had clean drinking-water available and accessible to all at all times and in all locations, had drinking-water safely stored in a clean bucket/tank with cover and tap, had water tanks cleaned annually, had an emergency water tank available, and had hot water available in the health centres. On the other hand, meeting the target for indicators related to the availability and functionality of water supply was high in both types of healthcare centres, and even higher in primary care centres, reaching 100 per cent.

Area	Number of indicators assessed	Type of health centre				Total (N = 33)	
		Primary (N = 11)		Comprehensive (N = 22)			
		Mean %	SD	Mean %	SD	Mean %	SD
Water	14	55.2	15.7	64.9	20.2	61.7	19.1
Medical waste and sanitation	16	39.2	20.2	54.0	24.3	49.1	23.8
Hygiene							
Hand hygiene	5	54.5	37.0	69.1	27.4	64.2	31.1
Environmental cleanliness and disinfection	11	61.2	19.5	66.9	12.4	65.0	15.1
Management	10	27.3	28.0	49.1	31.3	41.8	31.6
Infection prevention and control programme							
Basic indicators	7	29.9	30.3	45.5	30.4	40.3	30.8
Guidelines in IPC unit	12	48.5	39.4	77.3	29.3	67.7	35.2
Training and education for the Infection Prevention and Control Unit	3	30.3	37.9	42.4	41.4	38.4	40.1
Healthcare-associated infection monitoring	3	24.2	36.8	53.0	33.6	43.4	36.8
Monitoring/auditing of infection control practices and outcomes	8	51.1	32.3	73.9	16.3	66.3	24.9
Personal protective equipment	9	46.5	24.8	70.7	21.3	62.6	25.0
Availability of hygiene materials	5	52.7	33.8	57.3	29.8	55.8	30.7
Training and education	4	34.1	35.8	50.0	40.1	44.7	38.9
Evaluation and feedback							
Basic indicators	2	63.6	45.2	77.3	33.5	72.7	37.7
Respiratory safety	5	14.5	20.2	50.9	34.2	38.8	34.6
Environmental cleaning	2	31.8	33.7	56.8	41.7	48.5	40.5
Sterilization of reusable devices	2	81.8	33.7	100	0.0	93.9	20.8
COVID-19 precautionary measures	17	42.8	23.1	53.2	19.9	49.7	21.3

Table 2.
The mean percentage of indicators that met the targets in each assessed area.

Fortunately, the percentage of healthcare centres that fully met the target was greater than the percentage of centres that partially met the target for almost all the indicators related to water.

4.4 Medical waste and sanitation

The targets for many indicators related to toilet provision were met by very few primary healthcare centres and relatively few comprehensive healthcare centres. In addition to the low percentage of centres that met targets for indicators pertaining to the number, functionality, and monitoring of toilets, there were few, if any, toilets that serve people with special needs, or toilets designed to meet menstrual hygiene needs. The difference in the percentage of centres that met the targets for

Water	Primary centres (N = 11)				Comprehensive (N = 22)				Total (N = 33)			
	Partially meet target		Meet target		Partially meet target		Meet target		Partially meet target		Meet target	
	n	%	n	%	n	%	n	%	n	%	n	%
	2	18.2	1	9.1	4	18.2	6	27.3	6	18.2	7	21.2
Water services available at all times and of sufficient quantity for all uses	2	18.2	5	45.5	2	9.1	17	77.3	4	12.1	22	66.7
A clean drinking-water is available and accessible for staff, patients and healthcare providers at all times and in all locations/wards	2	18.2	5	45.5	6	27.3	14	63.6	8	24.2	19	57.6
Drinking-water is safely stored in a clean bucket/tank with cover and tap	5	45.5	5	45.5	7	31.8	14	63.6	12	36.4	19	57.6
Water tanks are cleaned annually	0	0.0	4	36.4	0	0.0	10	45.5	0	0.0	14	42.4
Emergency water tank is available	0	0.0	2	18.2	0	0.0	13	59.1	0	0.0	15	45.5
All water end points (i.e., taps) in the health centre are connected to an available and functioning water supply	0	0.0	10	90.9	5	22.7	17	77.3	5	15.2	27	81.8
Water services are available throughout the year (i.e., not affected by seasonality, climate change-related extreme events or other constraints)	0	0.0	11	100	0	0.0	22	100	0	0.0	33	100
Water storage is sufficient to meet the needs of the health centre for two days	0	0.0	11	100	0	0.0	21	95.5	0	0.0	32	97.0
Water is treated and collected for drinking with standards that meet WHO performance standards	0	0.0	8	72.7	3	13.6	15	68.2	3	9.1	23	69.7
Drinking-water has appropriate chlorine residual (0.2 mg/L or 0.5 mg/L in emergencies) or 0 *E. coli*/100 ml and is not turbid	0	0.0	7	63.6	3	13.6	17	77.3	3	9.1	24	72.7
The health centre water supply is regulated according to national water quality standards	0	0.0	9	81.8	0	0.0	21	95.5	0	0.0	30	90.9
Hot water is available in the health centre	4	36.4	3	27.3	13	59.1	4	18.2	17	51.5	7	21.2
Water heating indicator is available	0	0.0	4	36.4	0	0.0	9	40.9	0	0.0	13	39.4

Table 3.
Percentage of health centres that meet the target for each indicator of 'Water' according to the type of health Centre.

indicators pertaining to toilets was obvious between comprehensive and primary healthcare centres (**Table 4**).

Some targets were met by most primary and comprehensive healthcare centres, such as wastewater management (72.7 per cent and 77.3 per cent, respectively), and disposal of domestic waste (90.9 per cent and 100 per cent, respectively). However, the percentage of primary centres that met the target for indicators like sorting of waste and the availability of a trained liaison officer for waste management were higher than comprehensive healthcare centres.

4.5 Hygiene

4.5.1 Hand hygiene

Hand hygiene indicators were generally good at both the primary and the comprehensive healthcare centres; there were more centres that fully met the target than centres that partially met the target (**Table 5**). Over 70 per cent of healthcare centres were reported to have functioning and adequately available hand-hygiene stations that were supplied with water and soap. However, almost half of the centres had clearly displayed sign boards for hand hygiene (posters), had functioning hand-hygiene stations in waste disposal areas, and had regular hand-hygiene compliance activities.

4.5.2 Environmental cleanliness and disinfection

The target for many indicators for cleanliness and disinfection were met by most healthcare centres (**Table 6**). The percentage of primary healthcare centres that met the target was close to the percentage for comprehensive healthcare centres, but were quite different for centres that partially met the target. Two indicators —'record of cleaning' and 'laundry facilities'—were met by few centres only, and one-third of healthcare centres provide at least two pairs of gloves, apron, and boots for each cleaning and waste disposal staff member.

4.6 Management

Less than half of healthcare centres met the target for indicators related to the management of WASH, except for the availability of 'a dedicated WASH or IPC coordinator' and 'a written job description that is clear and legible for all staff' which were achieved by 57.6 per cent of centres. An annual planned budget for the centre that includes WASH infrastructure and service was available at 15.2 per cent of centres only, with none of the primary healthcare centres having completely met the target. However, there was a higher percentage of healthcare centres that completely met the target than those that partially met the target, except for few indicators in the primary healthcare centres like the availability of an annual budget, a protocol for operation and maintenance, and the availability of cleaners and WASH maintenance staff (**Table 7**).

4.7 Infection prevention and control programme

4.7.1 Basic indicators

One-third of primary healthcare centres (36.4 per cent) and two-thirds of comprehensive healthcare centres (63.6 per cent) have an IPC programme. Nonetheless, an IPC team or focal person was not available at most healthcare centres (**Table 8**). IPC objectives were clearly defined in 42.4 per cent of the health centres. Although the leadership in most healthcare centres shows full commitment to support the IPC programme in the centre, most centres lack the ability to support an appropriate

Medical waste and sanitation	Primary centres (N = 11)				Comprehensive (N = 22)				Total (N = 33)			
	Partially meet target		Meet target		Partially meet target		Meet target		Partially meet target		Meet target	
	n	%	n	%	n	%	n	%	n	%	n	%
Number of available and usable toilets in the health centre for patients	1	9.1	5	45.5	2	9.1	16	72.7	3	9.1	21	63.6
Toilets are clearly separated for staff and patients	4	36.4	2	18.2	6	27.3	12	54.5	10	30.3	14	42.4
Toilets are clearly separated for male and female	2	18.2	1	9.1	3	13.6	14	63.6	5	15.2	15	45.5
At least one toilet provides the means to meet menstrual hygiene needs	1	9.1	3	27.3	2	9.1	11	50.0	3	9.1	14	42.4
At least one toilet meets the needs of people with special needs (reduced mobility)	0	0.0	0	0.0	2	9.1	10	45.5	2	6.1	10	30.3
Functioning hand-hygiene stations within 5 metres of the toilets	0	0.0	4	36.4	2	9.1	8	36.4	2	6.1	12	36.4
Record of toilet cleaning is visible and signed by the cleaners each day	5	45.5	1	9.1	6	27.3	6	27.3	11	33.3	7	21.2
Wastewater is safely managed through the use of on-site treatment (i.e., septic tank, followed by drainage pit) or sent to a functioning sewer system	1	9.1	8	72.7	1	4.5	17	77.3	2	6.1	25	75.8
Greywater (i.e., rainwater or wash water) drainage system is in place that diverts water away from the health centre (i.e., no standing water) and also protects nearby households	0	0.0	3	27.3	2	9.1	4	18.2	2	6.1	7	21.2
Toilets are adequately lit, including at night	2	18.2	7	63.6	5	22.7	15	68.2	7	21.2	22	66.7
A trained liaison officer is responsible for the management of healthcare waste in the health centre	2	18.2	6	54.5	7	31.8	10	45.5	9	27.3	16	48.5
There are functional waste collection containers in close proximity to all waste generation points for non-infectious (general) waste, infectious waste, and sharps waste	4	36.4	5	45.5	9	40.9	13	59.1	13	39.4	18	54.5
Wastes are correctly sorted at all waste generation points	1	9.1	9	81.8	5	22.7	14	63.6	6	18.2	23	69.7
Functional burial pit/fenced waste dump or municipal pick-up available for disposal domestic waste	0	0.0	10	90.9	0	0.0	22	100	0	0.0	32	97.0
Protocol or standard operating procedure (SOP) for safe	2	18.2	2	18.2	2	9.1	13	59.1	4	12.1	15	45.5

Medical waste and sanitation	Primary centres (N = 11)				Comprehensive (N = 22)				Total (N = 33)			
	Partially meet target		Meet target		Partially meet target		Meet target		Partially meet target		Meet target	
	n	%	n	%	n	%	n	%	n	%	n	%
management of healthcare waste clearly visible and legible												
Appropriate protective equipment for all staff in charge of waste treatment and disposal	6	54.5	3	27.3	10	45.5	5	22.7	16	48.5	8	24.2

Table 4.
Percentage of health centres that meet the target for each indicator of "medical waste and sanitation" according to the type of health Centre.

Hand hygiene	Primary centres (N = 11)				Comprehensive (N = 22)				Total (N = 33)			
	Partially meet target		Meet target		Partially meet target		Meet target		Partially meet target		Meet target	
	n	%	n	%	n	%	n	%	n	%	n	%
Functioning hand-hygiene stations are adequately available at all care points	2	18.2	8	72.7	2	9.1	20	90.9	4	12.1	28	84.8
Functioning hand-hygiene stations are adequately available at all care points and supplied with water, liquid soap, or alcohol-based hand rub	1	9.1	8	72.7	4	18.2	18	81.8	5	15.2	26	78.8
There are sign boards for hand hygiene (posters) clearly displayed in an understandable manner in key areas	4	36.4	5	45.5	5	22.7	13	59.1	9	27.3	18	54.5
Functioning hand-hygiene stations are available in waste disposal areas	2	18.2	4	36.4	1	4.5	12	54.5	3	9.1	16	48.5
Hand-hygiene compliance activities are undertaken regularly	1	9.1	5	45.5	5	22.7	13	59.1	6	18.2	18	54.5

Table 5.
Percentage of health centres that meet the target for each indicator of 'hand hygiene' according to the type of health Centre.

IPC system, such as a microbiological laboratory (33.3 per cent) or an early-detection system (15.2 per cent).

4.7.2 Guidelines in IPC unit

A higher percentage of comprehensive healthcare centres met the targets compared to primary healthcare centres for all indicators of the IPC guideline (**Table 9**). Almost 48.5 per cent of health centres have policies and procedures for disease

Environmental cleanliness and disinfection in the health centre	Primary centres (N = 11)				Comprehensive (N = 22)				Total (N = 33)			
	Partially meet target		Meet target		Partially meet target		Meet target		Partially meet target		Meet target	
	n	%	n	%	n	%	n	%	n	%	n	%
The exterior of the health centre is well-fenced, kept generally clean (free from solid waste, stagnant water, no animal and human feces in or around the health centre premises, etc.)	2	18.2	8	72.7	0	0.0	21	95.5	2	6.1	29	87.9
There is a container assembly area managed by the municipality	0	0.0	10	90.9	0	0.0	19	86.4	0	0.0	29	87.9
General lighting sufficiently powered and adequate to ensure safe provision of health care including at night (mark if not applicable)	5	45.5	6	54.5	5	22.7	16	72.7	10	30.3	22	66.7
Floors and work surfaces are clean	1	9.1	10	90.9	1	4.5	20	90.9	2	6.1	30	90.9
Appropriate and well-maintained materials for cleaning (i.e., detergent, mops, buckets, etc.) are available	3	27.3	8	72.7	2	9.1	19	86.4	5	15.2	27	81.8
At least two pairs of household cleaning gloves, one pair of overalls or apron, and boots in a good state are available for each cleaning and waste disposal staff member	2	18.2	4	36.4	3	13.6	7	31.8	5	15.2	11	33.3
At least one member of staff can demonstrate the correct procedures for cleaning and disinfection and apply them as required to maintain clean and safe rooms	1	9.1	8	72.7	2	9.1	14	63.6	3	9.1	22	66.7
A mechanism exists to track supply of IPC-related materials (such as gloves and protective equipment) to identify stock-outs	1	9.1	7	63.6	1	4.5	15	68.2	2	6.1	22	66.7
Record of cleaning is visible and signed by the cleaners each day	1	9.1	1	9.1	2	9.1	5	22.7	3	9.1	6	18.2
Health centre's laundry is available to wash linen from patient beds between each patient	0	0.0	2	18.2	2	9.1	7	31.8	2	6.1	9	27.3
The health centre has sufficient natural ventilation and, where the climate allows, large opening windows, skylights and other vents to optimize natural ventilation	1	9.1	10	90.9	3	13.6	19	86.4	4	12.1	29	87.9

Table 6.
Percentage of health centres that meet the target for each indicator of 'environmental cleanliness and disinfection in the health Centre' according to the type of health Centre.

outbreak management and a preparedness system, 45.5 per cent have policies and procedures for antibiotic usage, 48.5 per cent of health centres had trained healthcare workers on the new or updated IPC guidelines, and 57.6 per cent of

Management	Primary centres (N = 11)				Comprehensive (N = 22)				Total (N = 33)			
	Partially meet target		Meet target		Partially meet target		Meet target		Partially meet target		Meet target	
	n	%	n	%	n	%	n	%	n	%	n	%
WASH FIT or other quality improvement/management plan for the health centre is in place, implemented and regularly monitored	1	9.1	3	27.3	3	13.6	10	45.5	4	12.1	13	39.4
An annual planned budget for the centre is available and includes funding for WASH infrastructure, services, personnel and the continuous procurement of WASH items	2	18.2	0	0.0	4	18.2	5	22.7	6	18.2	5	15.2
An up-to-date diagram of the health centre management structure is clearly visible and legible	0	0.0	4	36.4	2	9.1	12	54.5	2	6.1	16	48.5
Adequate cleaning and WASH maintenance staff are available	7	63.6	3	27.3	9	40.9	12	54.5	16	48.5	15	45.5
There is a protocol for operation and maintenance, including procurement of WASH supplies, that is visible, legible and implemented	3	27.3	1	9.1	1	4.5	8	36.4	4	12.1	9	27.3
Regular department-based audits are undertaken to assess the availability of hand rub, soap, single-use towels and other hygiene resources	4	36.4	4	36.4	3	13.6	12	54.5	7	21.2	16	48.5
New healthcare personnel receive IPC training as part of their orientation programme	3	27.3	2	18.2	2	9.1	13	59.1	5	15.2	15	45.5
Healthcare staff are trained on WASH/IPC each year (at least)	2	18.2	2	18.2	4	18.2	9	40.9	6	18.2	11	33.3
The health centre has a dedicated WASH or IPC coordinator	0	0.0	6	54.5	0	0.0	13	59.1	0	0.0	19	57.6
All staff have a job description written clearly and legibly, including WASH-related responsibilities, and are regularly appraised on their performance	1	9.1	5	45.5	1	4.5	14	63.6	2	6.1	19	57.6

Table 7.
Percentage of health centres that meet the target for each indicator of 'management' according to the type of health Centre.

health centres regularly monitor the implementation of at least some of the IPC guidelines in the health centre.

Further, there was a large difference between the percentage of primary healthcare centre and comprehensive healthcare centres that met the target for the following indicators: the availability of policies and procedures for transmission-based precautions (45.5 per cent versus 86.4 per cent), policies and procedures for prevention of infection during treatment (36.4 per cent versus 77.3 per cent), and

Infection prevention and control programme: Basic indicators	Primary centres (N = 11)				Comprehensive (N = 22)				Total (N = 33)			
	Partially meet target		Meet target		Partially meet target		Meet target		Partially meet target		Meet target	
	n	%	n	%	n	%	n	%	n	%	n	%
Have an IPC programme at the health centre	0	0.0	4	36.4	4	18.2	14	63.6	4	12.1	18	54.5
The health centre has a full-time ICP team or a specialist	3	27.3	3	27.3	10	45.5	7	31.8	13	39.4	10	30.3
IPC team or the focal person have dedicated time for IPC activities	1	9.1	2	18.2	8	36.4	10	45.5	9	27.3	12	36.4
IPC objectives are clearly defined in the health centre	2	18.2	2	18.2	6	27.3	12	54.5	8	24.2	14	42.4
Does the senior leadership team in the health centre show clear commitment and support for the IPC programme?	0	0.0	7	63.6	0	0.0	16	72.7	0	0.0	23	69.7
Does the health centre have microbiological laboratory support (either on or off site) for routine day-to-day use?	1	9.1	3	27.3	1	4.5	8	36.4	2	6.1	11	33.3
The health centre has an early-detection system and deals with potentially contagious individuals at early meeting points	0	0.0	2	18.2	0	0.0	3	13.6	0	0.0	5	15.2

Table 8.
Percentage of health centres that meet the target for each indicator of 'infection prevention and control programme: Basic indicators' according to the type of health Centre.

monitoring the implementation of at least some of the IPC guidelines (27.3 per cent versus 72.7 per cent).

4.7.3 Training and education for the infection prevention and control unit

Although 60.6 per cent of health centres have an employee who leads the IPC training, healthcare workers, cleaners or other workers receiving training in IPC is reported by few centres (27.3 per cent); primary (18.2 per cent) or comprehensive (31.8 per cent). However, some centres were reported to have partially met the target; about one-third of centres met the target for receiving training regarding IPC for healthcare workers (39.4 per cent) and cleaners (33.3 per cent) (**Table 10**).

4.7.4 Healthcare-associated infection monitoring

Surveillance was mainly conducted for epidemic-prone infections, as indicated by almost two-thirds of healthcare centres (60.6 per cent). Furthermore, surveillance for colonization or infections caused by multidrug-resistant pathogens was conducted by about one-fifth of healthcare centres (21.2 per cent), and about a half of them (48.5 per cent) conducted surveillance for infections that may affect healthcare workers in clinical, laboratory, or other settings, like the hepatitis virus (**Table 11**).

Guidelines in IPC unit	Primary centres (N = 11)				Comprehensive (N = 22)				Total (N = 33)			
	Partially meet target		Meet target		Partially meet target		Meet target		Partially meet target		Meet target	
	n	%	n	%	n	%	n	%	n	%	n	%
The health centre has policies and procedures for standard precautions	0	0.0	7	63.6	0	0.0	19	86.4	0	0.0	26	78.8
The health centre has policies and procedures for hand hygiene	0	0.0	8	72.7	0	0.0	19	86.4	0	0.0	27	81.8
The health centre has policies and procedures for transmission-based precautions	0	0.0	5	45.5	0	0.0	19	86.4	0	0.0	24	72.7
The health centre has policies and procedures for outbreak management and preparedness system	0	0.0	4	36.4	0	0.0	12	54.5	0	0.0	16	48.5
The health centre has policies and procedures for prevention of infection during treatment	0	0.0	4	36.4	0	0.0	17	77.3	0	0.0	21	63.6
The health centre has policies and procedures for disinfection and sterilization	0	0.0	6	54.5	0	0.0	19	86.4	0	0.0	25	75.8
The health centre has policies and procedures for healthcare worker protection and safety	0	0.0	6	54.5	0	0.0	19	86.4	0	0.0	25	75.8
The health centre has policies and procedures for injection safety	0	0.0	8	72.7	0	0.0	20	90.9	0	0.0	28	84.8
The health centre has policies and procedures for waste management	0	0.0	7	63.6	0	0.0	19	86.4	0	0.0	26	78.8
The health centre has policies and procedures for antibiotic usage	0	0.0	3	27.3	0	0.0	12	54.5	0	0.0	15	45.5
Healthcare workers receive specific training related to new or updated IPC guidelines introduced in the health centre	0	0.0	3	27.3	0	0.0	13	59.1	0	0.0	16	48.5
The implementation of at least some of the IPC guidelines in the health centre are regularly monitored	0	0.0	3	27.3	0	0.0	16	72.7	0	0.0	19	57.6

Table 9.
Percentage of health centres that meet the target for each indicator of 'guidelines in IPC unit' according to the type of health Centre.

4.7.5 Monitoring/auditing of infection control practices and outcomes

The targets for some infection control practices were well met by most comprehensive healthcare centres. For instance, monitoring of cleaning and disinfection was performed in 100 per cent of comprehensive healthcare centres and monitoring alcohol-based hand rub was performed in 95.5 per cent of them. In contrast, a low percentage of primary healthcare centres met the target for any indicator, except for disinfection and alcohol-based hand rub monitoring indicators, which were at 81.8 per cent each (**Table 12**).

Training and education for the Infection Prevention and Control Unit	Primary centres (N = 11)				Comprehensive (N = 22)				Total (N = 33)			
	Partially meet target		Meet target		Partially meet target		Meet target		Partially meet target		Meet target	
	n	%	n	%	n	%	n	%	n	%	n	%
There are personnel with the IPC expertise (in IPC and/or infectious diseases) who lead IPC training	0	0.0	6	54.5	0	0.0	14	63.6	0	0.0	20	60.6
The number of times healthcare workers receive training regarding IPC in the health centre	3	27.3	2	18.2	10	45.5	7	31.8	13	39.4	9	27.3
Number of times cleaners and other personnel directly involved in patient care receive training regarding IPC in the health centre	4	36.4	2	18.2	7	31.8	7	31.8	11	33.3	9	27.3

Table 10.
Percentage of health centres that meet the target for each indicator of 'training and education for the infection prevention and control unit' according to the type of health Centre.

Healthcare-associated infection monitoring	Primary centres (N = 11)				Comprehensive (N = 22)				Total (N = 33)			
	Partially meet target		Meet target		Partially meet target		Meet target		Partially meet target		Meet target	
	n	%	n	%	n	%	n	%	n	%	n	%
Surveillance is conducted for colonization or infections caused by multidrug-resistant pathogens based on the local epidemiological situation	0	0.0	2	18.2	0	0.0	5	22.7	0	0.0	7	21.2
Surveillance is conducted for epidemic-prone infections, e.g., norovirus, influenza, tuberculosis (TB), severe acute respiratory syndrome (SARS), and COVID-19	0	0.0	4	36.4	0	0.0	16	72.7	0	0.0	20	60.6
Surveillance is conducted for infections that may affect healthcare workers in clinical, laboratory, or other settings, e.g., hepatitis B or C, human immunodeficiency virus (HIV), and influenza	0	0.0	2	18.2	0	0.0	14	63.6	0	0.0	16	48.5

Table 11.
Percentage of health centres that meet the target for each indicator of 'healthcare-associated infection monitoring' according to the type of health Centre.

Monitoring of transmission-based precautions to prevent the spread of multidrug-resistant organisms (MDRO) was conducted by about one-quarter of primary healthcare centres (27.3 per cent) and one-fifth of comprehensive healthcare centres (22.7 per cent).

4.7.6 Personal protective equipment

There was a considerable wide range of difference for PPE indicators in the percentage of healthcare centres that met the target. Some indicators such as 'HCP

Monitoring/auditing of infection control practices and outcomes	Primary centres (N = 11)				Comprehensive (N = 22)				Total (N = 33)			
	Partially meet target		Meet target		Partially meet target		Meet target		Partially meet target		Meet target	
	n	%	n	%	n	%	n	%	n	%	n	%
Hand-hygiene compliance (using the WHO hand-hygiene observation tool or equivalent) is monitored regularly	0	0.0	2	18.2	0	0.0	12	54.5	0	0.0	14	42.4
Transmission-based precautions and isolation to prevent the spread of multidrug-resistant organisms (MDRO) are monitored regularly	0	0.0	3	27.3	0	0.0	5	22.7	0	0.0	8	24.2
Cleaning of the health centre is monitored regularly	0	0.0	7	63.6	0	0.0	22	100	0	0.0	29	87.9
Disinfection and sterilization of medical equipment/instruments are monitored regularly	0	0.0	9	81.8	0	0.0	22	100	0	0.0	31	93.9
Consumption/usage of alcohol-based hand rub or soap is monitored regularly	0	0.0	9	81.8	0	0.0	21	95.5	0	0.0	30	90.9
Waste management is monitored regularly in the health centre	0	0.0	6	54.5	0	0.0	18	81.8	0	0.0	24	72.7
Monitoring and feedback of IPC processes and indicators are performed in a "blame-free" institutional culture aimed at improvement and behavioral change	0	0.0	2	18.2	0	0.0	10	45.5	0	0.0	12	36.4
For all employees, there is an easily available, up-to-date list of reportable diseases (to the MoH)	0	0.0	7	63.6	0	0.0	20	90.9	0	0.0	27	81.8

Table 12.
Percentage of health centres that meet the target for each indicator of 'monitoring/auditing of infection control practices and outcomes' according to the type of health Centre.

do not wear the same gown for the care of more than one patient' and 'wearing protection for the mouth, nose, and eyes during procedures that are likely to generate splashes or sprays of blood or other body fluids' were met by 36.4 per cent and 39.4 per cent of centres, respectively. Comparatively, other indicators, such as 'wearing gloves' and 'replacing gloves after each patient' were met by 90.9 per cent and 81.8 per cent of centres, respectively, as illustrated in **Table 13**. A higher percentage of comprehensive healthcare centres met the target compared to primary healthcare centres for all indicators.

4.7.7 Availability of hygiene materials

As seen in **Table 14** only one-quarter of healthcare centres (24.2 per cent) reported the availability of a single-use towels at each sink. However, most healthcare centres of both types reported the availability of soap at each sink (81.8 per cent). Alcohol-based hand rub was available in 57.6 per cent of health centres. On the other hand, less than half of centres (42.4 per cent) have a dedicated budget

Personal protective equipment	Primary centres (N = 11)				Comprehensive (N = 22)				Total (N = 33)			
	Partially meet target		Meet target		Partially meet target		Meet target		Partially meet target		Meet target	
	n	%	n	%	n	%	n	%	n	%	n	%
Healthcare providers (HCP) that use personal protective equipment (PPE) receive training on how to use them properly	0	0.0	2	18.2	0	0.0	14	63.6	0	0.0	16	48.5
Compliance in using PPE is routinely reviewed and monitored	0	0.0	2	18.2	0	0.0	13	59.1	0	0.0	15	45.5
Suitable and sufficient PPE is easily accessible by healthcare providers	0	0.0	5	45.5	0	0.0	14	63.6	0	0.0	19	57.6
HCP wear gloves for potential contact with blood, body fluids, mucous membranes, non-intact skin, or contaminated equipment	0	0.0	9	81.8	0	0.0	21	95.5	0	0.0	30	90.9
HCP do not wear the same pair of gloves for the care of more than one patient	0	0.0	9	81.8	0	0.0	18	81.8	0	0.0	27	81.8
HCP wear proper gowns to protect skin and clothing during procedures or activities where contact with blood or body fluids is anticipated	0	0.0	6	54.5	0	0.0	19	86.4	0	0.0	25	75.8
HCP do not wear the same gown for the care of more than one patient	0	0.0	1	9.1	0	0.0	11	50.0	0	0.0	12	36.4
HCP wear mouth, nose, and eye protection during procedures that are likely to generate splashes or sprays of blood or other body fluids	0	0.0	4	36.4	0	0.0	9	40.9	0	0.0	13	39.4

Table 13.
Percentage of health centres that meet the target for each indicator of 'personal protective equipment' according to the type of health Centre.

for the procurement of hand-hygiene products (e.g., alcohol-based hand rubs) or any other way to ensure its availability.

4.8 Training and education

The targets for two training indicators are met by one-third of healthcare centres (33.3 per cent): receiving 'training regarding hand hygiene' and 'training assessors to verify compliance with hand hygiene'. The target for the other two indicators are met by more than half of centres: 'instructions on hand hygiene' (54.5 per cent), and 'safe injection training' (57.6 per cent). In addition, comprehensive healthcare centres met the target at a higher percentage—partially or completely—than primary healthcare centres (**Table 15**).

4.9 Evaluation and feedback

4.9.1 Basic indicators and respiratory safety

Most healthcare centres reported that hand hygiene is performed correctly (84.8 per cent) and regular reviews are done to assess the availability of hand-hygiene

Availability of hygiene materials	Primary centres (N = 11)				Comprehensive (N = 22)				Total (N = 33)			
	Partially meet target		Meet target		Partially meet target		Meet target		Partially meet target		Meet target	
	n	%	n	%	n	%	n	%	n	%	n	%
Alcohol-based hand rub is available in the health centre	5	45.5	6	54.5	9	40.9	13	59.1	14	42.4	19	57.6
Liquid soap is available at each sink	2	18.2	9	81.8	3	13.6	18	81.8	5	15.2	27	81.8
Single-use towels are available at each sink	4	36.4	2	18.2	11	50.0	6	27.3	15	45.5	8	24.2
There is a dedicated budget for the procurement of hand-hygiene products (e.g., alcohol-based hand rubs) or any other way to ensure its availability	0	0.0	5	45.5	0	0.0	9	40.9	0	0.0	14	42.4
Supplies needed for adherence to hand hygiene (e.g., soap, water, paper towels, alcohol-based hand rubs) are readily available to healthcare providers in patient-care areas	0	0.0	7	63.6	0	0.0	17	77.3	0	0.0	24	72.7

Table 14.
Percentage of health centres that meet the target for each indicator of 'availability of hygiene materials' according to the type of health Centre.

Training and education	Primary centres (N = 11)				Comprehensive (N = 22)				Total (N = 33)			
	Partially meet target		Meet target		Partially meet target		Meet target		Partially meet target		Meet target	
	n	%	n	%	n	%	n	%	n	%	n	%
Healthcare workers receive training regarding hand hygiene in the health centre	1	9.1	3	27.3	12	54.5	8	36.4	13	39.4	11	33.3
Posters or instructions on hand hygiene in health care are displayed to all healthcare workers	2	18.2	6	54.5	6	27.3	12	54.5	8	24.2	18	54.5
There is a system in place to train assessors to verify compliance with hand hygiene	1	9.1	2	18.2	6	27.3	9	40.9	7	21.2	11	33.3
Healthcare providers who prepare and/or administer parenteral drugs receive training in safe injection practices	1	9.1	4	36.4	4	18.2	15	68.2	5	15.2	19	57.6

Table 15.
Percentage of health centres that meet the target for each indicator of 'training and education' according to the type of health Centre.

materials (60.6 per cent), as shown in **Table 16**. One-quarter of centres reported that they review the availability of hand-hygiene materials (24.2 per cent), but not regularly.

Evaluation and feedback: Basic indicators and respiratory safety	Primary centres (N = 11)				Comprehensive (N = 22)				Total (N = 33)			
	Partially meet target		Meet target		Partially meet target		Meet target		Partially meet target		Meet target	
	n	%	n	%	n	%	n	%	n	%	n	%
Hand hygiene is performed in the health centre correctly	0	0.0	8	72.7	0	0.0	20	90.9	0	0.0	28	84.8
At department level, regular reviews are conducted (at least annually) in order to assess the availability of soaps, hand sanitizers, single-use towels, and other hand-hygiene resources	2	18.2	6	54.5	6	27.3	14	63.6	8	24.2	20	60.6
The health centre has policies and procedures for dealing with people who exhibit signs and symptoms of respiratory infections, starting from the point of admission to the health centre and continuing for the duration of the follow up	0	0.0	2	18.2	0	0.0	11	50.0	0	0.0	13	39.4
Face masks are offered upon admission to the health centre to cough patients and other people with symptoms, at least, during periods of increased respiratory tract infection in the community	0	0.0	1	9.1	0	0.0	5	22.7	0	0.0	6	18.2
Space is provided in waiting rooms, and people with symptoms of respiratory infections are encouraged to sit as far away from others as possible	0	0.0	0	0.0	0	0.0	14	63.6	0	0.0	14	42.4
The health centre educates healthcare providers on the importance of infection prevention measures to contain respiratory secretions to prevent the spread of respiratory diseases	0	0.0	2	18.2	0	0.0	16	72.7	0	0.0	18	54.5
Signboards and posters are displayed on entrances with instructions for patients with symptoms of respiratory infection in order to practice respiratory hygiene/cough etiquette (covering the mouth/nose when coughing or sneezing, using and disposing of tissues), and perform hand hygiene	0	0.0	3	27.3	0	0.0	10	45.5	0	0.0	13	39.4

Table 16.
Percentage of health centres that meet the target for each indicator of 'evaluation and feedback: Basic indicators and respiratory safety' according to the type of health Centre.

Less than half of healthcare centres met the target for indicators related to respiratory safety, except for educating healthcare providers on the importance of infection prevention measures, which was met by 54.5 per cent of the centres. This overall low percentage of meeting the target was attributed to the low percentage of primary healthcare centres that met the target, which was lower than 20 per cent for most indicators, as demonstrated. It is noteworthy to mention that none of the primary healthcare centres met the target for providing space in waiting rooms or encourage people with symptoms of respiratory infections to sit apart from others. However, the target for this indicator was met by 63.6 per cent of comprehensive healthcare centres.

4.9.2 Environmental cleaning and sterilization of reusable devices

About two-thirds of healthcare centres (63.6 per cent) met the target for using disinfectants according to manufacturer's instructions, and one-third (33.3 per cent) met the target for wearing PPE by staff involved in cleaning. However, cleaning of devices and packaging after cleaning were properly done by all comprehensive healthcare centre (100 per cent) and 81.8 per cent of primary healthcare centres (**Table 17**).

4.10 COVID-19 precautionary measures

The percentage of healthcare centres that met the target, partially or completely, varied widely among the different COVID-19 precautionary measures (**Table 18**). A low percentage of centres met the targets for some indicators, like emergency training of staff, or checking the temperature and breathing of staff or patients before entering the centre (18.2 per cent, each). On the other hand, a high percentage of centres met the targets for other indicators, like the requirements of washing hands frequently (81.8 per cent) or wearing masks (93.9 per cent). More comprehensive healthcare centres, compared to primary centres, met the targets for all

Evaluation and feedback: Environmental cleaning and sterilization of reusable devices	**Primary centres (N = 11)**				**Comprehensive (N = 22)**				**Total (N = 33)**			
	Partially meet target		**Meet target**		**Partially meet target**		**Meet target**		**Partially meet target**		**Meet target**	
	n	**%**	**n**	**%**	**n**	**%**	**n**	**%**	**n**	**%**	**n**	**%**
Cleaners and disinfectants are used in accordance with manufacturers' instructions (e.g., dilution, storage, shelf-life, contact time)	0	0.0	6	54.5	0	0.0	15	68.2	0	0.0	21	63.6
HCP engaged in cleaning wear appropriate PPE to prevent exposure to infectious agents or chemicals (PPE can include gloves, gowns, masks, and eye protection)	0	0.0	1	9.1	0	0.0	10	45.5	0	0.0	11	33.3
Devices are thoroughly cleaned according to manufacturers' instructions and visually inspected for residual dirt prior to sterilization	0	0.0	9	81.8	0	0.0	22	100	0	0.0	31	93.9
After cleaning, the tools are packaged appropriately for sterilization	0	0.0	9	81.8	0	0.0	22	100	0	0.0	31	93.9
The health centre has an emergency team	2	18.2	3	27.3	6	27.3	6	27.3	8	24.2	9	27.3

Table 17.
Percentage of health centres that meet the target for each indicator of 'evaluation and feedback: Environmental cleaning and sterilization of reusable devices' according to the type of health Centre.

COVID-19 precautionary measures	Primary centres (N = 11)				Comprehensive (N = 22)				Total (N = 33)			
	Partially meet target		Meet target		Partially meet target		Meet target		Partially meet target		Meet target	
	n	%	n	%	n	%	n	%	n	%	n	%
All health-centre staff are trained in the emergency programme	2	18.2	1	9.1	6	27.3	5	22.7	8	24.2	6	18.2
Health workers receive special training regarding COVID-19	0	0.0	4	36.4	0	0.0	12	54.5	0	0.0	16	48.5
All employees are asked to distance themselves from the rest of the staff, unless treating patients requires closer proximity	3	27.3	6	54.5	6	27.3	16	72.7	9	27.3	22	66.7
All employees are required to wash their hands frequently	3	27.3	7	63.6	2	9.1	20	90.9	5	15.2	27	81.8
All employees are required to adhere to wearing masks at all times	1	9.1	10	90.9	1	4.5	21	95.5	2	6.1	31	93.9
Health workers in the health centre receive regular tests for COVID-19	3	27.3	4	36.4	10	45.5	7	31.8	13	39.4	11	33.3
Patient appointment times are staggered and distances maintained, as a response to COVID-19 outbreak	5	45.5	3	27.3	13	59.1	5	22.7	18	54.5	8	24.2
Patients are required to wear a mask when they are in the health centre	2	18.2	7	63.6	4	18.2	18	81.8	6	18.2	25	75.8
Patients are required to maintain distance throughout their stay in the health centre	2	18.2	7	63.6	3	13.6	18	81.8	5	15.2	25	75.8
Temperature and breathing problems are checked for all patients before entering the health centre	1	9.1	3	27.3	3	13.6	3	13.6	4	12.1	6	18.2
Temperature and breathing problems are checked for all healthcare workers before entering the health centre	1	9.1	3	27.3	3	13.6	3	13.6	4	12.1	6	18.2
Medical staff treating COVID-19 permitted to socialize with the rest of the health-centre staff	1	9.1	4	36.4	6	27.3	12	54.5	7	21.2	16	48.5
Instructions given to health-centre staff with COVID-19 symptoms, like fever and coughing	4	36.4	6	54.5	7	31.8	12	54.5	11	33.3	18	54.5
There is a monitoring and registration record for all workers infected with the virus	0	0.0	4	36.4	0	0.0	9	40.9	0	0.0	13	39.4
All cases with COVID-19 are transferred to the hospital assigned to treat them.	0	0.0	4	36.4	0	0.0	16	72.7	0	0.0	20	60.6
All cases of COVID-19 are reported to the Ministry of Health	0	0.0	4	36.4	0	0.0	16	72.7	0	0.0	20	60.6

Table 18.
Percentage of health centres that meet the target for each indicator of 'COVID-19 precautionary measures' according to the type of health Centre.

indicators of COVID-19 precautionary measures, except for regular testing for COVID-19 and distancing and spacing the timings of appointments. However, these two indicators were met by only one-third (33.3 per cent) and one-quarter of healthcare centres (24.2 per cent), respectively. Moreover, three out of four healthcare centres (75.8 per cent) reported asking patients to wear masks and maintain distances, as shown in **Table 18**. It is interesting that only 60.6 per cent of healthcare centres reported COVID-19 cases to the Ministry of Health.

5. Conclusions

Based on the findings of this assessment, we could identify health facilities that fully met the targets and those that partially met or did not meet the targets. A wide range of performance was noted, and clear differences between facilities in meeting the targets were observed. Thus, healthcare policy makers are urged to develop WASH and IPC national policies and guidelines that set targets for all public and private healthcare facilities in the country. It is essential that healthcare providers in Jordan translate local and national IPC policies into their daily and regular practice. However, IPC policies should be enforced during the COVID-19 pandemic to control the spread of the virus. Developing and implementing a national IPC Action Plan (2021–2024) will assist the integration of IPC practices into the Jordanian healthcare system, which also identify, amend, and correct non-compliance practices with IPC standards. The action plan should be supervised by a national IPC unit, affiliated with, or as part of, the Ministry of Health.

Furthermore, stakeholders and policy makers are urged to institute a quality surveillance system through which standard precautions and transmission-based precautions can be implemented. This surveillance system assists healthcare facilities across Jordan to manage infections through early detection of patients with infectious diseases, immediate implementation of containment measures including the use of PPE and isolation; and measures required to control the spread of COVID-19.

The implementation of the surveillance system and WASH/IPC standards are possible only through capacity building with proper training that is carried out, based on international recommendations, like the WHO recommended procedures for PPE and WASH, for example.

Digital health solutions to enhance healthcare providers' skills and knowledge on WASH and IPC policies could be promising during the COVID-19 pandemic. Such digital health solutions can be designed to train healthcare providers to demonstrate evidence-based practices of infection control and to promote hygiene messages among patients to protect themselves and their families. However, the optimum benefits of precautionary measures and the sustainability of WASH and IPC targets are not achieved without the serious commitments from leaders and managers from all levels (national, provincial, and organizational). Skilful health management is necessary to officially mandate WASH and IPC practices and to provide and maintain necessary human and financial resources to conduct IPC activities. Moreover, medical leadership are expected to show tangible support and act as role models to drive a patient-safety culture, supporting WASH and IPC and all relevant subsequent actions.

Acknowledgements

Authors would like to acknowledge the technical and financial support from UNICEF Jordan Country office and Middle Eastern and Northern Africa Regional Office.

Author details

Yousef Khader[1*], Mohamad Alyahya[2] and Rami Saadeh[1]

1 Department of Public Health, Faculty of Medicine, Jordan University of Science and Technology, Irbid, Jordan

2 Department of Health Management and Policy, Faculty of Medicine, Jordan University of Science and Technology, Irbid, Jordan

*Address all correspondence to: yskhader@just.edu.jo

References

[1] The World Health Organization (WHO) and United Nations Children's Emergency Fund, Water, sanitation and hygiene in health care facilities-urgent needs and actions, Meeting Report, UNICEF, 2015, <www.who.int/water_sanitation_health/facilities/wash-in-hcf-geneva.pdf?ua=1>, last accessed 20 May 2021.

[2] Madge, P., et al., Prospective controlled study of four infection-control procedures to prevent nosocomial infection with respiratory syncytial virus. Lancet, 340 (8827), 1992,pp. 1079–1083.

[3] Ershova, K., et al., Implementing an infection control and prevention program decreases the incidence of healthcare-associated infections and antibiotic resistance in a Russian neuro-ICU. Antimicrobial Resistance and Infection Control, 7(1), 2018, pp. 1–11.

[4] Abdelrahman, M.A., et al., Knowledge of nosocomial infection control practices among radiographers in Jordan. Radiography, 23(4), 2017, pp. 298–304.

[5] Al-Rawajfah, O.M. and A. Tubaishat, A concealed observational study of infection control and safe injection practices in Jordanian governmental hospitals. American Journal of Infection Control, 45 (10) 2017, pp. 1127–1132.

[6] United Nations Department of Economic and Social Affairs Disability, THE 17 GOALS – Sustainable Development, 2020, <https://sdgs.un.org/goals>, last accessed 20 May 2021.

[7] United Nations Department of Economic and Social Affairs Disability, Goal 6 – Department of Economic and Social Affairs, 2020, <<https://sdgs.un.org/goals/goal6>, last accessed 20 May 2021.

[8] World Health Organization, Interim guidance April 2020: Water, sanitation, hygiene and waste management for the COVID-19 virus, WHO, April 2020, p. 1–9.

[9] Prüss, A., et al., Estimating the burden of disease from water sanitation and hygiene at a global level. Environmental Health Perspectives, 110 (5), 2002, pp. 537–542.

[10] Khader, Y.S., Water, sanitation and hygiene in Jordan's healthcare facilities. Int J Health Care Qual Assur, 30(7), 2017, pp. 645–655.

[11] The United Nations, Water, Sanitation and Hygiene, UN-Water, 2020, <www.unwater.org/water-facts/water-sanitation-and-hygiene>, last accessed 20 May 2021.

[12] United Nations Children's Emergency Fund, Water, Sanitation and Hygiene – Access to safe water and sanitation for every child, UNICEF Jordan, Amman, 2020, <www.unicef.org/jordan/water-sanitation-and-hygiene>, last accessed 20 May 2021.

[13] United Nations Children's Emergency Fund, Water, Sanitation and Hygiene (WASH) – Safe water, toilets and good hygiene keep children alive and healthy, UNICEF, 2020, <www.unicef.org/wash/3942_4456.html>, last accessed 20 May 2021.

[14] Bhowmick, G., et al., Coronavirus disease 2019 (COVID-19) outbreak: some serious consequences with urban and rural water cycle. npj Clean Water, 3, 2020.

[15] Anaissie, E.J., S.R. Penzak, and M.C. Dignani, The hospital water supply as a source of nosocomial infections: a plea for action. Arch Intern Med, 162 (13), 2002, pp. 1483–1492.

[16] Stuckey, M., et al., Water management and monitoring practices in hospitals—United States, 2018. Infection Control and Hospital Epidemiology, 41 (S1), 2020, pp. s83-s84. doi:10.1017/ice.2020.577.

[17] Chawla, S.S., et al., Water availability at hospitals in low- and middle-income countries: implications for improving access to safe surgical care. J Surg Res, 205(1), 2016, pp. 169–178.

[18] Patrício, A.L., et al., Rethinking and optimising plastic waste management under COVID-19 pandemic: Policy solutions based on redesign and reduction of single-use plastics and personal protective equipment. Science of The Total Environment, 742, January 2020.

[19] Castro Filho, E.C., et al., Gastrointestinal endoscopy during the COVID-19 pandemic: an updated review of guidelines and statements from international and national societies. Gastrointestinal Endoscopy, 92(2), 2020, pp. 440–445.

[20] Young, B.E., et al., Epidemiologic Features and Clinical Course of Patients Infected with SARS-CoV-2 in Singapore. JAMA – Journal of the American Medical Association, 323 (15), 2020, pp. 1488–1494.

[21] Zhang, J.C., S.B. Wang, and Y.D. Xue, Fecal specimen diagnosis 2019 novel coronavirus–infected pneumonia. Journal of Medical Virology, 92(6), 2020, pp. 680–682.

[22] Ahmed, W., et al. First confirmed detection of SARS-CoV-2 in untreated wastewater in Australia: A proof of concept for the wastewater surveillance of COVID-19 in the community. The Science of the total environment, 728, 2020, 138764. doi:10.1016/j.scitotenv.2020.138764

[23] The Center for Disease Control and Prevention, Water, Sanitation and Environmentally-related Hygiene, CDC, 2020, <www.cdc.gov/healthywater/hygiene/index.html>, last accessed 20 May 2021.

[24] Erasmus, V., et al., Systematic Review of Studies on Compliance with Hand Hygiene Guidelines in Hospital Care. Infection Control and Hospital Epidemiology, 31(3), 2010, pp. 283–294.

[25] Przekwas, A., and Chen, Z., Washing hands and the face may reduce COVID-19 infection. Medical hypotheses, 144, 2020, 110261. doi: 10.1016/j.mehy.2020.110261

[26] Wiedenmayer, K., et al., Impact of hand hygiene intervention: A comparative study in health care facilities in Dodoma region, Tanzania using WHO methodology. Antimicrobial Resistance and Infection Control, 9(1), 2020, pp. 1–9.

[27] Tomczyk, S et al. Testing of the WHO Infection Prevention and Control Assessment Framework at acute healthcare facility level. The Journal of hospital infection, 105(1), 2020, pp. 83-90. doi:10.1016/j.jhin.2019.12.016

[28] Aghdassi, S.J.S., et al., Evaluating infection prevention and control programs in Austrian acute care hospitals using the WHO Infection Prevention and Control Assessment Framework. Antimicrobial Resistance and Infection Control, 9(1), 2020, pp. 1–9.

[29] Maina, M., et al., Extending the use of the World Health Organisations' water sanitation and hygiene assessment tool for surveys in hospitals – from WASH-FIT to WASH-FAST. PLoS ONE, 14(12), 2019, pp. 1–15.

[30] Patel, K., et al., Assessment of water, sanitation and hygiene in HCFs:

Which tool to follow? Rev Environ Health, 34(4), 18 December 2019, pp. 435–440.

[31] World Health Organization, The burden of health care-associated infection worldwide, WHO, 2017, <www.who.int/infection-prevention/publications/burden_hcai/en>, last accessed 20 May 2021.

[32] World Health Organization, Water and Sanitation for Health Facility Improvement Tool (WASH FIT), WHO, 2017, <https://apps.who.int/iris/bitstream/handle/10665/254910/9789241511698-eng.pdf;jsessionid=CBA30FFCCFC3CD66C0827B5C38BCDDF9?sequence=1>, last accessed 20 May 2021.

[33] The World Health Organization, WHO Guidelines on core components of IPC programmes at the national and acute health care facility level, WHO, 2016,< http://apps.who.int/iris/bitstream/handle/10665/251730/9789241549929-eng.pdf?sequence=1>, last accessed 20 May 2021.

[34] The Center for Disease Control and Prevention, Guide to Infection Prevention for Outpatient Settings: Minimum Expectations for Safe Care, CDC, 2014, <www.cdc.gov/hai/settings/outpatient/outpatient-care-guidelines.html>, last accessed 20 May 2021.

[35] World Health Organization, Essential environmental health standards in health care, WHO, 2008, <http://apps.who.int/iris/bitstream/handle/10665/43767/9789241547239_eng.pdf?sequence=1>, last accessed 20 May 2021.

Section 7

Occupational Health and Safety in Primary Care

Chapter 16

Strategies to Enhance Compliance to Health and Safety Protocols within the South African Mining Environment

Livhuwani Muthelo, Tebogo Maria Mothiba and Rambelani Nancy Malema

Abstract

Occupational health focuses on promotive and preventive and curative health. The occupational health practitioners have the responsibility to guide management and employees on the occupational legislative obligations aiming to safeguard legal compliance at the workplace. Additionally, it is the responsibility of the health professionals within the mining industry to provide primary, secondary and tertiary prevention strategies to improve the health and safety of workers. However, the prevalence of work-related diseases such as noise induced hearing loss, silicosis and the occurrence of accidents in the mining industry is an alarming factor. Systematic review method was adopted to identify and screen relevant citations. This book chapter aims to review and discuss existing literature on health and safety strategies to enhance safety compliance within the South African mining industry.

Keywords: Compliance, Health and Safety, Mining, Clinic

1. Introduction

Worldwide, the mining sector is classified as the most dangerous work and customarily ranks within the top 3 occupations for related diseases and fatal accidents [1–7]. The complete health of the miners includes physical, social, and psychological, including protection from injury or any occupational disease [8]. Whereas safety is associated with the physical mining environment and interventions done to reduce exposure to risk [8]. Within the context of this review, the authors are concerned that if mining remains unsafe as occupational health practitioners how can we improve and make sure a healthy and safe workplace? Smith et al. highlighted the necessity for mining corporations to accommodate international and national safety and health laws and laws, but there's a requirement to implement preventative strategies to accommodates those standards and laws [1]. In Africa, though several African states have comprehensive laws regarding activity health and safety standards and hours of labor, systems to make sure compliance, their observance is usually weak and under-resourced in several organizations [9, 10]. According to the African Union's Mining Vision and Bocoum, a lot stays to be done to carry mining practices. Policies, regulatory capacity, and services associated with mine health need to be massively progressed, and standardized carrier shipping models want to be set up each nationally and domestically [10, 11].

The SA mine health and safety council have introduced pointers for compliance with the Mine Health and Safety Act (29 of 1996) [12]. However, the high rate of sub-standard performance has shown that accessible rules and policies have not led to the anticipated result [13]. Governmental and trade executives, policymakers, and material scientists voiced issues and conducted various reports stating matters and the risks of an offer crisis. Positively safety rules are necessary to form a healthy and safe work atmosphere, but it's of significant importance to explore the social relations within the employment context (organization), the individual factors (beliefs, attitudes, and behavior), and also the cultural processes that contribute to non-compliance with health and safety standards within the mining trade [14]. Given these gaps, there is an obligation to identify the ways that may enhance compliance with health and safety standards. Muchiri emphasized the necessity and the duty for the occupational health and safety professionals, employers, workers, agencies, and alternative stakeholders to incessantly develop and implement multi-faceted OSH ways [9]. Within the context of this review, compliance shall refer to the proper practice of the staff and also the organization following the health and safety standards within the mining industry [14].

2. Objectives

This review aims to analyze the present state of compliance with the health and safety regulations/standards, among the South African Mining industry and to highlight the importance of the implementation of preventative strategies through the occupational health clinic. The review additionally provides insights upon that a part of health and safety legislation standards would like an improvement. in addition, this review intends to create clear links between the studies and also the activity health and safety legislation and also the conclusions, confirm any controversies, weaknesses, and gaps with the compliance in the mining industry and generate information and data on the world strategies that may be used for compliance and making property health and safety atmosphere within the mining industry. This review adds worth to existing electronic databases through the integration of analysis results.

3. Systematic literature review method

The review adopted the systematic review technique that enabled the reviewers to discover and investigate the systematic evidence of both qualitative and quantitative research, government and private documentation, and also the laws bearing on occupational health and safety compliance. The subsequent systematic steps as outlined by Cronin, et al.; Ramdhani et al. were applied to cut back literature-review errors and bias and to supply a clear, structured, and comprehensive summary of the obtainable literature (**Figure 1**) [15, 16].

Step 1: Defining the research question.

As per Hempel, Xenakis, and Danz it's important to layout the requests to be addressed in occupational safety and health systematic review to recognize the point and extent of the survey [17]. Additionally forming the inquiries can coordinate the reader on the sort of information looked still up in the review. The examination question was illustrated through the conversation with the supervisor

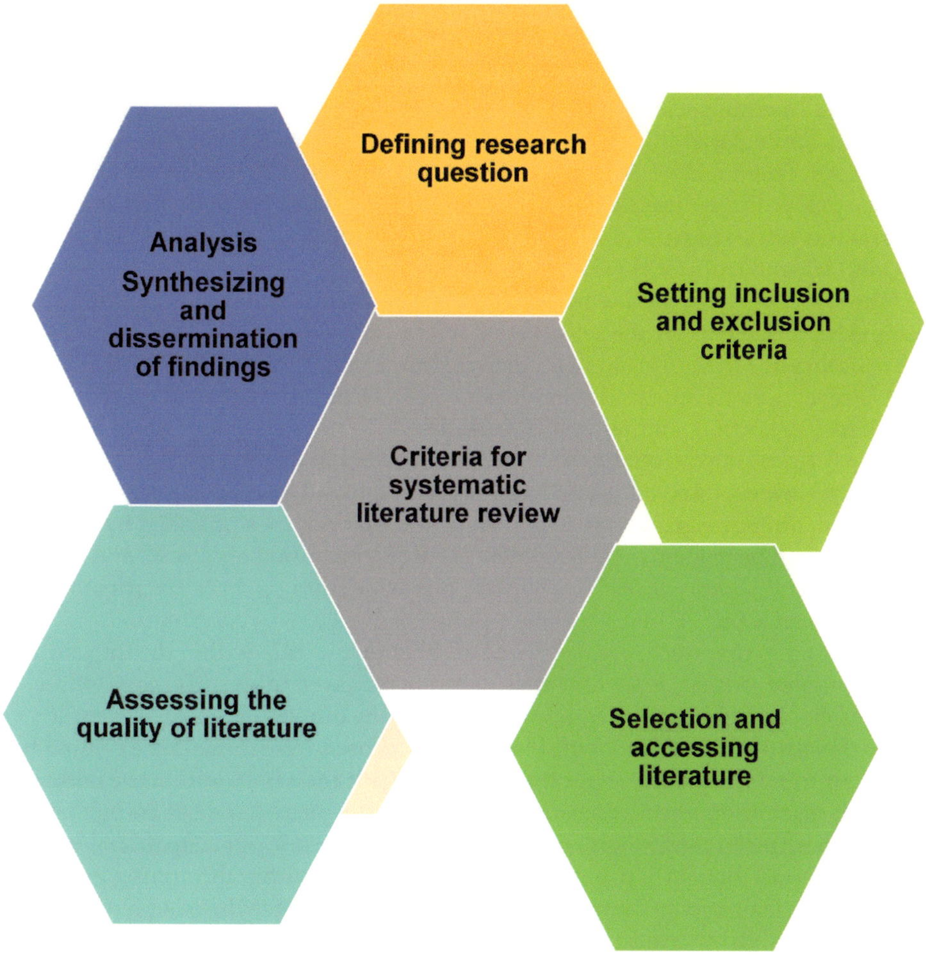

Figure 1.
Systematic review steps adopted from: (Ramdhani et al., Hempel, Xenakis & Danz).

and co-supervisor, meeting with the master's word related wellbeing specialists to affirm that the audit has significance to genuine difficulties. The examination question was: What is the current situation with compliance with the health and safety guidelines /principles among the SA mining exchange and what are the procedures, which will be created to affirm the compliance with the health and safety enactment/norms among the SA mining industry?

Step 2: Setting for inclusion and exclusion criteria.

Shamseer, Moher Clarke, et al. laid out that setting for incorporation and prohibition measures guarantees that the survey is led in a coordinated manner [18]. Also, it accommodates the straightforwardness of how the qualities and restrictions were surveyed. Furthermore, the conceptual model in the current study guided the researcher through the review to explore the defined study question. The PICO (population, intervention, comparison, and outcome) format was followed [19]. The conceptual model defined the population which was the mine occupational health practitioners, satety representatives, occupational health clinics, miners, the mining organizational and the mine management, interventions, in this case, was the legislation, standards, and the preventative strategies that guide the employees to comply with the health and safety.

Step 3: Conducting a literature search.

The online database literature search enclosed a mixture of South African and international government OHS legislation, policies, standards, reports from the labor departments and international labor workplace, the qualitative, quantitative, and mixed- methods scientific journal articles, conference proceedings. Seven databases are enclosed PUBMED, EBSCOHOST, SEMATIC SCHOLAR, GOOGLE SCHOLAR, domain EDU, SAFE WORK AUSTRALIA. gray literature including conference proceedings, dissertations, theses, government information, and committee reports was retrieved from searches in web OF SCIENCE, ILO, WHO. HSELINE, NIOSHTIC, and from OSH UPDATE.

The search strategy adopted Boolean operators combined sets of keywords, using AND/OR terms for the selection of articles and reports [20]. The terms from the subsequent 7 categories were accustomed to search the articles and gray literature (Prevention, Compliance, health and safety, Occupational health practitioner, standards, legislation, and mining) (**Table 1**).

Step 3: Assessing the quality of literature included in the review.

This review enclosed all the articles, reports obtained when databases were integrated, duplicate articles were removed, and extra articles provided by content specialists had been identified. Secondary sources, including textbooks and review articles or descriptions or outlines by someone aside from the first investigator, were removed [20].

Only studies that were revealed between 1994 to July 2021 within the English peer- reviewed journal, report, or websites were reviewed to identify gaps within the compliance with the health and safety within the mining industry. Moreover, abstracts solely were not enclosed. The studies enclosed were those that explored the compliance and the preventative strategies for health and safety within the mining industry. in addition, the studies, that reported on the present state of compliance with the health and safety legislation and standards, the role of occupational health clinics and practitioners in promoting health and safety within the mining industry, and also the occupational interventions/strategies to reinforce the compliance.

Step 4: Analyze, synthesize and disseminate the findings.

The studies which have been protected were clustered and prepared by using ideas, which emerged as themes. To offer enough substance to a topic, standards from at the least 3 articles had been required. Five thematic domains emerged from the literature. Six thematic domains emerged from the literature: Global laws, legislation, and standards on health and safety compliance within the mining industry; African countries mining health and safety compliance literature; health and safety compliance literature within the South African mining industry; Legislations; preventative strategies to improve the health and safety compliance within the mining industry and occupational health practitioners role in improving health and safety standards compliance.

Step 4: Analyze, synthesize and disseminate the findings.

The analysis and synthesis process is shown below **Figure 2**.

Occupational health and safety- related search terms	**Mining health, medical surveillance, mining safety, occupational health, safety behavior, safety culture**
Health and safety compliance search terms	Adherence, legislations, guidelines, standards, policy, preventative strategies
Occupational health search terms	Occupational health practitioners, health and safety representatives, occupational diseases, occupational injury, and accidents, safety culture
Mining health strategies related search terms	Prevention levels, occupational health interventions,

Table 1.
Search terms.

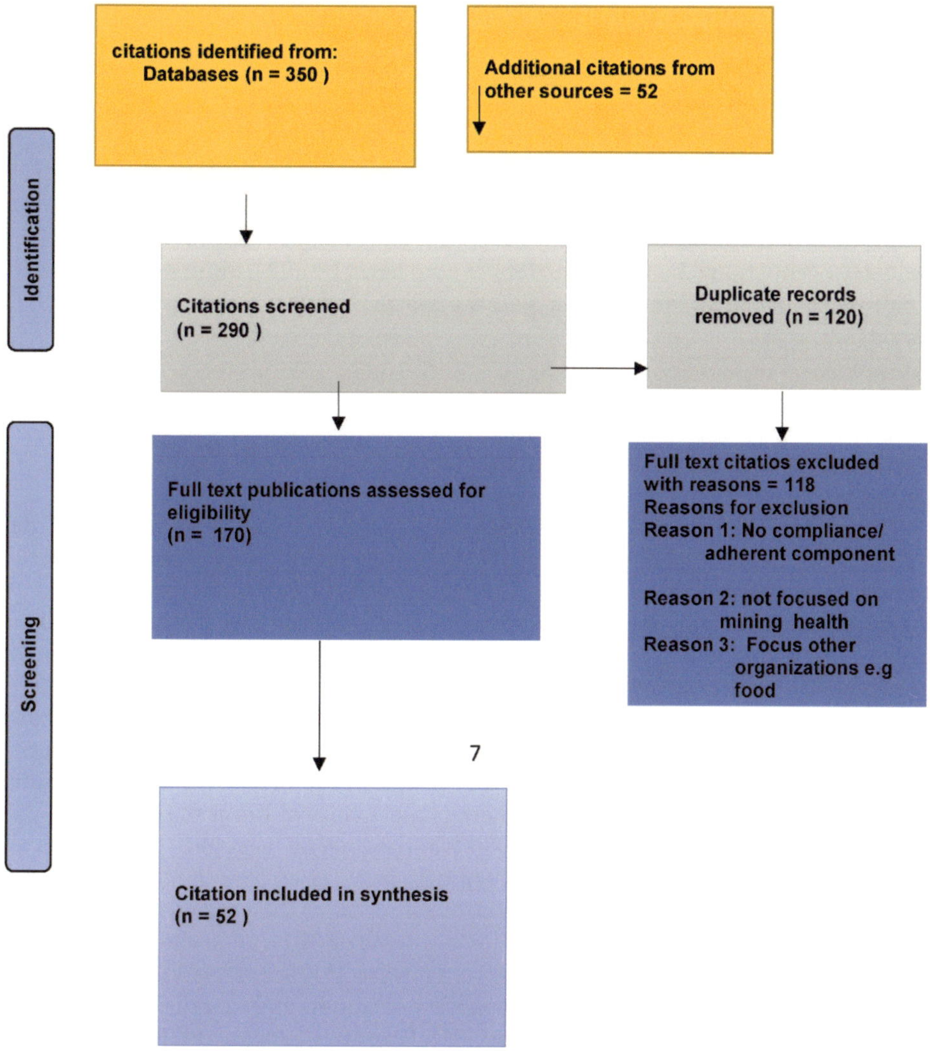

Figure 2.
A flow diagram (literature).

4. Occupational health and safety compliance in mining

Health and Safety compliance is the volume to which personnel adheres to health and safety standards, techniques, jail responsibilities, and wishes. It's furthermore accomplice diploma absence of injuries and incidents within the geographic component [21]. The majority of mine fitness and safety government international agree that the fundamental causes of mine accidents and fatalities are dangerous conditions, terrible control, and mainly non-compliance with the health and protection standards [22]. Furthermore, Vassem, Fortunato, Bastos, and Balassiano documented that the excessive incidence charge of accidents inside the mining enterprise calls for the information of interpersonal family members within the employment context (corporation), the individual factors (beliefs, attitudes, and behavior) that contribute to non-compliance with health and safety standards within the mining industry [23]. On the opposite hand the venture with the implementation of occupational legislation and requirements is that miners understanding of occupational regulation is confined and adherence is as a result impaired [24]. Therefore, to make certain compliance with fitness and safety requirements occupational fitness occupational health practioners have a duty to increase cognizance of health risks that impact the people' health and safety, as well as the measures which can mitigate the dangers [25].

The SA mining industry is under the spotlight with an increase in accidents and fatalities. In 2019 SA reported a total of 2406 injuries and 51 deaths in the mining industry [26]. This are a serious concern considering that In 2016, the chamber of mines signed a declaration of actions pledge as a change to improve the mining industry occupational health and safety to zero harm by 2024, aiming to generate a culture change in an industry that will transform the behavior of people at all levels [27].

5. Global laws, legislation, and standards on health and safety compliance within the mining industry

Occupational health and safety standards plays important role in guiding all the miners on health and safety-related issues focusing more on prevention. However though there are available standards, the occurrence of injuries and occupational diseases remains to be a challenge worldwide. The literature revealed that globally in every 15 seconds a miner dies [28, 29]. World Health Organization (WHO)outlined occupational health and safety as 'the advancement and maintenance of the most significant level of physical, mental and social health of miners in all occupations by preventing health risks and controlling danger and the adaption of work to miners and their positions [30]. Furthermore, it is of utmost importance to note that a safe and healthy working environment influences the quality of life at the individual level to substantial impacts on public health at the societal level [30].

Globally, the health and safety of the miners have raised serious concerns. In the United States (US) the former chief executive director of the upper big branch coal mine was sentenced to a year in prison for the death of 38 miners who were killed after a coal explosion [31]. He was convicted for a workplace safety violation by putting profits of the company ahead of the safety of miners and creating a culture of non-compliance within the organization [31]. Dragan, Georges, and Mustafa's study in Canada indicated that cultural factors within the organization especially from the management focusing on performance and efficiency and neglecting safety plays a key role in creating conditions for triggering major accidents [32]. More particularly from the administration with more emphasis on the execution and productivity and dismissing the safety and wellbeing of miners.

Different countries have laws and regulations in place at the workplace aiming to protect the health and safety of individuals in their occupations. Occupational health and safety laws across nations share many similarities highlighting that the health and safety of employees must be secured through the assessment, analysis, adjustment and reducing the risks and hazards for illness and injury at the workplace [33, 34]. Occupational health and safety compliance shapes the required or desirable behavior in the workplace. Furthermore, compliance is linked to the safety culture or climate in the organization, which is believed to shape employee behavior through expectations [35].

Statute law may uphold extra obligations, start explicit obligations, and structure government bodies with the power to direct work environment wellbeing and medical problems. As set by Spada and Burgherr; Mabika, reinforcing the wellbeing controller is required, upheld by the authoritative approaches [36, 37]. Such drives can save the existence of mine accidents and occupational diseases in both developed and undeveloped countries [37]. United Kingdom (UK) is one of the created nations with a fruitful record of wellbeing and safety practices in the mine. As indicated by Uyanusta Kucuk and Ilgaz, wellbeing and safety laws in the UK have been in existence for more than 200 years [38]. Moreover, the laws came because of political reactions to social issues emerging from the unsettling influences of the industrial revolution [38]. Among other enactments, the mines and safety act 1954 was the broadest safety enactment in the UK. The demonstration set down legal obligations on mine chiefs and offered.

6. African countries mining health and safety compliance literature

A triangulation study led by Kheni and Braimah; Mustapha, Aigbavboa, and Thwala conducted in Ghana looking at the institutional and lawful conditions identifying with health and safety management referred to helpless coordination of activities related to health and safety standards, absence and unwanted degree of consistency with significant H&S enactment as the serious issues [39, 40].

The greater part of the African nations is known for deprived safety and health practices [41, 42]. Takala and Saarela featured that low-pay nations in Africa and Asia have recorded raised paces of injuries and fatalities contrasted with created nations, for example, Europe and America [43]. Besides, it has been assessed that 54000 fatality related to occupational accidents happen in Sub-saharan Africa yearly contrasted with 16000 fatalities in Europe and America. Boniface, Maseru, Munthali and Lett study results on Occupational injuries and fatalities in Tanzania highlighted the requirement for improving health and safety principles systems in the mines [44].

7. Health and safety compliance literature within the South African mining industry

The South African mining industry does not have a good reputation for health and safety due to recurrent accidents and fatalities. One of the largest mining companies in SA with a major interest in both platinum and gold mining (Sibanye) outlined that one of the causes of fatalities was non-compliance by miners and management as people try to take shortcuts [45]. On the contrary, the union representatives within the mining industry blame the high pressure to reach production targets means that miners remain in unsafe working conditions and environment [39].

The South African mining Act, 1996 (Act 29 of 1996) was endorsed to improve health and safety performance and great emphasis was placed on adherence to mine standards [46]. Furthermore, different types of legislation were passed to assist in the transformation6and "improvement of the safety standards in the mining sector, among others, the Skills Development Act of 1998 (SDA), Broad-Based Black Economic Empowerment Act, 2013 (BBEEA), (Minerals Petroleum Resources and Development Amendment Bill 2013 (MPRDAB), Compensation for Occupational Injuries and Diseases Act, 1997 (COIDA), Occupational Diseases in Mines and Works Amendment Act, 2002 (ODMWAA), Labour Relations Act, 1996 (LRA), Basic Conditions of Employment Act of 1997, Mining Charter 2010, and the Constitution of the Republic of South Africa, 1996".

The Society for Mining, Metallurgy and Exploration (SME) Mining Engineering Handbook, expresses that all mining tasks are needed to adhere to local, provincial, and governmental guidelines that indicate mine health and safety guidelines and norms, environmental protection, and work relations. The nature, degree, and toughness of these guidelines, at last, administer the mining activity [45].

Lack of emphasis on the promotion of health of mine-workers made the Commission to endorsed to improve the state of the safety standards in the mining sector, among others, the enactment of a new Mine Health and Safety Act 29 of 1996 (hereinafter referred to as MHSA), which started operating from January 1997.140 The Act (MHSA) has established a council known as Mine Health and Safety Council (MHSC), that contemplates the status of health and safety in the mining sector, recommends policy and legislation, commissions' research, and offers suitable advice to the Minister of Mineral Resources.

The Department of mineral resources and energy South Africa is responsible to promote and regulate the minerals and mining sector in SA. Furthermore, the Department also has the responsibility to ensure that all the mining companies in SA follow and comply with the health and safety legislation. They also have an obligatory role to take action when the mining companies do not implement and comply with the regulations. Laws and standards. The mineral resource department can close/terminate the mining activities or take the mining companies to the Court of Justice if they fail to comply. The following regulations guide all the mines in SA on health and safety.

8. Mine health and safety act (MHSA, act no 29 of 1996)

The MHSA regulates the mining sector focusing on the health requirements in the mining industry.

8.1 Objectives of the act

The goals of this act are to accommodate the wellbeing of the workers and different people at mines: support consistent with the standards of health and safety; take into account the execution of health and safety measures; accommodate suitable frameworks of the employee, employer, and state participation in health and safety matters; build up delegate three-sided organizations to audit enactment, advance wellbeing and upgrade appropriately designated research; accommodate compelling observing frameworks and assessments, to guarantee that there are examinations and requests to further develop health and safety; advance preparing and HR improvement; manage businesses' and workers' obligations to recognize hazards and prevent, control and limit the danger to health and safety; settle in the option to decline to work in hazardous conditions, and to offer impact to the public worldwide law commitments of the Republic identifying with mining health and safety [12].

8.2 The role of the occupational medical practitioner (OMP) in ensuring the health and safety of employees in the mine

Section 13 of MHSA outlines the legal requirement for all the mining organizations in SA to have an OMP either on a full-time or part-time basis. The OMP has legal duties and ethical duties when ensuring the overall health of the miners [12, 28, 46]. They play a major role in preventative medicine, determining the fitness and ensuring that every person in the mine (both the employer and the miners undergo medical surveillance. Medical surveillance is a scheduled program that includes medical examinations, conducting different tests depending on the job that the miner applied for such tests includes audiometry, spirometry, and vision screening. The purpose of medical surveillance is to ensure that all the miners are fit to perform their duties without endangering their health and safety. Medical problems that may arise due to workplace exposure are also identified [12, 28]. The occupational medical practitioner must ensure that the medical surveillance must be suitable and be planned in such a way that it affords the miners to gain knowledge that can be used to the information that employees can use to eradicate, govern and reduce risks and hazards related to health and safety [28, 46]. This is achieved through continuous health education providing information to the miners relaxed to their medical results e.g. education related to audiometric test results on hearing loss. Medical surveillance includes the following types of medical examinations:

- Pre-placement/baseline medical examination

It is a legal requirement for all mining organizations to conduct a pre-placement examination to be done before the miner can be appointed and placed in a job. The examination assists in the assessment of the miner's suitability for the position applied and also the work environment that will be exposed to. More importantly pre-employment is also done to ensure the safety of the miners and others ensuring that the new employee does not pose risk [28].

- Periodic medical examination

This examination is done every year or six months depending on the risk that the miner is exposed to. The examination I also done if the exposure risk increase or there is deterioration noted in the test results, when the miner is transferred from one department to another, after being involved in a serious injury or sickness [28].

- Exit medical examination

This examination is performed before the miners leave their current employment. It s a legal requirement for the miners to produce their exit fitness certificate to their new employer. The exit medical examination safeguards the organization against future medical claims. The records are kept for 40 years [28].

9. The occupational health and safety act (OHS act No 85 of 1993) as amended by the occupational health and safety amendment Act (OHS act NO 181 of 1993)

9.1 Objective of the act

The target of the demonstration is to accommodate the wellbeing and safety of miners at work, particularly regarding the utilization of apparatus (South Africa, 1993). Moreover, the Act accommodates the safety of miners against dangers to wellbeing and safety emerging from or regarding the exercises of people at work. This act recognized settled an advisory council on occupational and safety [47]. The overall obligations of the business and the miners in the work environment are likewise specified [47].

9.2 The role of health and safety representatives in ensuring compliance

All the mines must appoint a health and safety team including health and safety representatives where there are 20 or more employees. Whereas if the mine has 100 or more miners the health and safety committee should be established. The health and safety representatives have the following major roles to play in ensuring the safety of the miners:

- Review health and safety measures whether they are effective or not
- Identifying possible hazards and the occurrence of incidents
- They represent all the miners concerning health and safety and investigates all the complaints related to the safety of miners.
- They do workplace inspections to identify potential health and safety risks
- They participate in the inspection of the mine by the inspectors and provide safety- related information when needed.
- They form part of the health and safety committee and participate in the internal health and safety audit.
- They also investigate health and safety accidents [28, 47].

9.3 Occupational health practioner role in health and safety standards compliance

According to the Mine Health and Act (29 of 1996), all organizations must employ a practitioner who is in the position of qualification in occupational medicine recognized by the Interim National Medical and Dental Council of South Africa or the South African Interim Nursing Council [12]. The occupational health practitioners are the largest single group of the multidisciplinary health care team at the workplace. Therefore, OHN is the frontline in protecting and promoting the health of the working population.

The occupational health practitioner is gifted in injury or diseases preventative skills and interventions. The OHP might recognize the requirement for, survey, and plan mediations to, alter working conditions, frameworks of work, or change working practices to decrease the danger of exposure to hazards [48]. Moreover, OHP experts are skilled in thinking about factors, like human conduct and habits about real working practices. They additionally team up in the origination, and rectification of work factors, decision, and quality of protective equipment, protection of miners from injury and illnesses, just as giving guidance in issues concerning the assurance of the climate [28, 48]. The OHP close relationship with the workers, and involvement with the management, they are in a decent situation to distinguish early changes in unsafe working practices, recognize miners challenges over health and safety, and present these to management in an independent objective manner can be the catalyst for changes in the workplace that lead to primary prevention by present these to the executives in a free target way can be the motivation for changes in the work environment that lead to essential counteraction [48].

The occupational health professionals inform on a wide reach concerning medical problems, and especially on their relationship to working capacity, wellbeing, and safety at work or where alterations to the work or workspace can be made to assess the changing wellbeing status of representatives [28]. In many regards, organizations are not exclusively worried about just those conditions that are straightforwardly brought about by work however, they need occupational health professionals to assist with attending to any wellbeing related issues that might emerge that may impact the miner's participation or execution at work, and numerous representatives like this degree of help being given to them at the work environment since it is so advantageous for them [43]. Specifically, the improvement of medical care administrations for miners at the workplace. With regards to this survey, the OHP plays a significant part in guaranteeing the health and safety of the miners through primary, secondary, and tertiary avoidance [49].

10. Preventative strategies

Different scholars have acknowledged that there is a gap in the literature on the management of compliance with the health and safety strategy. Moreover, scholars have also raised a concern that the impact of legal non-compliance is even more scarce in the literature [49, 50]. Previous research done by Tibane and Niemand on challenges experienced by employees relating to safety compliance emphasized the importance of the development of strategies to reduce safety threats caused by poor compliance as a result of unsafe acts [51]. The question is that if they are safety regulations available and miners are aware of the dangers, what is the rationale behind poor compliance with the health and safety standards [52, 53].

The strategies are aimed at can be named preventive and treatment mediations. Precaution mediations are typically presented to every one of the excavators helping them to take on well- being conduct and sound way of life unconstrained and without incidental effects fuming them to search for help. On the other hand, Bagherpour et al. argue that preventive strategies need to be applied before the incidents, but preparative adjustments must be implemented both before and after the occurrence [6]. Preventive interventions, accordingly, are named as a primary, secondary, or tertiary counteraction.

Preventative strategies are normally offered to all the miners assisting them to adopt a safe behavior and healthy lifestyle spontaneous and without side effects seething them to look for help. More importantly, the literature revealed that compliance with health and safety law involves the development and implementation of an effective health and safety preventative system and building a positive health and safety culture at work [54]. Preventive mediations, thusly, are named as primary, secondary, or tertiary prevention [55].

10.1 Primary preventive strategies

In occupational health primary, preventative strategies are aimed at eradicating risks and exposures at the workplace before they occur. This level of prevention is important because the effect has not yet occurred yet the extent of the risk is visible [56]. In the occupational health clinic, primary prevention focuses on health promotion and protection within the context of a safe and healthy work environment [21]. This is achieved through continuous health education, conducting medical surveillance, and monitoring of chronic diseases thereby enhancing employees' morale and maintaining optimal health. However, in the mining sector, the following health promotion programs are essential to promote good health and to prevent occurrences of accidents and diseases, this may include such elements as continuous health education on health and safety-related topics such as noise-induced hearing loss, chronic disease monitoring, and management, accident prevention, the importance of personal protective equipment's, medical surveillance to identify and prevent the occurrences of health- related illnesses that might be caused by the work environment. Part of primary prevention is the assessment of health risks, this is achieved through continuous inspection by the occupational health practitioners and the safety team to identify and observe the work environment and working practices that might put the miner's health at risk [21, 47]. More importantly, the health promotion activities have the potential to change the miner's health practices such as choice of a healthy diet, exercising more frequently to prevent occurrences of chronic diseases. Additionally, the primary prevention activities have the potential to reduce the incidence of injuries and accidents because miners will be having more knowledge on health-related risks that might endanger their lives.

The implementation of an educational and training programme in the mine with a specific focus on creating a culture of safety among miners and more focus on safe working conditions can therefore help overcome the challenges of non-compliance [55, 56]. Moreover, since the mining environment is considered hazardous, all the mining organization needs to conduct medical surveillance as a primary preventative strategy as stipulated by Mine Health and Safety Act (29 of 1996) [12]. The medical surveillance is done before employment, annually or bi- annually and when the miner leaves the company, this is done according to the exposure levels in a different occupation and remedial actions are initiated based on the fitness status [28].

10.2 Secondary prevention

In secondary prevention, the main aim of occupational health is to diminish the impact of sickness or injury that has effectively occurred [47]. Additionally, this level of prevention put more emphasis on reinforcement and decreasing the reaction to the occupational disease or illness caused by the mining environment, thereby intensifying resistance through the provision of treatment [55]. This is achieved by distinguishing and regarding illness or injury at the earliest opportunity to end or slow its progression, encouraging safety strategies to prevent re-injury or recurrence, and implementing programs to return people to their original health and function to prevent long-term problems [56]. The secondary interventions include a regular medical examination and screening tests such as audiometry, spirometry, and vision screening. During the screening process, once the deterioration is identified further interventions such as referral to the specialist and recommendations for the removal of a miner to the occupation which will not have a further effect on the identified problem are done. The chronic disease management programme also forms part of the primary prevention strategy by constantly monitoring compliance through blood pressure and blood glucose monitoring to ensure compliance. Moreover, secondary prevention also included the advocacy to place a miner in a suitably modified work so injured or ill workers can return safely to their jobs [56].

10.3 Tertiary prevention

In occupational health, tertiary anticipation intends to diminish the effect of a continuous sickness or injury that has enduring impacts. This is finished by assisting individuals with overseeing long-haul, frequently complex medical issues and injury (for example ongoing sicknesses, long-lasting impedances) to work on however much as could reasonably be expected their capacity to work, their satisfaction, and their future [56]. Secondary prevention activities in the mining environment include a Hearing conservation program to support and rehabilitate those who have already lost their hearing due to noise exposure. These activities include modification of personal protective equipment, job placement to a less noisy area zone. The miners are also referred to a different specialists such as the audiologist, occupational speech therapy for rehabilitation purposes. This assists the miners to adapt to new jobs and also in their changed health status so that they can cope.

DOI: http://dx.doi.org/10.5772/intechopen.100264

11. Conclusion

The results of this review revealed that there are limited studies addressing the interventions to improve safety compliance. Furthermore in South Africa though there are several legislations to guide in safety and health compliance is still documented as poor with more focus on production. This review also demonstrated that combination of primary, secondary, and tertiary mediations is fundamental to accomplish a significant level of prevention and adherence in mining safety. The role of the OSH professional within the mining organization focusing more on addressing the challenges of none adherence requires further attention. None of the studies identified in the present review focused on the role of the OSH professional in ensuring compliance with the health and safety standards. Occupational health and safety is a human right issue that has got to be given legal, social, and ethical concerns. In SA there's a requirement for the SA mining business to make an OHS culture that's strong enough to manage most of OHS problems at each the national and sector levels.

Author details

Livhuwani Muthelo*, Tebogo Maria Mothiba and Rambelani Nancy Malema
University of Limpopo, South Africa

*Address all correspondence to: livhuwani.muthelo@ul.ac.za

References

[1] Smith, NM, Ali, Bofinge RCD & Collins N. Human health and safety in artisanal and small-scale mining: an integrated approach to risk mitigation. *Journal of Cleaner Production*. 2016. 129. 43- 52. https://doi.org/10.1016/j.jclepro.2016.04.124

[2] Beth, AA. Assessment of Occupational Safety Compliance in Small scale Gold Mines in Siaya Country Nairobi. Masters (Geography and Environmental Studies) dissertation. Nairobi: University of Nairobi. 2018. From: *erepository.uonbi.ac.ke › bitstream › handle › Beth_Asses...*

[3] International Labour Organization (ILO). Mining : a hazardous work. 2015. https://www.ilo.org› topics › WCMS_356567 › lang—en

[4] Sanmiquel, L, Bascompta, M, Rossell,JM, Anticoi, HF & Guash, E. Analysis of Occupational Accidents in Underground and Surface Mining in Spain Using Data-Mining Techniques. 2018. International Journal of Environmental Research and Public health. 15(3), 462; **h**ttps://doi.org/10.3390/ijerph150304621.

[5] Yarahmadi, R.; Bagherpour, R.; Khademian, A. Safety risk assessment of Iran's dimension stone quarries (Exploited by diamond wire cutting method). Saf. Sci. **2014**, 63, 146-150. DOI:10.1016/j.ssci.2013.11.003.

[6] Bagherpour, R.; Yarahmadi, R.; Khademian, A. Safety risk assessment of Iran's underground coal mines based on preventive and preparative measures. Hum. Ecol. Risk Assess. **2015**, 21, 2223-2238. doi: 10.1080/10807039.2015.1046418

[7] Hämäläinen, P.; Takala, J.; Leena, K. Global estimates of occupational accidents. Saf. Sci. **2006**, 44, 137-156. doi:10.1016/j.ssci.2005.08.017.

[8] Qasim, M., Bashir, A. Anees, M.M. Ghani, M.U. Khalid, M. Hanan, F. and Malik, J. Occupational Health, Safety and Risk Analysis in large scale industry of Lahore. *Bulletin of Energy Economics. 2014,* 2(4), 113-118. http://www.tesdo.org/JournalDetail.aspx?Id=4

[9] Muchiri, F. Occupational safety and health issues in Africa. 2009. From: *www.occhealth.co.za/?/download/articles_182_1050/...safety...health...in+Africa*.

[10] Bocoum, B. The importance of health and Safety at African mine Site. World Bank Group. www.worldbank.org/en/topic/ health/brief/tuberculosis-control.

[11] African Union. 2009. "African Mining Vision." AU Summit of Africa Heads of State, Addis Ababa, Ethiopia, February. http://www.africaminingvision.org/about.html.

[12] South Africa. *Mine Health and Safety Act*, no. 29, 1996. From: http://www.dmr.gov.co.za/legislation/summary/30-mine-health-and-safety/530-mhs-act-29-of-1996.Html.

[13] Kleyn, G., & du Plessis, J.J.L. (2016). *Sub-standard practices: Effects on safety performance in South African gold mines* www.scielo.org.za/pdf/jsaimm/v116n4/05.pdf.

[14] Vassem,A.S., Fortunato,G., Bastos, S.A.P, & Balassiano,M. Factors that make up safety culture a look at mining industry. *Gest. Prod., São Carlos*. 2017. 24 (4): 719-730. https://doi.org/10.1590/0104-530X1960-16

[15] Cronin P, Ryan F, Coughlan, M (2008) 'Undertaking a literature review: A step-by-step approach', *British Journal of Nursing* 17(1):38-43. doi: 10.12968/bjon.2008.17.1.28059

[16] Ramdhani, A., Ramdhani, M. A., & Amin, A. S. Writing a literature review research paper: A step- by-step approach. *International Journal of Basic and Applied Science*,. 2014,*1*(3), 47-56.

[17] Hempel, S. Xenakis, L & Danz, M. Systematic Reviews for Occupational Safety and Health Questions.

[18] Shamseers, L, Mohers, D, Clarke et al. Preferred reporting items for systematic review and meta-analysis protocols (PRISMA-P) 2015: elaboration and explanation. *BMJ* 2015; 349 doi: doi:10.1136/bmj.g7647

[19] Aslam, S & Emmanuel, P. Formulating a researchable question: A critical step for facilitating good clinical research Indian J Sex Transm Dis AIDS. 2010 Jan-Jun; 31(1): 47-50. doi: 10.4103/2589- 0557.69003.

[20] Coughlan, M., Cronin, P & Ryan, F. (2013) *Doing literature review in nursing, health and social care*. London: Sage publications.

[21] Neal, A., Griffin, M.A., Hart, P.M. (2000). Impact of organizational climate on safety and individual behaviour. *Safety Science.* 54:946 – 953.

[22] Kleyn, G., & du Plessis, J.J.L. (2016). *Sub-standard practices: Effects on safety performance in South African gold mines* www.scielo.org.za/pdf/jsaimm/v116n4/05.pdf

[23] Vassem,A.S., Fortunato,G., Bastos, S.A.P, & Balassiano,M. Factors that make up safety culture a look at mining industry. *Gest. Prod., São Carlos*, 2017. 24 (4): 719-730.

[24] Mogale L. Pilusa, Mataniele S. Mogotlane. Worker knowledge of occupational legislation and related health and safety benefits. *Curationis.* 2018; 41(1): 1869.

[25] Michell K.E. (2011). *A practical approach to occupational health nursing*, South African Society of Occupational Health Nursing Practitioners, Johannesburg.

[26] Minister Gwede Mantashe. 2019. Mine Health and Safety statistics. https://www.gov.za/speeches/2019-mine-heatlh-and...

[27] Chamber of mines. 2016. Safety Minerals Council South Africa. www.mineralscouncil.org.za/reports/2016/download/CM-IR16-focus-safety.pdf.

[28] Hatting, SP & Acutt, J. (2016). *Occupational Health: Management and Practice for health Practitioners*. 5th edition. Cape Town: Juta & Company Ltd.

[29] Pilusa, M.L. & Mogotlane, M.S., 2018, 'Worker knowledge of occupational legislation and related health and safety benefits', *Curationis* 41(1), a1869. https://doi.org/10.4102/curationis.v41i1.1869

[30] Mogale L. Pilusa, Mataniele S. Mogotlane. (2018). Worker knowledge of occupational legislation and related health and safety benefits. *Curationis.* 2018; 41(1): 1869.

[31] Wagner, L. (2016). *The two way breaking news. Former Coal Executive Don Blankenship Sentenced to 1 year in Prison*. Available at: https://www.npr.org/.../former-coal-executive-don-blankenship-sentenced-to-1-year-in-... (Accessed March 2018).

[32] Dragan, K., Georges,L., & Mustafa, K. Organization: A new focus on mine safety improvement in a complex operational and business environment. *International Journal of Mining Science and Technology. 2017*. 27: 617-625. https://doi.org/10.1016/j.ijmst.2017.05.006

[33] Mojapelo, T.J. & Kok, L. (2017) 'Adherence to occupational health and safety standards: the case of a South

African steel processing company', *African Journal of Governance and Development* 6(1), 51-71.

[34] Luchini, BG & London, L. Global Occupational Health: Current Challenges and the Need for Urgent Action. Annals of health. 2014. 2:251-256 https://doi.org/10.1016/j.aogh.2014.09.006

[35] Lingard, H. Blismas, N. & Cooke, T. 2011. Co-workers response to occupational health and safety: An overlooked dimension of group-level safety climate in the construction industry. *Engineering, Construction and Architectural Management.* (18) 2: 159-175.

[36] Mabika, B. 2018. Improving Workers' Safety and Health in the Zimbabwean Mining and Quarrying Industry. Ph.D. Thesis.Walden University.

[37] Spada, M., & Burgherr, P. (2016). An aftermath analysis of the 2014 coal mine accident in Soma, Turkey: Use of risk performance indicators based on historical experience. Accident Analysis & Prevention, 87, 134-140. doi: 10.1016/j.aap.2015.11.020.

[38] Uyanusta Kucuk, F. C., & Ilgaz, A. (2015). Causes of coal mine accidents in the world and Turkey. Turkish Thoracic Journal/Türk Toraks Dergisi, 16(1), 9-14. doi: 10.5152/ttd.2015.0

[39] Kheni, N.A., & Braimah, C. Institutional and Regulatory frameworks for health and safety administration: study of the construction industry of Ghana. *International Refereed Journal of Engineering and Science*. 2014. 3 (2):24-34.

[40] Mustapha, Z., Aigbavboa, C. & Thwala, D.T. Conceptualized integrated health and safety compliance model for the Ghanaian construction industry. *International Journal of Advanced Technology and Engineering Studies.* 2015. 4 (2): 33-48.

[41] Baum, F. E., Sanders, D. M., Fisher, M., Anaf, J., Freudenberg, N., Friel, S., Sen, A. (2016). Assessing the health impact of transnational corporations: Its importance and a framework. Global Health, 12(1), 27. doi: 10.1186/s12992-016-0164-x.

[42] Gyekye, S. A., & Salminen, S. Age and workers' perceptions of workplace safety: A comparative study. *The International Journal of Aging & Human Development.* 2009. 68(2), 171-184.

[43] Takala J, Saarela KL. 2006. Global estimates of occupational accidents. Saf Sci. 44(2):137-156. [Google Scholar]

[44] Boniface, R, Maseru, L, Munthali, V & Lett, R. Occupational injuries and fatalities in a tanzanite mine: Need to improve workers safety in Tanzania. Pan African Journal. 2013;16:120.

[45] Guild, R, Ehrlich, RI, Johnston, JR & Ross, MH. 2001. *Handbook of Occupational Health Practice in the South African Mining Industry*. Johannesburg: The Safety in Mines Research Advisory Committee (SIMRAC).

[46] South Africa. (1996). *Mine health and safety Act*, no. 29, 1996. From: http://www.dmr.gov.co.za/legislation/summary/30-mine-health-and-safety/530-mhs-act-29-of- 1996.Html

[47] South Africa. (1993). *Occupational health and safety Act*, no. 85, 1993. www.labour.gov.za/.../legislation/regulations/occupational-health-and-safety/Regulation

[48] World Health Organization (WHO). The Role of the Occupational Health Nurse in Workplace Health Management. 2001. https://www.who.int/occupational_health/regions/en/...

[49] Jacinito, C, Soares, CG, An overview of occupational accidents notification systems within the enlarged EU. Work. 2011. 39(4):369-78. DOI:10.3233/ WOR-2011-1187

[50] F. Salguero-Caparrós, M.C. Pardo-Ferreira, M. Martínez-Rojas, J.C. Rubio-Romero, Management of legal compliance in occupational health and safety. A literature review, Safety Science. 2020. 111-118. https://doi.org/10.1016/j.ssci.2019.08.033.

[51] Tibane, M .& Niemand, L ."Investigation into Challenges Faced by Employees in Implementing a Safety Strategy in a South African Platinum Mine" *International Journal of Research in Business Studies and Management. 2017.* 4: I2 http://dx.doi.org/10.22259/ ijrbsm.0402005

[52] Shibambu, O.P. *Implementation and enforcement of safety standards in the mining industry SA: challenges and prospects.* Masters (development and management law) Mini-dissertation. Limpopo. University of Limpopo. 2017. ulspace.ul.ac.za/bitstream/ handle/10386/1900/... · PDF file

[53] Maseko, M.M. *Effects of non-compliance with the occupational health and safety act (no. 85 of 1993) among the food and beverage industries in selected provinces of South Africa*. PHD (Health sciences) dissertation. Pretoria : University of SouthAfrica 2016...From: uir.unisa.ac.za/bitstream/ handle/10500/21042/ thesis_maseko_mm.pdf?sequence..

[54] Smith PG, Morrow RH, Ross DA. 2015. Field Trials of Health Interventions: A Toolbox. 3rd edition.

[55] Lowry, J. Betty Neuman Theorist. 2011. sites.jmu.edu/nursing463/.../ Betty-Neuman-Nursing- Theorist.pptx.

[56] Peters, RH. Strategies For Improving Miners' Training. Department of Health and Human Services Centers for Disease Control and Prevention National Institute for Occupational Safety and Health. 2002. https://www.cdc.gov/ niosh/mining/UserFiles/works/pdfs/ IC9463.pdf · PDF file

Chapter 17

Early Occupational Therapy Intervention: Patients' Occupational Needs

Margherita Schiavi, Barbara Volta, Gilda Sandri, Erica Keeling and Maria Teresa Mascia

Abstract

The occupational therapy management involves the assessment of the individual's specific needs. This kind of assessment facilitates the therapeutic relationship and boosts the person's motivation, as he or she feels valued and heard. Early-stage collection of information about meaningful activities for the individual helps them project themselves outside the context of illness. Collecting occupational need at an early stage, permits "Engagement", which means participating in activities even without actually doing them. An occupational therapy model called "Personal Environment Occupation Model" suggests that already at an early stage we should make the environment and occupations meaningful to the person in order to maximise the patient's performance. An observational study on stroke patients shows how people have personal occupational needs beyond simple self-care, including productive life and leisure time, already in the subacute phase. A further study is underway to demonstrate the effectiveness of early occupational therapy intervention, including complex patients regardless of diagnosis and taking into account their need for care and disability in order to promote their participation and maximise their autonomy.

Keywords: occupational therapy, assessment, activity daily log, Canadian occupational performance measure, engagement, personal environment occupation model

1. Introduction

The occupational therapy (OT) treatment is a "client-centred" rehabilitation approach based on the occupational needs of the person as a unique individual. People identify with their occupations [1]; the loss of these occupations causes a decline in the perception of self-efficacy and depression.

During the acute phase of the illness, the medical team's main focus is on the person's state of health in its organic and physical components. Occupational therapy, in this early phase, brings the focus back to the individual's entire being and his or her position at the centre of the rehabilitation intervention. It has been shown that focusing rehabilitation on occupations that are meaningful to the person can improve their quality of life [1].

2. Relevance of assessment in occupational therapy

Occupational therapy focuses on occupations, i.e., everything a person does from the morning when they wake up until the evening when they go to sleep. This involves many different activities that each person does in his or her own unique way. Rehabilitation to occupations therefore means having individualised goals. The OT treatment is indeed individualised and varied.

There are no treatment protocols but reference models that guide the therapist in defining the objectives and setting the treatment. Goal setting is based on the person's needs, taking into account the value the person places on the activities and their perception of the urge to recover them. The occupational therapist will negotiate treatment goals with the patient based on occupations that are meaningful to the person.

It is therefore necessary to be able to identify occupational needs, which is why it is important to use assessment tools and outcome measures. Assessing needs in a pre- and post-intervention phase of OT means monitoring the change in the person, and thus verifying the impact and effectiveness of the treatment itself. Assessing also means tailoring the treatment to the person's characteristics, needs and wishes. The evaluation serves to establish goals that are a priority for the individual. The most important part is the individual's perceived functioning and disability, regardless of the diagnosis. Finally, evaluation means being able to show the results of one's work to the scientific community, sharing experiences and promoting evidence-based practice.

2.1 Occupational therapy assessment characteristics

Both performance in everyday life and occupational problems encountered can be assessed. The focus of the evaluation in occupational therapy remains on the needs of the person. This evaluation is done using a variety of tools, semi-structured interviews, collection of stories, or similar, all aimed at getting to know the person and establishing a good therapeutic relationship. The advantage is that the person feels listened to, at the centre of their treatment, welcomed and projected into his or her reality even outside the context of the illness. This has a positive impact on treatment compliance and motivation. The more motivation/desire a client has to engage in activities, the better he/she will be able to cope with the impairment [2].

2.2 Some occupational therapy-specific evaluation tools

Among the most widely used tools in Occupational Therapy is the Canadian occupational performance measure (COPM) [3]. COPM is a semi-structured interview, which allows the analysis of the areas of self-care, productivity and leisure time of the person, identifying problems that may arise within the normal routine. In addition to being a cognitive tool that helps to establish the therapeutic relationship, it also helps the patient and therapist to establish, or rather to negotiate, the objectives of the occupational therapy treatment. It is also an outcome measure as it scores the patient's subjective perception of the performance of the activities and the degree of satisfaction in performing them.

The post-treatment evaluation makes it possible to understand if the objectives have been achieved or if it is necessary to modify the action plan. By providing this evaluation with two measurement times (an initial and a final one) it allows to understand if the treatment leads to a clinically significant result for the patient, that is a real positive change in daily activities and autonomy. This instrument is non-dependent from the pathology, it can be administered to the person or to the patient's caregiver. Another tool is the daily diary (Activity Daily Log). The Activity Daily Log allows the person to collect his/her occupations reflecting on the time spent performing them and the emotions felt while doing so. The collection of these activities will serve as a starting point for goal setting. It is a widely used tool for orthopaedic patients [4] and patients with chronic fatigue [5].

Both tools allow an assessment aimed at collecting the person's own needs and guarantee a person-centred practice, favouring the therapeutic relationship.

2.3 Results of a study on the occupational needs of complex sub-acute patients

The cross-sectional observational study "Occupational therapy for complex inpatients with stroke: identification of occupational needs in post-acute rehabilitation setting" [6] identifies the characteristics and occupational needs of stroke inpatients who are considered as "complex", focusing on function and ability, regardless of diagnosis. In this study, the occupational therapist identified occupational needs through the COPM.

The results found that the enrolled patients were dependent in basic activities of daily living (ADLs), limited in instrumental ADLs and easily fatigued. Their occupational needs were related to self-care (75%) and, to a lesser extent, productivity (15%) and leisure time (10%). According to the results of the inpatient survey, the rehabilitation process should primarily address self-care needs, followed by productivity and leisure time activities.

Despite the small sample size, this study described the patterns of occupational needs in complex stroke patients and pointed out that, although to a lesser extent than self-care needs, productivity and leisure issues also arise in the early post-acute phase.

Client-centred rehabilitation programmes must address self-care needs, as well as focusing on the recovery of family and social roles, both in the productive and leisure sectors.

Addressing these needs helps the patient to project himself into the home dimension, boosting motivation, recovering his role in the community and occupying time in a meaningful way.

2.4 Early occupational therapy: engagement and personal environment occupation model

Having explained the relevance of the needs assessment, it is important to underline that taking care of patients in the acute phase is crucial because occupational therapy has the peculiarity not only to engage the person in doing activities, but also simply to make him/her participate in the activity. If it is not possible to carry out the activity in practice, the person can be engaged, giving him or her the role of coordinator of the activity, which is physically carried out by another person, who performs it according to the given instructions. The performance of occupation may provide a means to engagement; however, it is not necessary for engagement, acknowledging that an individual may engage in occupation passively [7].

This concept is defined in literature as "Engagement".

Engaging in occupations that are meaningful to the person is seen as a fundamental prerequisite for good health and well-being [7] and it is the basis of the Occupational Therapy practice [8].

The concept of occupational engagement first emerged in the work of Wilcock in 1993 [8], who described occupational engagement as something that goes beyond performing occupations in the physical sense, including engagement in the occupation on a mental and spiritual level.

The conceptual model personal environment occupation model (PEO) [9] is an excellent tool to be used at an early stage to promote the recovery of the maximum level of autonomy of the person by making the best use of his or her resources. This model explains that the rehabilitation process must necessarily start from the analysis of the characteristics of the individual, understood as a physical, emotional and psychological being ("P"). It is then necessary to analyse the significant occupations for the person (O) and finally the context in which the occupations are normally carried out (E). From the intersection of this information we obtain the "occupational performance" (**Figure 1**).

If one of these areas is reduced, the intersection with the others is also reduced, which means that the performance may no longer be possible or may not be satisfactory for the person performing it. At the reduction of the person's area (P), which occurs when a deficit and/or illness appears, the model stresses the importance of expanding the other areas (environment and occupation) to allow the person to maintain his/her occupational performance and as much as possible a satisfactory routine (graphically maintain an area of intersection between the three circles, namely performance, **Figure 2**).

In the case of the acute phase, therefore, it is essential to expand the area of the environment, which is the only area that can have a significant impact on performance, reducing disability. Expanding the area of the environment (E) can mean eliminating physical barriers, favouring accessibility, or educating and training the population to favour the reception of a person with disabilities, reducing the difficulty of social integration and promoting participation (**Figure 3**).

Expanding the area of occupations means considering whether, in order to improve performance, it may be necessary to do the activity differently, to use strategies or aids, or simply to train oneself to perform the activity more efficiently and effectively.

This model underlines the importance of addressing treatment to environments and occupations that the health care system fails to take into account very often, focusing, almost uniquely, on resolving the deficit and pathology or reducing the effects caused by it, which is important but not the only aspect to provide the person with the highest possible quality of life.

2.5 Future scope of occupational therapy

In order to promote the motivation and engagement of the person, it seems useful to include an early assessment not only in neurological patients, but also in

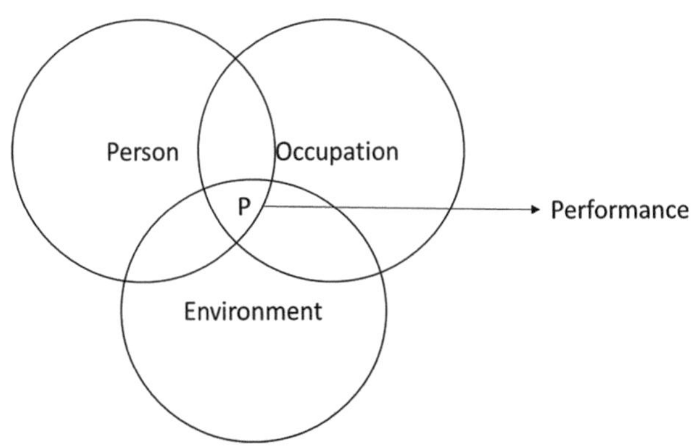

Figure 1.
Personal environment occupation model.

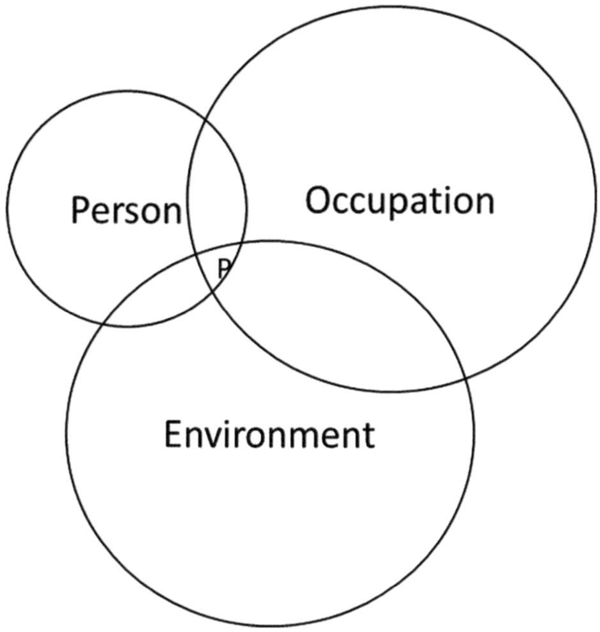

Figure 2.
Reduction of the person's area (P).

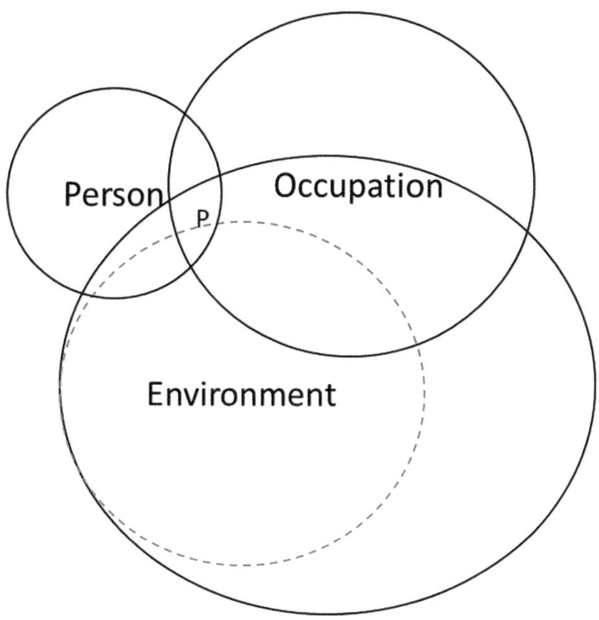

Figure 3.
Expanding the area of the environment (E).

patients with other diseases. For referral to the specific assessment of the occupational therapist, the complexity criterion could be used. According to the agency for healthcare research and quality (AHRQ), the patient described as complex "is a person with two or more chronic diseases, in which each of the conditions present is able to influence the outcome of the care of the other coexisting conditions in various ways: limitation of life expectancy, increased morbidity, interactions between drug therapies, and the impossibility of full use of appropriate treatment due to contraindications" [10]. The measurability of this criterion seems to us to be expressed by the rehabilitation complexity scale extended (RCS-E) [11].

Our experience described in Section 2.3 is extending the selection of patients on the basis of their RCS-E score, extending the sample under examination regardless of pathology.

Sharing the early assessment of occupational needs with the specialists in the care team can avoid a delay in the rehabilitation programme.

3. Conclusion

Occupational therapy at an early stage is necessary to set up a client-centred treatment that reflects the person's occupational needs, impacting on their motivation and compliance in the rehabilitation treatment. Of fundamental importance is the detection of the person's occupational problems and performance difficulties in the person's meaningful activities. This is carried out through specific tools such as the COPM and the daily diary.

Engagement is crucial to encourage participation at an early stage.

Through the PEO model we can decrease disability already in the acute phase, regardless of health conditions, by enabling occupational performance by implementing the "environment" and "occupation" areas.

A study on the occupational needs of "complex" patients in the subacute phase is under way.

Conflict of interest

The authors declare no conflict of interest.

Acronyms and abbreviations

OT	Occupational therapy
COPM	Canadian occupational performance measure
ADL	Activities of daily living
PEO	Personal environment occupation model
RCSE	Rehabilitation complexity scale extended

Author details

Margherita Schiavi[1*], Barbara Volta[1], Gilda Sandri[2], Erica Keeling[3] and Maria Teresa Mascia[2]

1 Department of Health Professions, Azienda USL—IRCCS di Reggio Emilia, Reggio Emilia, Italy

2 Rheumatology Unit, University of Modena and Reggio Emilia, Modena, Italy

3 University of Modena and Reggio Emilia, Modena, Italy

*Address all correspondence to: margherita.schiavi@unimore.it

References

[1] Hammell KW. Dimensions of meaning in the occupations of daily life. Canadian journal of occupational therapy. Revue canadienne d'ergotherapie. 2004;**71**(5):296-305. DOI: 10.1177/000841740407100509

[2] Kennedy P, Evans M, Sandhu N. Psychological adjustment to spinal cord injury: The contribution of coping, hope and cognitive appraisals. Psychology, Health & Medicine. 2009;**14**(1):17-33. DOI: 10.1080/13548500802001801

[3] Baptiste S, Carswell A, McColl MA, Polatajko H, Pollock N. Canadian Occupational Performance Measure (COPM). Ottawa, ON, Canada: Canadian Association of Occupational Therapists (CAOT); 2014

[4] Hiraga Y, Hisano S, Nomiyama K, Hirakawa Y. Effects of using activity diary for goal setting in occupational therapy on reducing pain and improving psychological and physical performance in patients after total knee arthroplasty: A non-randomised controlled study. Hong Kong Journal of Occupational Therapy. 2019;**32**(1):53-61. DOI: 10.1177/1569186119849117

[5] Jason LA, Timpo P, Porter N, Herrington J, Brown M, Torres-Harding S, et al. Activity logs as a measure of daily activity among patients with chronic fatigue syndrome. Journal of Mental Health. 2009;**18**(6):549-556. DOI: 10.3109/09638230903191249

[6] Schiavi M, Costi S, Pellegrini M, Formisano D, Borghi S, Fugazzaro S. Occupational therapy for complex inpatients with stroke: Identification of occupational needs in post-acute rehabilitation setting. Disability and Rehabilitation. 2018;**40**(9):1026-1032. DOI: 10.1080/09638288.2017.1283449

[7] Polatajko HJ, Townsend EA, Craik J. Canadian Model of Occupational Performance and Engagement (CMOPE). In: Townsend EA, Polatajko HJ, editors. Enabling occupation II: Advancing an occupational therapy vision for health, well-being & justice through occupation. Vol. 23. Ottawa, ON: CAOT Publications ACE; 2007

[8] Wilcock A. A theory of the human need for occupation. Journal of Occupational Science. 1993;**1**(1):17-24

[9] Law M, Cooper B, Strong S, Stewart D, Rigby P, Letts L. The person-environment-occupation model: A transactive approach to occupational performance. Canadian Journal of Occupational Therapy. 1996;**63**(1):9-23

[10] Sevick MA, Trauth JM, Ling BS, et al. Patients with Complex Chronic Diseases: Perspectives on supporting self-management. Journal of General Internal Medicine. 2007;**22**(Suppl 3): 438-444. DOI: 10.1007/s11606-007-0316-z

[11] Turner-Stokes L, Scott H, Williams H, et al. The Rehabilitation Complexity Scale–extended version: Detection of patients with highly complex needs. Disability and Rehabilitation. 2012;**34**(9):715-720

Section 8

Telehealth and Telemedicine in Primary Care

Chapter 18

Telephone Consultations by Medical Scheme Patients Consulting General Medical Practitioners, South Africa

Michael Mncedisi Willie, Neo Nonyana and Sipho Kabane

Abstract

Background: The COVID-19 climate has seen a shift in the manner that patients seek care. Lockdown measures and COVID-19 regulations, and the fear of contracting the virus at a health care facility has also changed health seeing behaviour among patients. The COVID-19 climate has seen a significant increase in the utilisation of virtual platforms to consult with providers. **Objectives:** The objective of this chapter was to conduct the descriptive analysis of telephonic consultations by members of medical schemes who consulted general medical practitioners. **Methods:** The study entailed a descriptive analysis of medical scheme claims data for the 2020 review period. The inclusion criteria were all National Pharmaceutical Product Interface (NAPPI) codes associated with a telephonic consultation consulting general medical practitioners. The ICD-10 code primary diagnosis was used to describe the diagnosis. The study mainly focused on outpatient patients with service dates between March and December 2020. **Results:** The analysis covered claims data from a total of 12 medical schemes. The schemes analysed accounted for 1,6 million lives. The total number of telephonic consultations was 17 237. The mean (SD) claimed amount for telephone consultation for a general medical practice consult was R282[1] (SD = 20). This was slightly lower than the scheme tariff of R287[2] (SD = 19). The study found that most telephonic consults were for Acute bronchitis, unspecified; Acute upper respiratory; Emergency use of U07.1 (Confirmed diagnosis); Emergency use of U07.2 (Suspected Diagnosis); Follow-up examination; Special screening. **Conclusion:** The study found evidence of patients utilising telephonic consultations for general medical practitioner services. The effect of COVID-19 in this respect was seen in the three main primary diagnoses that were associated with the consult, Acute upper respiratory, Emergency use of U07.1 (confirmed diagnosis) and Emergency use of U07.2 (suspected diagnosis). Even though the average telephonic consult was claimed at just under R300[3], few general medical practitioners claimed between R400[4] and R500[5] which were higher than the industry average. There is a need to develop telephone consult guidelines at industry level, these should also address reimbursement rate differentials.

1 14.2 British Pound (GBP)

2 14 British Pound (GBP)

3 15.1 GBP

4 20.1 GBP

5 25.2 GBP

Keywords: Telephonic consultation, general medical practitioners, medical schemes, South Africa

1. Introduction

The COVID-19 epidemic has adversely affected health systems globally. The utilisation of technology and other innovative channels to link up with patients has evolved drastically over the past 12 months. COVID-19 regulations and the fear of contracting the virus at a health care facility has also changed health seeing behaviour among patients. There has been a plateau in teleconsultations since the end of the lockdown in France (on May 11, 2020), but the amount remains higher than before, stabilising at 150,000 per week [1]. Temporary disruptions in routine and non-emergency medical care access and delivery have been observed in the US and worldwide during COVID-19 [2]. The authors estimated that 40.9% of adults had avoided the use of medical care services during the pandemic. The study further depicts that 12.0% of adults also avoided urgently or emergency care, and just under a third of adults (31.5%) avoided routine care. A study comparing health facility visits from March to May 2020 with in-person visits during the same period in 2019, the results showed a reduction of 52% and 47% of emergency department visits and hospital admissions was observed compared to in-person visits ($p < 0.01$) [3]. The study also found that, of 120 patients surveyed, 95% were satisfied/very satisfied with the telephone visits.

1.1 Virtual consultations during emergencies

According to authors such as Martos-Pérez *et al.* and Downes *et al.*, telephone consultations could ease up the overburdened healthcare system [3–5]. A study by Bokolo found that telemedicine and virtual software as one of the contributing factors to the decrease in the number of visits to emergency rooms [6]. Accordingly, outpatient in-person visits can be converted to telephone visits [3].

1.2 Arguments against virtual consultations

Furthermore, there were challenges and obstacles cited in the use of virtual consultations. McGrail, Ahuja and Leaver, [7] conducted a systematic review on the view against the use of the telephone for virtual consultations [7]. The author concluded that patient consultations platforms such as telephones might allow minor problems to be dealt with without a face-to-face visit, In particular for acute illness. The author further depicts that even though these platforms may be cost savings, they may miss rare but serious conditions [7]. Another study by Car *et al.* showed that remote consultations were perceived as being less "information-rich" than face-to-face consultations, and technical issues were common [8]. Furthermore, there was no credible evidence to guide clinicians on when to use phone or video consultations.

2. Background

The utilisation of technology and other innovative channels used to link up with patients has evolved over the past ten (10) years. However, this has been accelerated eminently during COVID-19 [6, 9]. Lockdown restrictions and regulations, fear of contracting the virus at a health care facility has also changed health seeing behaviour among patients. The use of virtual platforms such as telephones for consultations has also been well received by physicians, who have used them widely, and they have been highly rated by patients [9]. A survey conducted in 2020 of 120 patients surveyed showed that 95% were satisfied/very satisfied with the telephone visits [3]. The study also surveyed 26 physicians and found that 84.6% of them considered telephone visits were useful to prioritise patients.

2.1 Virtual consultation- general practitioners

Virtual consultations (also called telemedicine consultations) have been in place for decades, with many healthcare systems advocating a digital-first approach, even before the COVID-19 pandemic [7, 10]. The has, however, further accelerated the use k [11, 12]. At the beginning of the pandemic, many health professionals, including General Practitioners (GPs), specialists and others, resorted to the use of video consultations to reduce patient flow in their practices and facilities as a risk measure to limit infectious exposures [8].

The General Practitioner (GP) data for England shows a rapid increase in telephone consultations relative to face-to-face consultations [12]. The authors found that the number of telephone consultations increased from more than 850 thousand to more than 2 million per week between March 2 and May 18 2020, while the number of video consultations was higher in March than in April or May when it was around 10,000 per week [12]. Richardson *et al.,* a large proportion of teleconsultations (96 percent) in France found) were billed by private practitioners, with GPs billing 80 percent of all teleconsultations, followed by psychologists (6 percent), paediatricians (2 percent), gynaecologists (1.3 percent), dermatologists (1.1 percent), and endocrinologists (1.1 percent) (1.1 percent). In the Netherlands, teleconsultations are expanding, with 72 percent of GPs surveyed said they had begun using video consultations with patients in 2020.

2.2 Funding of telephone consultations – Medical schemes

Update and use of technology have also been evident in medical schemes, where some medical schemes continue to fund these. However, not all medical schemes[6] fund telephone consultations related to COVID-19 [5, 9]. Medscheme affiliated or contracted schemes provide some evidence of schemes that do fund telephone consultation with effect in 2020. According to their newsletter publication, the administrator, in partnership with their affiliate solution providers, has developed a digital platform to facilitate virtual consultations [13]. The **Table 1** below depicts various rates for various schemes. The fees range between R281 and R437.

2.3 Legislative requirements

There are legislative restrictions on the use of virtual consultations [9]. Some of these have made the implementation of virtual consultation in low-income countries difficult. Some present challenges are related to data security and privacy requirements [8]. A number of countries have also evolved and developed protocols and guidelines for adopting video consultations. These developments and improvements have taken a leapfrog jump in countries like the UK and the US. Clinicians in many developed countries are working closely with regulators in terms of compliance to standards on the use of non-medical, electronic platforms and applications such as Skype, WhatsApp, and FaceTime in addition to medical ones [8].

[6] A **medical scheme** is a non-profit organisation, governed by a board of trustees, and must be registered with the Council for **Medical Schemes**.

Scheme name	2020 tariff rates
AECI	R287.00
Barloworld	R283.40
Bonitas	R281.60
Fedhealth	R281.50
Horizon	R293.70
Hosmed	R325.40
MBMed	R282.70
Medshield	R436.60
Nedgroup	R287.00
Parmed	R279.80
Polmed	R268.80
SABC	R282.00
Sasolmed	R281.60

Source: [13].

Table 1.
Telephone consultation fees – Medscheme affiliated schemes tariff rates.

3. Objectives

The primary objective of this study was to conduct a descriptive analysis of general medical practitioner telephonic consultations by members of medical schemes.

4. Methods

4.1 Study design

The study entailed a descriptive analysis of medical schemes claims data for the 2020 review period.

4.2 Setting

Medical schemes, which are also called health insurance companies operating in the private health sector in South Africa, are non-profit organisations governed by a board of trustees and must be registered with the Council for Medical Schemes (CMS). The CMS is a statutory body which is a Section 31 entity that regulates medical schemes in South Africa. There are two types of medical schemes, which are open and restricted medical schemes. Open membership schemes must accept anyone who wants to become a member [14]. Restricted membership schemes can restrict who may become a member, and they are typically employer or union based [14]. The schemes that were included in the analysis were those that submitted data as per circular 29 of 2020: Claims information for beneficiaries treated for COVID-19 of the CMS [15]. Theschemes covered in the analysis represented approximately

1,6 million lives, and this counted for 18% of all lives covered by medical schemes in 2019. The CMS annual reports twere used to source the data [16].

4.3 Unit of measures

The unit of measurement for the amount of the claim was measured in rand terms (**R: ZAR**). As of May 2020, the equivalent value was:

- 1 **ZAR** to GBP = 0.0502
- 1 ZAR = 0.07077 USD

4.4 Inclusion criteria

The inclusion criteria were all National Pharmaceutical Product Interface (NAPPI) codes. These are unique product identifier for a given surgical product, medical appliance, consumable product, pharmaceutical product or other medicinal product. The inclusion criteria were all NAPPI codes associated with a telephonic consultation consulting general medical practitioners. The ICD-10 code primary diagnosis was used to describe the diagnosis. The study mainly focused on outpatient patients with service dates between March and December 2020. A laboratory-confirmed (RT – PCR assay) COVID-19 was used to identify the COVID-19 case as per the World Health Organisation [17, 18] guidelines and definition. Inclusion criteria for COVID-19 admissions were patients that had a laboratory-confirmed (RT – PCR assay) COVID-19. An emergency ICD-10 code of U07.1 COVID-19, virus identified, is assigned to a diagnosis of COVID-19, confirmed by laboratory testing. An emergency ICD-10 code of 'U07.2' COVID-19, virus not identified, is assigned to a clinical or epidemiological diagnosis of COVID-19, where laboratory confirmation is inconclusive or not available. Both U07.1 and U07.2 may be used for mortality coding (cause of death).

5. Results

The analysis covered claims data from a total of 12 medical schemes. The schemes analysed accounted for 1,6 million lives. The total number of telephonic consultations was 17 237. The mean (SD) claimed amount for telephone consultation for a general medical practice consult was R282[7] (SD = 20). This was slightly lower than the scheme tariff of R287[8] (SD = 19) (**Table 2**).

Figure 1 below depicts the proportion of consultations per month. The results depicted a peak in the proportion of consultations in July and December, with July accounting for 33 percent and 22 percent of consultations in July and December, respectively. This phenomenon was consistent with COVID-19 infection rates at a national level in South Africa.

The study found that most telephonic consults were for Acute bronchitis, unspecified; Acute upper respiratory; Emergency use of U07.1 (Confirmed diagnosis); Emergency use of U07.2 (suspected diagnosis); Follow-up examination; Special screening. **Table 3** below further depicts that average consults for an acute respiratory

[7] 14.2 GBP

[8] 14.4 GBP

	Mean (SD)	Median (IQR)
Claimed amount per telephone consultation	R282.7 (20.9)	R282 (R279 - R285)
Scheme Tariff Amount	R286.7 (19.2)	R283 (R282 - R289)

Table 2.
Summary statistics: Claimed amount vs. scheme tariff amount- general medical practice telephone consultations. (1 R: 1 ZAR = 0.0503 GBP).

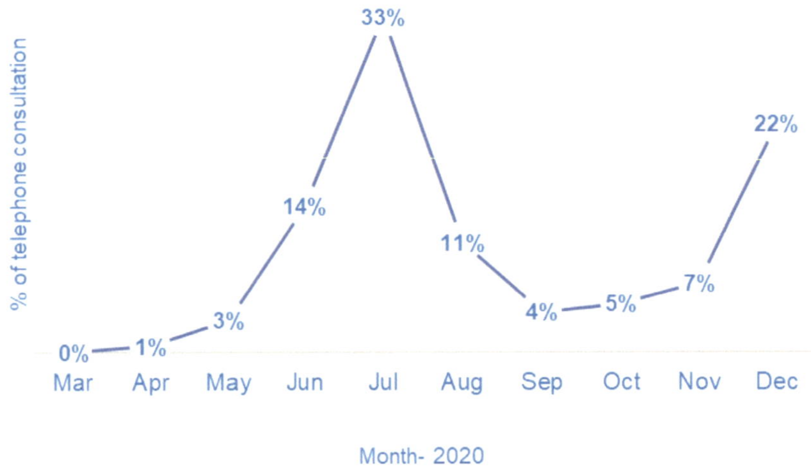

Figure 1.
Total number of telephone consultations per month to general medical practitioners.

consult were higher at R298 (SD = 103). However, there was variability in this regard. The average claim amount for a COVID-19 confirmed diagnosis was lower than the suspected diagnosis at R284 (SD = 27) and R288 (SD = 83), respectively.

Figure 2 below depicts a Box and Whisker plot of the average claim amount for the general medical practitioner telephonic consultations. The findings depict that the most prevalent telephone consults were mainly for general medical practice, specialist family medicine depicting outliers. The average claim amount per telephonic consults for other specialist telephonic consults for Independent Practice Specialist Obstetrics and Gynaecology was higher than R400. Their results also showed some evidence of telephone consultation for non-consulting specialists such as Urologists and Paediatrics Independent Practice Specialist though the volumes were not as significantly high.

ICD-10 primary ICD-10 code description	N	Mean	Std Dev
Acute bronchitis, unspecified	28	R284	R11
Acute upper respiratory	75	R298	R103
Emergency use of U07.1 (confirmed diagnosis)	968	R284	R27
Emergency use of U07.2 (suspected diagnosis)	1,192	R288	R83
Follow-up examination	30	R280	R16
Special screening exam	40	R283	R9

Table 3.
Summary statistics: Claimed amount per ICD-10 primary ICD-10 code description- general medical practice telephone consultations. (1 R: 1 ZAR = 0.0503 GBP).

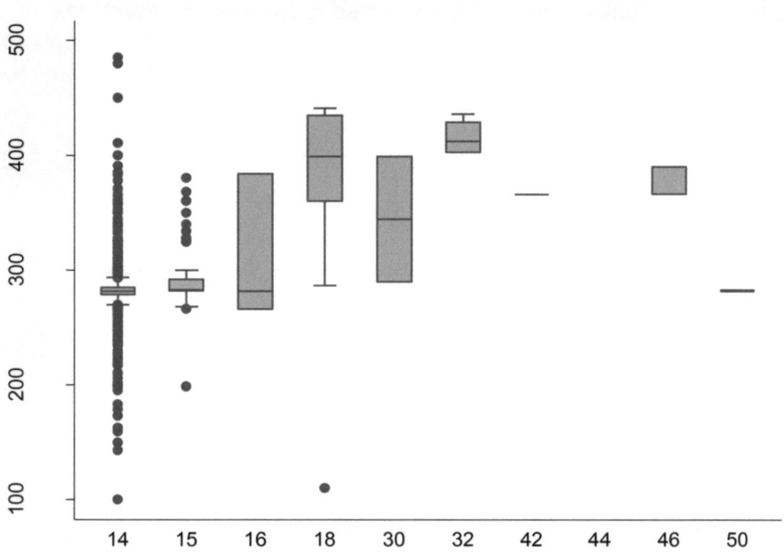

Figure 2.
Box and whisker plot - telephonic consultations (claimed amount) by discipline. (14 = general medical practice; 15 = specialist family medicine; 16 = independent practice specialist obstetrics and Gynaecology; 18 = independent practice specialist medicine; 30 = otorhinolaryngology; 32 = Paediatrics independent practice specialist; 42 = surgery independent practice specialist; 44 = cardio thoracic surgery; 46 = urology; 50 = group practices).

6. Discussion

The objective of this paper was to explore and assess telephone consultations among members of medical schemes in South Africa. This study found that telephone consultations were mainly for general medical practice services with an average claimed amount of less than R300 per telephone consultation. The average claimed amounts in this study were within the ER Consulting estimates of between R270 and R330 (ER Consulting, 2020). The amount claimed for virtual consultations ranged between R281 and R437, and these were similar to rates depicted earlier in this study [13]. The study also found telephone consults among specialist services, and these had an average claimed amount higher than R400, reflecting the specialist level of care by these specialists which attract higher reimbursement rates. A study conducted in Frace found that a large proportion of teleconsultations (96 percent) were billed by private practitioners [12]. This study also explored the average claim amount per general medical practice telephone consultation on six different diagnoses. The study found similarities among these average claims per telephone consultation, which also included follow-up examination and special screening exam. A notable feature of the findings was that the average claim amount for an acute upper respiratory telephone consult was higher than COVID-19 confirmed diagnosis or COVID-19 suspected primary diagnosis consultation. There are currently no pricing guidelines across various specialists and practitioner telephone consultations in South Africa, at least at the time of writing this Chapter. According to Hammersley *et al.*, remote consultations are perceived to be less "information-rich" than face-to-face consultations, and technical issues were common [19]. Hobbs *et al.* found that telephone consultations were usually shorter than face-to-face consultations (mean duration 5.4 minutes compared with 9.22 minutes [20]. A study by Hewitt, Gafaranga and McKinstry found no underlying contrasts between the communicative practices used in face-to-face and telephone consultations [21]. Further research is projected to further investigate the varying reimbursement rates for various specialist groups and other disciplines relative to a face-to-face consultation. Future research should also seek to develop guidelines on telephonic consultations and assess value add to patients.

7. Conclusion

The study found evidence of patients utilising telephonic consultations for general medical practitioner services. The effect of COVID-19 in this respect was seen in the primary diagnoses associated with the consult, Acute upper respiratory, Emergency use of U07.1 (confirmed diagnosis) and Emergency use of U07.2 (suspected diagnosis). The average claim amount for a telephonic consultation was lower than R300, and few general medical practitioners claimed between R400 and R500 which was higher than the industry average. There is a need to develop telephone consult guidelines at industry level, these should also address reimbursement rates differentials. Furthermore, the guidelines should potentially cover both provider and patient conduct. There is a need to also develop guidelines on how these are adjudicated, validated, and funded at the scheme level.

8. Limitations

This study mainly used secondary data collected from the CMS, which was transactional data; as a result, essential information on telephone consultation characteristics were not considered. Information such as frequency of calls to the provider, average call time, and mode or type of device used to contact the provider was not available and thus not included in the study. Future research should consider telephone consultation characteristic and patient perspective.

Conflict of interests

The authors have declared that no competing interest exists.

Authors contributions

The authors drafted and proofread the article.

Author details

Michael Mncedisi Willie*, Neo Nonyana and Sipho Kabane
Policy Research and Monitoring, Council for Medical Schemes, South Africa

*Address all correspondence to: m.willie@medicalschemes.co.za

References

[1] Domenico D, Pullano L, Sabbatini G *et al.* Impact of lockdown on COVID-19 epidemic in Île-de-France and possible exit strategies. BMC Med **18,** 240 (2020). https://doi.org/10.1186/s12916-020-01698-4

[2] Czeisler M.É., Marynak, K., Clarke, K.E., *et al.* (2020). Delay or avoidance of medical care because of COVID-19–related concerns — United States. MMWR Morb mortal weekly report - 2020;69:1250-1257. DOI: http://dx.doi.org/10.15585/mmwr.mm6936a4external icon.

[3] Martos-Pérez, F. *et al.* (2021). The value of telephone consultations during the COVID-19 pandemic. An observational study, *QJM: An International Journal of Medicine*, 2021; hcab024, https://doi.org/10.1093/qjmed/hcab024.

[4] Downes, M.J., Mervin, M.C., Byrnes, J.M. *et al.* (2017). Telephone consultations for general practice: A systematic review. Syst Rev *6*, 128 (2017).https://doi.org/10.1186/s13643-017-0529-0.

[5] Mills, J., Coffey, J., and Draper, R. (2021). Telephone consultations. InnovAiT. 2019;12(1):43-44. doi:10.1177/1755738018806327

[6] Bokolo, A. (2021). Exploring the adoption of telemedicine and virtual software for the care of outpatients during and after the COVID-19 pandemic. Ir J Med Sci 190, 1-10 (2021). doi:10.1007/s11845-020-02299-z.

[7] McGrail, K.M., Ahuja, M.A. and Leaver, C.A. (2017). Virtual visits and patient-centred care: results of a patient survey and observational study. *J Med Internet Res* 2017;19:e177. DOI: 10.2196/jmir.7374 pmid: 28550006.

[8] Car J, Koh GC, Foong PS, Wang CJ. Video consultations in primary and specialist care during the covid-19 pandemic and beyond. BMJ. 2020 Oct 20;371:m3945. doi: 10.1136/bmj.m3945. PMID: 33082127.

[9] Willie, M.M. (2021). Telephone consultations by medical scheme patients for Covid-19 related Diagnosis-2020, South Africa. Progress in Medical Sciences, 5 (1), 1-5.DOI: 10.5455/pms.20211020

[10] Greenhalgh, T., Vijayaraghavan, S., Wherton, J. *et al.* (2016). Virtual online consultations: advantages and limitations (VOCAL) study. British Medical Journal. 6:e009388. doi: 10.1136/bmjopen-2015-009388 pmid: 26826147.

[11] Kalenzi C. (2020). Telemedicine can be a COVID-19 game-changer. Here's how. World economic forum. May 13 2020. Available at: https://www.weforum. Org/agenda/2020/05/telemedicine-covid-19-gamechanger/

[12] Richardson, E., Aissat, D., Williams, G.A. and Fahy, N. (2020). Keeping what works: Remote consultations during the COVID-19 pandemic. Eurohealth, 26 (2), 73 - 76. World Health Organization. Regional Office for Europe. https://apps.who.int/iris/handle/10665/336301.

[13] Medscheme. (2020). Telephonic and Virtual consultation codes offered by Medscheme in light of the COVID-19 nationwide public health emergency. COVID-19 Update. Available at: https://www.saheart.org/cms/attachment/155.

[14] Medical Schemes Act 131 of 1998. (1998). Regulations. Available from: https://www.gov.za/sites/default/files/a131-98.pdf. Accessed May 18 2021.

[15] Council for Medical Schemes (CMS).(2020). Circular 29 of 2020: Claims Information for Beneficiaries Treated for COVID-19 of the CMS.

Council for Medical Schemes. South Africa. Pretoria. Available at: https://www.medicalschemes.co.za/latest-publication/circular-29-of-2020/

[16] Council for Medical Schemes (CMS).(2019).Annual report 2019-2020. Council for Medical Schemes. Pretoria. South Africa

[17] World Health Organization. (2020a). Media Statement: Knowing the Risks for COVID-19. [Online] Available at: <https://www.who.int/Indonesia/news/detail/08-03-2020-knowing-the-risk-for-covid-19> [Accessed 15 April 2021].

[18] World Health Organization. (2020b). *Emergency Use ICD Codes for COVID-19 Disease Outbreak.* Geneva: WHO. Available at: https://www.who.int/classifications/icd/covid19/en/.

[19] Hammersley V, Donaghy E, Parker R, McNeilly H, Atherton H, Bikker A, Campbell J, McKinstry B. Comparing the content and quality of the video, telephone, and face-to-face consultations: a non-randomised, quasi-experimental, exploratory study in UK primary care. Br J Gen Pract. 2019 Aug 29;69(686):e595-e604. doi: 10.3399/bjgp19X704573. PMID: 31262846; PMCID: PMC6607843.

[20] Hobbs, F.R., Bankhead, C., Mukhtar, T. *et al*. (2016). Clinical workload in UK primary care: A retrospective analysis of 100 million consultations in England, 2007-14. The Lancet. 387(10035): 2323-2330. DOI: 10.1016/S0140-6736(16)00620-6.

[21] Hewitt H., Gafaranga J. and Ministry B. (2010). British Journal of general practice. 60 (574): e201-e212. DOI: https://doi.org/10.3399/bjgp10X501831.

Chapter 19

Utilisation of Digital Health in Early Detection and Treatment of Pre-Eclampsia in Primary Health Care Facilities South Africa: Literature Review

Mxolisi Welcome Ngwenya, Livhuwani Muthelo, Masenyani Oupa Mbombi, Mamare Adelaide Bopape and Tebogo Maria Mothiba

Abstract

Gestational hypertension and pre-eclampsia are the most prevalent in Sub-Saharan Africa leading to undesirable perinatal and maternal outcomes. In South Africa, a high rate of maternal death was noted due to pre-eclampsia. However, the use of digital maternal health in South Africa has become of significance for reinforcement of health care. Digital health initiatives such as mobile health technologies were developed to improve better access to communities in low and middle-income countries. The implementation and practices of digital health seem to be growing expandable to achieve the UHC goals in the provision of care to all globally and nationally. This review aims to review existing literature on the use of digital maternal health to minimise admission of pre-eclampsia and early identification of gravid women who are at risk of developing pre-eclampsia.

Keywords: digital health, early detection maternal health, pre-eclampsia

1. Introduction

Maternal mortality remains a burden across the globe with 295,000 reported by the World Health Organisation. This burden continues to increase despite Primary Health Care (PHC) being are regarded as the cornerstone to curve the rise of maternal deaths due to pregnancy-related complications [1]. One of the leading causes of maternal death is reported to be pre-eclampsia [1]. Pre-eclampsia is the elevation of blood pressure (> 140 systolic mmHg and > 90 mmHg diastolic) after 20 weeks of gestation with a significant amount of protein in the urine in gravid women [2]. It accounts for approximately 5–11% of pregnancies and remains the leading cause of maternal and perinatal morbidity and mortality worldwide [3]. Also, it is reported to account for approximately 63,000 yearly maternal mortality worldwide [4].

Approximately 6% of pregnancies develop mild pre-eclampsia and 1 to 2% develop severe pre-eclampsia in the United Kingdom (UK) [5]. Furthermore, one in six women with a history of pre-eclampsia is predicted to be most likely to have pre-eclampsia in the next pregnancy. As a result, the development of digital health solutions such as mobile health initiative applications, telemonitoring and SAFE@HOME to diagnose and manage pre-eclampsia has been implemented and designed for use in health facilities and homes by health care providers and patients respectively. The digital health applications assist by providing recommendations on treatment, reassessment and referral [6, 7].

Digital Health is the utilisation of digital, mobile, and wireless technologies for health [8]. Digital Health innovation has become of significance in Sub-Saharan Africa for the reinforcement of health care [9]. Digital Health initiative such as telemonitoring was applied in Parkinstan to support women at risk of developing pre-eclampsia by close monitoring of blood pressure at home for earliest signs. The use of telemonitoring could lead to early detection of pre-eclampsia and the required need for treatment and admission of women with pre-eclampsia [10]. South Africa implemented mobile health initiatives such as Mom-Connect to improve foetal-maternal well-being at home by targeted communications to pregnant women with various disorders including pre-eclampsia [8].

2. Literature review methodology

The literature review is a survey of scholarly sources and a good literature review summarises, evaluates, synthesises and analyses to give a clear understanding knowledge of the proposed subject of the study [11]. The context of the study adopted a narrative literature review methodology. Narrative literature reviews identify and summarize the previously published studies, and avoid duplications; further seek new study areas [12]. The adopting of the narrative literature review methodology allowed the researcher to identify, evaluate, synthesise and critically analyse the published studies relevant to the topic of study. Moreover, the narrative literature review assisted with drafting an evidence-based global and national perspective picture underpinning the digital health utilisation by patients and health care providers.

2.1 Purpose of the literature review

The literature review aimed at retrieving current empirical evidence underpinning the utilisation of digital health in early detection and treatment of pre-eclampsia at primary health care facilities. Consequently, acquired informed knowledge on the providers' and patient's views of digital health challenges and barriers. Furthermore, the literature review was subjected to identify the extensive existence of research gaps of what is currently known to develop strategies to enhance the utilisation of digital health in early detection and treatment of pre-eclampsia at primary health care facilities. Making use of the practical evidence determined and identified through the literature review to expedite an ingenious background, comprehensive clinical judgement and standardised quality care for gravid women with pre-eclampsia. This was achieved by answering the following questions;

- What are the knowledge midwifery practitioners on utilisation of digital health at primary health care facilities?

- What is the knowledge of gravid women on utilisation of digital health?

- What are barriers to utilisation of the digital health by midwifery practitioners and gravid women?

2.2 Literature review sources identification

A thorough literature sources review was initiated as early from August 2021 using electronic databases with peer-reviewed journals such as PubMed, google scholar, science direct, paperpile and mendeley. Moreover, other sources were also reviewed through cross-referencing of other published articles. Lastly, websites and textbooks were reviewed to identify and synthesis the literature of relevance.

2.3 Selection of search terms

The selection of literature was achieved through using several key words and various combinations of words to select the appropriately relevant literature and exclude the irrelevant literature. Truncation, phrase searching, keywords searching and Boolean operators were adopted using the nesting logic to gather extensive literature relevant to the topic. Truncation and wild card searching permit the researcher to search the roots and portion of words with the variant endings; whilst Boolean operators are based on the Boolean algebra mostly used in databases and further provide the abilities to combine variant concepts to access the relevant items. AND, OR and NOT are the basic Boolean connectors [13]. Meanwhile, nesting is used to reveal search logic and the in order in which Boolean commands will be executed using parentheses.

2.3.1 Key words

The literature search was broadened by the use of; NOT, OR, AND, Vs, asterisk, exclamation mark and question mark. The literature search included keyword search, Boolean operators and truncation such as; (digital health AND utilisation), Digital health*, digital health vs. pre-eclampsia, digital health in primary health care facilities?, ((pre-eclampsia NOT eclampsia), (Pre-eclampsia AND primary health care facilities)), knowledge OR utilisation of digital health. Pre-eclampsia trends*, "digital health utilization in primary health care facilities", "Digital health". Each mechanism used with the key words search revealed an extensive literature and irrelevant literature was excluded (**Table 1**).

2.3.2 Inclusion criteria

The literature review included studies published from the year January 2010 to July 2021. Moreover, the quantitative, qualitative, mixed methods, narrative and systematic analysis were included in the literature. Lastly, the written English sources concentrating on and relevant to digital health utilisation in early detection and treatment of pre-eclampsia were included.

digital health-related terms	digital health methods, digital health in primary facilities, digital health in pregnancy, digital health vs. pre-eclampsia
utilisation of digital health-related terms	knowledge of digital health, implications of digital health
pre-eclampsia related terms	pathophysiology, perinatal and maternal outcomes

Table 1.
Key words search.

2.3.3 Exclusion criteria

Literature that was published before 2010 was excluded and not English-based was excluded. Moreover, literature irrelevant to digital health utilisation in early detection and treatment of pre-eclampsia were excluded (**Figure 1**).

2.4 Literature search findings

The findings of the literature search were as follows:

The literature has a total of 47 studies of which were qualitative, quantitative, mixed research methods, systematic review, meta-analysis review and narrative review. Other 11 kinds of literature were from websites, 3 were magister curations dissertations and 1 book was also reviewed. In addition, this literature review only included literature of relevance.

2.5 Identified themes

The thorough literature review identified the following themes of the current evidence underpinning digital health utilisation;

- Primary health care implications on maternal care
- Pre-eclampsia pathophysiology and implication
- Perinatal and maternal outcomes
- Early detection and treatment of pre-eclampsia
- Digital health in health and maternal care
- Purpose, implications and impact of digital health
- Challenges, barriers and knowledge of digital health

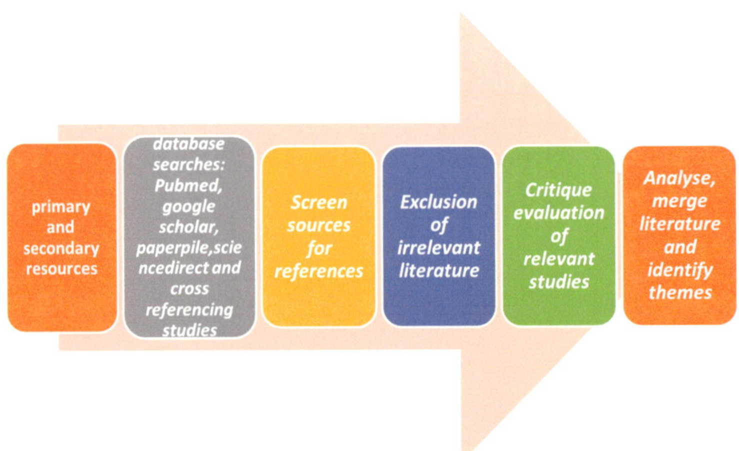

Figure 1.
Literature review process.

3. Primary health care implications on maternal care

Primary health care (PHC) is a whole of society approach to the well-being of persons that targets optimal health standards while warranting standardised quality and unbiased caretaking into consideration the individuals needs in the context of the prevention of illness such as pre-eclampsia and promotion of health, furthermore, interventions of the PHC across the developing countries expected to save approximately 60 millions of lives and possible upsurge the life expectancy by 3.7 years by the year 2030 [14].

The global health community endorsed an obligation to appoint PHC as a keystone to endeavour the sustainable development goals (SDGs) by the year 2030 [15]. However, with the achieved decrease in maternal mortality between 1990 and 2015 by 44 and 49% correspondingly. Hypertensive disorders in pregnancy (HDPs) pre-eclampsia included remain the cause of death accounting for 11 and 16% of maternal deaths and stillbirth amongst gravid women globally, respectively [15]. The aspects of classification, diagnosis and management of HDPs remains a disparity globally, therefore, leading to lack of consensus that hinders the aptitude not only to study the immediate rates of adverse effects of perinatal outcomes for the classified HDPs but also the long-term effects on the maternal and newborn's health that survived the condition [16].

A study to assess the quality of antenatal care (ANC) to detect and treat HDPs pre-eclampsia included in two-tier Nigerian establishments shown that PHC accomplished significantly worse than tertiary institutions in all elements of quality of care in assessment, diagnosis and treatment of HDPs, further substantiated that to provide optimal standard care PHC must seek to regenerate ANC programs through training to reduce disparity in quality of care [17]. A meta-analysis and systematic review of 34 studies in Etopia shown that the prevalence of HDPs and pre-eclampsia in Etopia were 6.82 and 4.74%. Showing that the prevalence of such conditions is relatively higher compared previously therefore further encouraging stakeholders and government to reinforce ANC practice to include identification of risk factors of HDPs at early ANC visits [17].

Approximately 78% of maternal deaths in South Africa at the secondary and tertiary level of care HDP emergencies such as pre-eclampsia emerged from PHC facilities and district hospitals. Moreover, such deaths were due to preventable factors at community health centres accounting for 60% of cases of maternal deaths as a result of the poor assessment, faults in diagnosing, delayed or no referrals to a higher level of care as well as non-adherence to treatment protocols and inadequate monitoring [18]. As a result of such maternal mortalities resulting from preventable factors, South Africa implemented a mobile health initiative such as mom connect to improve foetal-maternal well-being at home by targeted communications to pregnant with all kinds of disorders pre-eclampsia included and breastfeeding women via messages with the provision of information reflecting on their gestational age or postpartum period twice weekly [8].

4. Pre-eclampsia pathophysiology and implications

Pregnancy results in physiological adaptation in all the body system, however the failure of such adaptation could lead to a number of illnesses within the gravidas, such as pregnancy-induced by hypertension resulting from the failure of the trophoblast to invade the spiral arteries causing vasoconstriction and damage to the endothelial layer such as the impact on gravidas causes impact and compromise placental foetal unit likely to lead to negative perinatal outcomes [4]. Pre-eclampsia has multifaceted pathophysiology, abnormal placentation being the most primary cause [19]. The pathogenesis of pre-eclampsia progresses in 2 stages; being abnormal placentation in the first trimester and maternal syndrome in the second and third trimester characterised by the antiangiogenic factors. A non-conclusive number of theories has been proposed for placental dysfunction; being oxidative stress, abnormal natural killer cells, genetic and environmental factors [20]. The progressive stages are as follows;

Stage 1: Abnormal placentation

In normal placentation implantation, cytothrophoblasts invade the maternal spiral arteries, to form a maternal-foetal crossing point for nutrition and other functions. However, during pre-eclampsia development, there's a failure of the cytothrophoblast to migrate into the spiral arteries. This leads to incomplete spiral artery remodelling causing spiral artery narrowing causing oxidative stress and placenta ischemia [19, 20]. The placental ischemia will result in foetal complications such as intrauterine growth restrictions (IUGR) and intrauterine death (IUD). The oxidative stress due to decreased oxygen tension results in maternal peripheral endothelial cells dysfunction causing systemic inflammatory response leading to second stage namely; maternal syndrome [19–21].

Stage 2: Maternal syndrome

The effects of stage result in decreased blood flow to the maternal organs leading to multi-organs failure in the maternal systems. The biological assessment will then indicate vasospasm, coagulation cascade activation and decreased plasma levels [21]. As a result of the endothelial cell dysfunction, a hepatic system will be affected contributing to haemolysis, elevated liver enzymes and low platelet count (HELLP) syndrome, neurological system impairment (cerebral endothelial damage) causing neurological disorders [19]. Moreover, the endothelial dysfunction results in renal system impairment, i.e. acute kidney failure and proteinuria [22]. Lastly, the endothelial dysfunction promotes microangiopathic haemolytic anaemia and

Box 1 | Risk factors for pre-eclampsia from three systematic reviews[13,18,19]

- Chronic hypertension
- Antiphospholipid antibody syndrome
- Systemic lupus erythematosus
- Pre-gestational diabetes
- Chronic renal disease
- Multifetal pregnancy
- Pre-pregnancy BMI >30
- Previous stillbirth
- Nulliparity
- Maternal age >40
- Increased pre-pregnancy BMI
- Long inter-pregnancy interval (>5 years)
- Reduced school education
- Previous pre-eclampsia
- Assisted reproduction
- Previous intrauterine growth restriction
- Previous placental abruption

Figure 2.
pre-eclampsia risk factors [21].

hyperpermability linked with low albumin levels causing pulmonary and peripheral oedema [19]. Pre-eclampsia is associated with the number of risk factors as outlined in the table below (**Figure 2**) [21].

5. Perinatal and maternal outcomes of pre-eclampsia

Globally, approximately 10% of pregnant women develop hypertension during pregnancy and 2–8% of the pregnancies are complicated by pre-eclampsia [23]. Approximately 10–15% of direct maternal deaths leading to undesirable physiological changes in the kidneys, liver, brain, and clotting systems, further associated with poor foetal outcomes such as poor foetal growth and prematurity [24]. More than a half-million women died during pregnancy and childbirth across the globe in 2000 and 2002. It was also estimated that half of these maternal deaths occurred in Africa (251000) and about 48% in Asia (253000) [25].

In Sub-Saharan Africa (SSA), a meta-analysis of 13 studies in Etopia revealed that out of 5894 women diagnosed with hypertensive disorder 4% died and 13% had HELLP syndrome. Moreover, adverse perinatal outcomes were reported with perinatal death at 25% and prevalence of low birth weight at 37% [26]. Hence it is of recommendations to develop strategies and policies to enhance quality maternal health services [26]. As cited by [27] WHO estimates that the prevalence of pre-eclampsia in developing nations is seven times that of developed nations, furthermore, the rates of pre-eclampsia in African countries vary from 1.8 to 7.1%, with Nigeria prevalence varying from 2–16%.

Gestational hypertension and pre-eclampsia are the major causes of maternal and perinatal morbidity and mortality in low and middle-income countries [28]. Severe pre-eclampsia remains a major burden health problem is Sub-Saharan Africa leading to undesirable perinatal and maternal outcomes [29]. Gestational hypertension and pre-eclampsia are the most prevalent in Sub-Saharan Africa with 4.1 and 4.1%, respectively; these may be due to poor-seeking behaviour, present late and with advanced disease [30].

A prospective cohort study conducted at three South African tertiary hospitals to describe the maternal and perinatal outcomes on women with pre-eclampsia reported that hypertensive disorders remain a burden amongst pregnant women [31]. It was also reported that the incidence of pre-eclampsia is relatively in obese women and pregnant teenagers. Further reported that obese women and pregnant teenagers were more prone to pre-eclampsia complications such as perinatal deaths and preterm deliveries [31]. Furthermore, Nathan et al. further reported that out of 1547 women having pre-eclampsia 1% died, 0.3% had a stroke whilst approximately 9.5% progressively developed eclampsia and kidney injury at 17.6% [31]. Moreover, it was reported out of 1589 of the births were associated with perinatal deaths at 21 and 84.5% of stillbirths; 1308 of live births were preterm deliveries. A dissertation on factors contributing to stillbirth at Witbank hospital corroborated that hypertensive disorders pose a significant risk to the well-being of the mother and the foetus. It was reported that approximately 12% of the women admitted at Witbank hospital had stillbirths were due to hypertensive disorders in pregnancy [32].

6. Early detection and treatment of pre-eclampsia

Detection of early-onset pre-eclampsia can be achieved through effective screening as early as the first trimester. Moreover, screening can be achieved via certain methods such as maternal history screening by combination of maternal risk factors, placental growth factor, mean arterial blood pressure and uterine artery Doppler [33]. Digital health has been introduced in maternal health to help curve maternal mortalities rise due to preventable conditions such as pre-eclampsia. A retrospective study for early prediction of pre-eclampsia using machine learning through analysis of clinical and laboratory data in previous ANC visits; revealed that a significant set of features for prediction of pre-eclampsia were identified which shown significantly elevated prediction performances of the risk of pre-eclampsia [34]. Early detection of pre-eclampsia is a global burden that should be addressed. The study developed a wearable device to monitor women at risk of pre-eclampsia using the identified risk factors and blood monitoring the prototype yielded good results for identification of the biomedical signals. However, comparison of the methodology is still to be done with another facility [35].

Digital health can overcome access limiting factors and lack of trained HCP in low-resourced settings through mHealth solutions. Studies have evidently proven mHealth can benefit pre-eclampsia women through early detection and symptoms control. mHealth has a great potential for improving clinical practice as positive results were reported on maternal health improvement through digital health [28]. The use of digital health such as electronic health (eHealth) showed improved efficiency and suitability of care, moreover had an effect on mortality, readmissions, and total costs [36]. Furthermore, the use of digital health such as mobile technology through self-monitoring of blood pressure amongst women at risk of pre-eclampsia reduces perinatal and maternal mortalities and morbidities due to pre-eclampsia and reduces the number of hospitalisations [37].

7. Digital health in health and maternal care

Digital health is a comprehensive category entailing mobile health, electronic health, and telehealth and health data. It strengthens health systems through bringing such services directly to their homes and unprivileged communities; further map illness outbreaks and digital tool integration to make health care to be more productive and approachable [38]. Over the past 20 years, digital health technology has been splendidly growing to improve health and maternal health. Furthermore, the digital health technologies vary some are client-focused meaning they provide women enhanced capabilities to raise their health and risk consciousness, self-participated monitoring and management in preconception, antenatal and postnatal period. In addition, provides awareness of any pregnancy-related complications such as pre-eclampsia and treatment as well as lifestyle and health choices [39].

While some digital health technologies are provider-focused digital health technologies; they enable substantial management of obstetric complications during primary consultation, admission and referral process. Telemedicine and telecare are the common examples of digital systems that encompass access to specialist services behind the limitations of the clinic. In addition, the systems are developed for healthcare professionals and introduced into the high-risk patients, i.e. pre-eclampsia women [39]. Digital health innovations are not the replacements for the health system in place, however, they empower and enhance the components of the health systems to make an informed decisions and optimise health outcomes [40]. The national department of health (NDoH) on the national digital health strategy for South Africa for 2019–2024 (NDHSSA) substantiated that digital enable support for health sectors for a health life for the population through health systems strengthening to enable service delivery. Moreover, further enables effective patient care and personal empowerment needed to achieve universal health coverage (UHC), [41]. A case study to improve maternal health through digital health using mobile technology indicated that maternal mortality remains a burden across SSA. Corroborated that mobile communication encourage the provision of fast and accessible care. Moreover, it was found that digital health through mobile devices increase workplace efficiency and enable faster decision making amongst health care providers (HCP) [42].

In South Africa the public health system distorted to more comprehensive and cohesive health systems [43]. The use of public health services across the scale of care was highest in SSA. Approximately 94% of pregnant women attended ANC and 76% attended the recommended ANC visits showing active utilisation of such services to achieve the MDG 5. However, this use of public services was linked to digital health initiatives such as mom connect [43].

8. Purpose, implications and impact of digital health

Digital health primarily aims to provide widespread reachable and digestible information to all stakeholders. It provides high-quality information essential to researchers, patients, health care providers, social scientists, industries and government [44]. Digital health includes variants of sets such as mobile health, telehealth, telemedicine, health information technology, wearable devices and personalised medicine. Digital health can improve the diagnosing and treating of illnesses, further heightening the rendering of health care for each person [45]. The use of digital health can assist in reaching well-informed decisions with one's health and provide alternative options for facilitating prevention, early diagnosis of life-threatening diseases, and management of diseases outside the health care facilities. The stakeholder's implications with regards to utilisation of digital health were that optimise patient care and personalise individual's care through reduction of inefficiencies and costs, improved accessibility, optimal quality and more patient-oriented care [45, 46].

A qualitative perspective of community health workers on using health mHealth to improve health care delivery in India revealed that mHealth was accepted by community health workers because it sought of improving their status in their communities [47]. However, there was a mix of negative and positive perceptions surrounding the use and impact of the mHealth software such as underlying mistrust, socio-economic barriers in engagement and technological barriers in implementation [47].

9. Digital health methods

Approximately 3–10% of pregnancies are complicated by hypertensive disorders [48]. Around 30,000 women yearly due to hypertensive disorders in pregnancy [49]. This shows that the use of digital and telehealth can considerably benefit women at risk of hypertensive disorders and ensure early detection of symptoms and treat the symptoms and improve maternal and perinatal outcomes during and after pregnancy [28, 50]. A randomised controlled trial study to improve maternal and neonatal health in Bangladesh, corroborated that using digital health such as mobile can make great contributions in reducing maternal and neonatal mortalities

[51]. The digital methods below will be client-focused and provider-focused from global, SSA and South Africa.

However, below are the digital health methods used by various countries to strengthen the maternal digital health system for high risk and low-risk pregnancies;

9.1 Mobile initiatives

9.1.1 International

- Text4Baby

Text4baby is a mHealth initiative in the United States that provides timely messages to pregnant women and puerperia's with regards to their wellbeing. Furthermore, the mHealth addressed the prenatal and postnatal being of the women with messages addressing the pregnancy, labour, nutrition and when to reach health care [52]. Text4Baby is one of the patient education strategies to help curve the rise of maternal and perinatal morbidity and mortality due to pre-eclampsia [53].

- Smart mom

Smart mom is a Canadian mHealth initiative focused on prenatal education on pregnant women through text messages. Smart mom guide women throughout pregnancy by the provision of evidence-based information developed by experts in maternal and child health [54].

- Mobile4Health

In response to significantly high maternal mortality rates in Bangladesh due to maternal pregnancy-related conditions such as pre-eclampsia, the Mobile4Health initiative was developed. The mobile health initiative aimed to provide pregnant women with information via messages for self-care relating to their conditions and postpartum care [42].

9.1.2 Sub-Saharan Africa

- Pigia daktari

Pigia daktari is a Tanzanian telemedicine mobile app developed for use by HCP and patients to access specialised care especially for patients in communities with no specialised care. Moreover, it encourages the utilisation of referral systems and its user-friendly interactive box; it aims to identify and solve existing barriers to access and provide consistent and timely optimised health services [55].

- Wazazi Nipendeni

Wazazi Nipendeni is a mHealth initiative used by Tanzanian pregnant women to receive tailored messages with regards to pregnancy and gestational age as well as the health of their infant. The mHealth was implemented to reduce high Tanzania's maternal and infant mortality ratio [56].

9.1.3 South Africa

- Mom connect

Mom connect is a South African client-focused digital mHealth initiative utilised by pregnant women and puerperia's through any mobile device integrated with maternal and child health services via messages in all 11 official languages [57]. Mom connect has registered over more than 60% of gravid women nationally and registered approximately 1.7 million subscribers since 2014, maternal health service will improve maternal health services and most patients were enthusiastic about utilisation of the mHealth [58].

- Essential Medicine guidance

Essential medicine (EM) guidance is a provider-focused digital health app initiative that encompasses 12 local clinical guidelines and decision-making tools for HCP. Moreover, EM guidance assists the HCP in accurately diagnosing and management of conditions such as pre-eclampsia utilising South Africa's comprehensive evidence-based medicine sources [59].

9.2 Telemedicine and telehealth

- SAFE@HOME

SAFE@HOME is a digital health platform designed to monitor daily blood pressure monitoring and symptoms amongst women with chronic hypertension, history of pre-eclampsia and pre-eclampsia in the Netherlands [7]. The evaluation of the care telepath noted a significantly minimal admission amongst women of hypertension and suspected pre-eclampsia with the utilisation of the SAFE@ HOME tele monitoring. Moreover, telemonitoring of blood pressure amongst women is feasible in high-risk patient for early detection and has the potential to change antenatal care (ANC) [7].

9.3 Medical social media

Social media platforms are regarded as one of the digital health initiatives widely. A cross sectional study to determine how individuals used social media for evidence maternity care stated that women were highly engaged in utilising social media to access and share maternity information [60]. Furthermore, the utilisation of maternal health care services was significantly higher amongst women who were exposed to mass media across countries and such women were 46–86% likely to receive ANC [61].

A study conducted in Ota, Nigeria to identify sources of maternal health awareness and examine the means of access to maternal information corroborated that the internet was the most used source to access maternal health awareness services at 49% and followed by adverts and campaigns at 30.6% [62]. In addition, apps claim to sanction for greater convenience, connectivity and efficiency. Social media such as Facebook have many users and allow women to access and share information with other moms with regards to their pregnancy [63].

9.4 Digitised health record platforms

Digitised health records systems are technological innovations adopted by numerous health institutions. A study indicated that the use of electronic medical records for maternal and child care and health most like improve health care; as supported by the results that the women who had prenatal care visits with the HCP who adopted the electronic health record (EHR) were most likely to have well-child visits [64]. A qualitative analysis of the user of EHR in the maternity care environment described it as being favourably, whilst other midwives are shown limited understanding of the EHR [65]. However, a systematic review in South Africa to identify success factors for the implementation of EHRs identified social, technical and environmental barriers, i.e. lack of supporting infrastructure, political influence, legislation and regulations, user's training and commitment, and lack of structure implementation and management [66].

10. Challenges, barriers and knowledge of digital health

Despite the standard benefits and implications of digital health in clinical practice to diagnose, treat, disease management and prevention and wellness; challenges and issues arose such as doctors not having adequate information for prescription and use digital health technologies [46]. A perspective review on critical perspectives on digital health technologies reported a number of complexities on patients' perspective on the use of digital health such as telehealth; some patients felt that they had slight control over their doctors' decision to use technologies and wish to continue using the ordinary patient-doctor model [67]. A digital health: a path to validation review conducted in the United States of America (USA) stated that the concept of digital health continues to evolve and digital health technologies are being used worldwide in medicine to diagnose, treat and clinical decision support [68]. The impact of digital health technologies on optimising individuals' health and well-being is extraordinary as the technologies have transformed clinical practice from prevention to disease management and self-management [69]. However, despite the uprising of digital health in clinical practice, challenges were noted during the path to validation of digital health hindering the extensive implementation of evolving approaches such as health digital scorecard and requirements-driven approach [68]. Three challenges were noted namely; conceptual, financial and organisational and operational challenges.

In a study conducted in the United States, lack of technical support, lack of authentication of expertise and lack of expertise usability were the barriers to implementation of digital health by patients with hypertension [70]. There is a number of contributing factors hindering the implementation of electronic health (e-Health) programmes in Uganda such as poor coordination and communication, untrained health personnel, loss of network connection, lack of knowledge and skills about telehealth, illiterate community and people financial status [71]. A study in the implementation of digital health technology such as mHealth applications in Botswana aiming to reduce patients and HCP barriers inaccessibility to care and knowledge, respectively, indicated that numerous social and technical challenges were faced; such as cultural misalignment between the Information technology (IT) and HCP, unreliable IT, infrastructure accidental damage to mobile devices and malfunctioning mobile devices [72]. There are unravelling barriers in adoption of digital health at the primary health care level in African Countries by health care providers such as lack of technology knowledge, lack of innovation acceptance, limited knowledge and abilities of utilisation of digital health, absence of enthusiasm and poor organisational and management level [73]. Furthermore, study conducted in Iran shown significant poor knowledge of health care providers in utilisation of digital health and most probably due to lack of training [73].

Approximately 79% of pregnant women utilising mom connect in the year 2017 asked questions related to health and others were about disrespect and abuse from the midwifery practitioners, showing significant utilisation of digital health [58]. Further showing that improper communication amongst the midwifery practitioners and gravid women can further hinder the utilisation of digital health by gravid women. However, despite the improper communications, approximately 2.5 million pregnant women registered for the digital health initiate by 2019. Evidence shows effective usage of digital health amongst pregnant women [41]. The working conditions can hinder optimal midwifery care to the patient such as the implementation of digital health; this supported [74] that absenteeism, shortage of staff, work overload of staff and overcrowding of patients in healthcare facilities are contributing factors to perinatal morbidity and mortality. This significantly remains a major common barrier in the provision of standardised care such as improper teaching of pregnant women such as the utilisation of mom connect.

11. Conclusion

Despite the digital health initiatives and digital health methods utilisation growing expandable across the globe, the empirical evidence pertinent to digital health utilisation to maternal health services to early detect and treat pre-eclampsia was limited. The extensive literature review showed significant extensive existence of research gaps in digital health utilisation in maternal services. Therefore, it remains within the jurisdiction of the department of health and researchers to research beyond to identify facilitators and impediments of strengthening maternal digital health systems amongst high-risk pregnant women in South Africa, to develop quality standards and more evolved digital health initiatives supporting the maternal and child health. Moreover, for South Africa to achieve the UHC goals more context-rich digital health solutions need to be developed to improve the accessibility of services and further achieve the millennium developmental goal 5.

Author details

Mxolisi Welcome Ngwenya[1], Livhuwani Muthelo[1*], Masenyani Oupa Mbombi[1], Mamare Adelaide Bopape[1] and Tebogo Maria Mothiba[2]

1 Department of Nursing Science, University of Limpopo, South Africa

2 Faculty of Health Sciences Executive Dean's Office, University of Limpopo, South Africa

*Address all correspondence to: livhuwani.muthelo@ul.ac.za

References

[1] WHO. 2021. Available from: https://www.who.int/news-room/fact-sheets/detail/maternal-mortality

[2] Sellers PM. Seller's Midwifery. 3rd ed. Da Serra D, Dippenaar J. Cape Town: Juta 2018.

[3] Townsend R, O'Brien P, Khalil A. Current best practice in the management of hypertensive disorders in pregnancy. Integrated Blood Pressure Control. 2016;**9**:79

[4] Ross MG, Pierce JG. What is the Mortality Rate Associated With Ecclapsia? Medscape; 2019. Available from: https://emedicine.medscape.com/article/253960-overview

[5] National Health Services. 2018. Available from: https://www.nhs.uk/conditions/pre-eclampsia

[6] Dunsmuir DT, Payne BA, Cloete G, Petersen CL, Görges M, Lim J, et al. Development of mHealth applications for pre-eclampsia triage. IEEE Journal of Biomedical and Health Informatics. 2014;**18**(6):1857-1864

[7] van den Heuvel JF, Lely AT, Huisman JJ, Trappenburg JC, Franx A, Bekker MN. SAFE@ HOME: Digital health platform facilitating a new care path for women at increased risk of preeclampsia–A case-control study. Pregnancy Hypertension. 2020;**22**:30-36

[8] Mehl GL, Tamrat T, Bhardwaj S, Blaschke S, Labrique A. Digital health vision: Could MomConnect provide a pragmatic starting point for achieving universal health coverage in South Africa and elsewhere? BMJ Global Health. 2018;**3**(Suppl. 2):e000626

[9] Holst C, Sukums F, Radovanovic D, Ngowi B, Noll J, Winkler AS. Sub-Saharan Africa—the new breeding ground for global digital health. The Lancet Digital Health. 2020;**2**(4): e160-e162

[10] Feroz A, Saleem S, Seto E. Exploring perspectives, preferences and needs of a telemonitoring program for women at high risk for preeclampsia in a tertiary health facility of Karachi: A qualitative study protocol. Reproductive Health. 2020;**17**(1):1-7

[11] McCombes S. How to write a literature review [Thesis]. 2019. Retrieved 2021. Available at https://www.scribber.com/dissertation/litrature-review

[12] Ferrari R. Writing narrative style literature reviews. Medical Writing. 2015;**24**(4):230-235

[13] Coughlan M, Cronin P, Ryan F. Doing a Literature Review in Nursing, Health and Social Care. Los Angeles: SAGE Publications; 2013

[14] WHO. Primary Health Care. Switzerland: WHO; 2021. Available from: https://www.who.int/news-room/fact-sheets/detail/primary-health-care

[15] Warren CE, Hossain SMI, Ishaku S, Armbruster D, Hillman E. A primary health care model for managing pre-eclampsia and eclampsia in low-and middle-income countries. Reproductive Health. 2020;**17**(1):1-7

[16] Brown MA, Magee LA, Kenny LC, Karumanchi SA, McCarthy FP, Saito S, et al. Hypertensive disorders of pregnancy: ISSHP classification, diagnosis, and management recommendations for international practice. Hypertension. 2018;**72**:24-43

[17] Salomon A, Ishaku S, Kirk KR, Warren CE. Detecting and managing hypertensive disorders in pregnancy: A cross-sectional analysis of the quality of antenatal care in Nigeria. BMC Health Services Research. 2019;**19**(1):1-14

[18] Naidoo M, Pattinson RC. An approach to hypertensive disorders in pregnancy for the primary care physician. South African Family Practice. 2020;**62**(1):1-6

[19] Uzan J, Carbonnel M, Piconne O, Asmar R, Ayoubi JM. Pre-eclampsia: Pathophysiology, diagnosis, and management. Vascular Health and Risk Management. 2011;**7**:467

[20] Rana S, Lemoine E, Granger JP, Karumanchi SA. Preeclampsia: Pathophysiology, challenges, and perspectives. Circulation Research. 2019;**124**(7):1094-1112

[21] Burton GJ, Redman CW, Roberts JM, Moffett A. Pre-eclampsia: Pathophysiology and clinical implications. BMJ. 2019;**366**:l2381

[22] Kattah A. Preeclampsia and kidney disease: Deciphering cause and effect. Current Hypertension Reports. 2020;**22**(11):1-11

[23] WHO. WHO | Prevention and Treatment of Pre-Eclampsia and Eclampsia. Switzerland: WHO; 2011

[24] Luger RK, Kight BP. Hypertension in Pregnancy. Treasure Island, FL: StatPearls Publishing; 2017

[25] Li J, Luo C, Deng R, Jacoby P, de Klerk N. Maternal mortality in Yunnan, China: Recent trends and associated factors. BJOG. 2010;**114**:7

[26] Mersha AG, Abegaz TM, Seid MA. Maternal and perinatal outcomes of hypertensive disorders of pregnancy in Ethiopia: Systematic review and meta-analysis. BMC Pregnancy and Childbirth. 2019;**19**(1):1-12

[27] Osungbade KO, Ige OK. Public health perspectives of preeclampsia in developing countries: Implication for health system strengthening. Journal of Pregnancy. 2011;**2011**:481095. DOI: 10.1155/2011/481095

[28] Rivera-Romero O, Olmo A, Muñoz R, Stiefel P, Miranda ML, Beltrán LM. Mobile health solutions for hypertensive disorders in pregnancy: scoping literature review. JMIR mHealth and uHealth. 2018;**6**(5):e130

[29] Machano MM, Joho AA. Prevalence and risk factors associated with severe pre-eclampsia among postpartum women in Zanzibar: A cross-sectional study. BMC Public Health. 2020;**20**(1): 1-10

[30] Gemechu KS, Assefa N, Mengistie B. Prevalence of hypertensive disorders of pregnancy and pregnancy outcomes in Sub-Saharan Africa: A systematic review and meta-analysis. Women's Health (London). 2020;**16**. DOI: 10.1177/1745506520973105. PMID 33334273; PMCID: PMC7750906

[31] Nathan HL, Seed PT, Hezelgrave NL, De Greeff A, Lawley E, Conti-Ramsden F, et al. Maternal and perinatal adverse outcomes in women with pre-eclampsia cared for at facility-level in South Africa: A prospective cohort study. Journal of Global Health. 2018;**8**(2):20401

[32] Mhlophe C. Factors contributing to occurrence of stillbirths in a tertiary hospital (thesis). Pretoria: University of Pretoria; 2019

[33] Poon LC, Nicolaides KH. Early prediction of preeclampsia. Obstetrics and Gynecology International. 2014; **2014**:297397

[34] Marić I, Tsur A, Aghaeepour N, Montanari A, Stevenson DK, Shaw GM, et al. Early prediction of preeclampsia via machine learning. American Journal of Obstetrics & Gynecology MFM. 2020;**2**(2):100100

[35] Espinilla M, Medina J, García-Fernández ÁL, Campaña S, Londoño J. Fuzzy intelligent system for patients with preeclampsia in wearable devices. Mobile Information Systems. 2017;**2017**

[36] Keasberry J, Scott IA, Sullivan C, Staib A, Ashby R. Going digital: a narrative overview of the clinical and organisational impacts of eHealth technologies in hospital practice. Australian Health Review. 2017;**41**(6):646-664

[37] Ganapathy R, Grewal A, Castleman JS. Remote monitoring of blood pressure to reduce the risk of preeclampsia related complications with an innovative use of mobile technology. Pregnancy Hypertension: An International Journal of Women's Cardiovascular Health. 2016;**6**(4): 263-265

[38] WHO. Towards a Global Strategy on Digital Health. Switzerland: WHO; 2020. Available from: https://www.who.int/bulletin/volumes/98/4/20-253955/en/

[39] Mackintosh N, Gong SQ, Hadjiconstantinou M, Verdezoto N. Digital mediation of candidacy in maternity care: Managing boundaries between physiology and pathology. Social Science & Medicine. 2021:114299

[40] Government of Canada. Digital Health. Canada; 2020. Available from: https://www.grandchallenges.ca/see-our-impact/

[41] Department of Health. National digital health strategy for South Africa 2019-2024, Pretoria. 2019. Available from: https://www.bhfglobal.com/wpcontent/uploads/downloads/news/national%20digital%20health%20strategy%20for%20south%20africa%202019-2024a.pdf

[42] West DM. Using mobile technology to improve maternal health and fight Ebola: A case study of mobile innovation in Nigeria. Center for Technological Innovation at Brookings. 2015;**19**:308-312

[43] Pillay Y, Motsoaledi PA. Digital health in South Africa: Innovating to improve health. BMJ Glob Health. 2018;**3**(Suppl. 2):e000722

[44] Walsh L, Hyett N, Juniper N, Li C, Rodier S, Hill S. The use of social media as a tool for stakeholder engagement in health service management and quality improvement: A scooping review. Digital Health. 2021;7:2055207621996870

[45] Food Drug Administration. What is Digital Health? 2020. Available from: https://www.fda.gov/medical-devices/digital-health-center-excellence/what-digital-health

[46] Ronquillo Y, Meyers A, Korvek SJ. Digital Health. StatPearls: Statpearls Publishing; 2017

[47] Gopalakrishnan L, Buback L, Fernald L, Walker D, Diamond-Smith N, in addition to The CAS Evaluation Consortium. Using mHealth to improve health care delivery in India: A qualitative examination of the perspectives of community health workers and beneficiaries. PLoS One. 2020;**15**(1):e0227451

[48] Mol BW, Roberts CT, Thangaratinam S, Magee LA, De Groot CJ, Hofmeyr GJ. Pre-eclampsia. The Lancet. 2016;**387**(10022):999-1011

[49] Kassebaum NJ, Bertozzi-Villa A, Coggeshall MS. Global, regional, and national levels and causes of maternal mortality during 1990-2013: A systematic analysis for the Global Burden of Disease Study 2013. Lancet. 2014;**384**(9947):956-956

[50] Mercer L. Telehealth Enhances Management of Hypertensive Disorders During Pregnancy. United States: Health recovery solutions, 2021. Available from: healthrecoverysolutions.com

[51] Tobe RG, Haque SE, Ikegami K, Mori R. Mobile-health tool to improve maternal and neonatal health care in Bangladesh: A cluster randomized

controlled trial. BMC Pregnancy and Childbirth. 2018;**18**(1):1-7

[52] Whittaker R, Matoff-Stepp S, Meehan J, Kendrick J, Jordan E, Stange P, et al. Text4baby: Development and implementation of a national text messaging health information service. American Journal of Public Health. 2012;**102**(12):2207-2213

[53] Roberts JM, August PA, Bakris G, Barton JR, Bernstein IM, Druzin M, et al. Hypertension in pregnancy: Executive summary. Obstetrics and Gynecology. 2013;**122**(5):1122-1131

[54] Smart Mom. Smart Mom Health Education. Vancouver; 2021. Available from: https://local.infobel.ca/CA103986854/smartmom_mobile_health_education-vancouver.html

[55] Dar es Salaam. Aga Khan Health Services in Tanzania Launches First Digital Health App. Tanzania; 2021. Available from: https://www.akdn.org/press-release/aga-khan-health-services-tanzania-launches-first-digital-health-app

[56] Tanzania's Health Baby SMS Service Records 1M mHealth Registrations, Tanzania. 2015. Available from: https: hitconsultant.net/2015/10/13/Tanzania's Health Baby SMS service records 1M mHealth Registrations

[57] National Department of Health. 2014. Available from: http://www.health.gov.za/momconnect/

[58] Peter J, Benjamin P, LeFevre AE, Barron P, Pillay Y. Taking digital health innovation to scale in South Africa: ten lessons from MomConnect. BMJ Global Health. 2018;**3**(Suppl. 2):e000592

[59] EMguidance. 2021. Available from: https://emguidance.com/

[60] Dekker RL, King S, Lester K. Social media and evidence-based maternity care: A cross-sectional survey study. The Journal of Perinatal Education. 2016;**25**(2):105-115

[61] Fatema K, Lariscy JT. Mass media exposure and maternal healthcare utilization in South Asia. SSM-Population Health. 2020;**11**:100614

[62] Igbinoba AO, Soola EO, Omojola O, Odukoya J, Adekeye O, Salau OP. Women's mass media exposure and maternal health awareness in Ota, Nigeria. Cogent Social Sciences. 2020;**6**(1):1766260

[63] Johnson SA. "Maternal devices", social media and the self-management of pregnancy, mothering and child health. Societies. 2014;**4**(2):330-350

[64] Meghea CI, Corser W, You Z. Electronic medical record use and maternal and child care and health. Maternal and Child Health Journal. 2016;**20**(4):819-826

[65] Hawley G, Jackson C, Hepworth J, Wilkinson SA. Sharing of clinical data in a maternity setting: How do paper hand-held records and electronic health records compare for completeness? BMC Health Services Research. 2014;**14**(1):1-9

[66] Katurura MC, Cilliers L. Electronic health record system in the public health care sector of South Africa: A systematic literature review. African Journal of Primary Health Care & Family Medicine. 2018;**10**(1):1-8

[67] Lupton D. Beyond Techno-Utopia: Critical Approaches to Digital health Technologies. AG Basel, Switzerland: MDPI; 2015

[68] Mathews SC, McShea MJ, Hanley CL, Ravitz A, Labrique AB, Cohen AB. Digital health: A path to validation. NPJ Digital Medicine. 2019;**2**(1):1-9

[69] Kostkova P. Grand challenges in digital health. Frontiers in Public Health. 2015;**3**:134

[70] Palacholla RS, Fischer N, Coleman A, Agboola S, Kirley K, Felsted J, et al. Provider-and patient-related barriers to and facilitators of digital health technology adoption for hypertension management: Scoping review. JMIR Cardio. 2019;**3**(1):e11951

[71] Kiberu VM, Mars M, Scott RE. Barriers and opportunities to implementation of sustainable e-Health programmes in Uganda: A literature review. African Journal of Primary Health Care and Family Medicine. 2017;**9**(1):1-10

[72] Littman-Quinn R, Chandra A, Schwartz A, Fadlelmola FM, Ghose S, Luberti AA, et al. mHealth applications for telemedicine and public health intervention in Botswana. In: 2011 IST-Africa Conference Proceedings. Botswana: IEEE; 2011. pp. 1-11

[73] Ohia C, Ongolo-Zogo P, Fawole OI. Digital health information technology utilization for enhanced health services delivery in Africa: Unravelling barriers to adoption among Primary healthcare providers. South Eastern European Journal of Public Health (SEEJPH). 2021:2

[74] Mathebula MG. Factors contributing to high perinatal morbidity rates in Mankweng-Polokwane Complex of the Capricorn District, Limpopo Province, South Africa [thesis]. University of Limpopo Limpopo; 2016

Chapter 20

Evaluating A Mobile App for Data Collection in Occupational Therapy Practice

Tanja Svarre, Marie Bangsgaard Bang and Tine Bieber Lunn

Abstract

This study investigates the use of a mobile app for data collection in occupational therapy practice. Seven occupational therapists used a mobile app to collect data on housing-adaptation home visits for a period of two months. The occupational therapists documented five home visits on an online diary to document their use of the mobile app. Subsequently, a follow-up focus-group interview was conducted to discuss the diary results and elaborate on the use of the app in occupational therapy practice. The benefits of using the mobile app include the app's systematic approach, ease of navigation, and the automation of data collection steps. Limitations include the inability to capture the complexity of the practice. Thus, the occupational therapists to some extent experienced that the need to use the mobile app is an added task in therapists' daily work that did not reflect their current practice. Future transformations of paper-based tools must be conducted in a way that closely reflects the work processes in clinical practice. This study suggests that a digitized tool holds significant potential for developing clinical practice, but digitization does not change the issues or the complexity associated with the tool itself or the existing practice.

Keywords: mobile application, health information technology, workplace information, occupational therapy, practice studies

1. Introduction

The practice of occupational therapy naturally includes client-centered investigations of the clients' abilities and disabilities, as well as problems related to occupational performance. Occupational therapy involves the examination of external factors, such as the physical and social environment, along with personal factors, such as body function. A wide range of standardized and non-standardized assessment tools has been developed over the years as an important part of occupational therapists' work in this regard. To our knowledge, most of these assessments, including the ADL taxonomy [1], OSA [2], COPM [3], Mohost [4], and IPPA [5], only exist in paper form.

Health information technology (HIT) refers to the information technology used in the health domain and it is commonly associated with two lines of research: adoption and impact. Adoption studies focus on the level of adoption and barriers to the adoption of existing solutions, while impact studies center on the effect of the technology on the quality of the service, efficiency, or financial performance [6]. This study can be characterized as an adoption study.

M-health is a concept that is closely related to HIT. It denotes the use of mobile technology in the healthcare field [7] by patients, clinicians, and health professionals [8]. Applications have been developed for mobile phones and tablets to support information and time management, health-record maintenance and access, communication and consulting, referencing and information gathering, clinical decision making, patient monitoring, and medical education and training. A number of benefits have been identified in conjunction with m-health, including convenience, better clinical decision making, improved accuracy, increased efficiency, and enhanced productivity [9].

Occupational therapists are employed by all Danish municipalities. Notably, occupational therapists are the primary professionals involved in investigating the physical home environment of people with functional limitations. In this regard, they are responsible for identifying factors that hinder daily activities and for finding solutions to identified problems. In identifying these factors, the Housing Enabler tool is one of only a few assessment instruments that offer a valid, reliable, and systematic way to identify accessibility barriers in the dwellings of adults with functional limitations [10]. In occupational therapy practice, the demand to use information and communication technology (ICT) to document observations and share data creates a need to replace paper-based rating forms and assessments with digital solutions. In order to comply with this demand, we developed a mobile version of Iwarsson and Slaug's Housing Enabler assessment tool [10], which we hereafter refer to as the HE app. The purpose of developing this app was to transform the paper-based rating forms into a digital solution that could communicate with other ICT tools and documentation systems [11]. The development of the HE app was based on interactions with users and several usability tests [12].

The use of mobile technology in occupational therapy has only been covered to a minor extent in research [11]. In the present chapter, we investigate the use of the HE app for data collection in an occupational therapy clinical setting. Two recent studies have analyzed the acceptance and use of technology in occupational therapy interventions. Liu et al. [13] used a questionnaire to investigate the adoption of new technologies among occupational and physical therapists at a Canadian rehabilitation hospital. The study, which had 91 participants, showed that therapists see the potential for technology to help them reach their work goals and assist clients, but they have trouble finding the time to use it and they need more training in its use. Furthermore, Liu et al. [13] found that positive expectations about technology and its use increase intentions to use it in the future. Another study investigated the adoption of a web-based obesity prevention intervention program at commercial health centers in the Netherlands [14]. Clients were offered tailored feedback based on their own reports of their weight over time. Eight adopters and 12 non-adopters took part in semi-structured interviews. The study found that the main reasons for adoption were accessibility and correspondence with related activities. Similar findings emerged in a review study on general m-health by Sezgin and Yildinm [15], in which usability and ease of use were found to improve adoption. Notably, in the Dutch study, non-adoption was attributed to issues regarding time consumption, competitiveness with own interventions, and fear of falling profits [14]. Lastly, a study from 2007 investigated the use of the Housing Enabler tool in a Swedish municipality [16]. Twenty-five occupational therapists participated in the study and carried out 422 assessments using the tool. The purpose of the study was to analyze the implementation of the tool on PalmPilots in the municipality. Various methods were used to document the process, including diaries, e-mail correspondence, and meeting minutes, all of which were subjected to qualitative analysis. The study found that the utilization of technology in occupational therapy practice was demanding in terms of the amount of technical support needed and in other ways. The occupational therapists' initial expectations that the use of technology would reduce the time needed for the assessments were not met. At the same time, the potential to digitize professional communication was appreciated by the participants [16].

This chapter aims to examine the adoption of the HE app in Danish occupational therapy clinical practice. While this study is somewhat similar to the study by Fänge et al. [16], we assume that occupational therapists have become more accepting of the technology. Furthermore, tablets are now more widely used by the general public than was the case with the PalmPilot a decade ago. Our focus is on the practical benefits and challenges of using the HE application from the perspective of work processes. We use the findings to identify the ways in which the HE app example can inform the development of data-collection apps and add to best practices in this respect.

1.1 The HE app

After the publication of the paper describing the transformation of the HE assessment to a mobile app [11], further programming and development were carried out to improve the app. When the revised version was ready for testing in the field of occupational therapy, our aims were not only to create a final report but also to gain deeper insight into the use of the app in occupational therapy practice.

The HE app, which is in Danish, is available for Android from Google Play in Denmark. In order to ensure data security, users must have a personal login. The dwelling and client function profiles are registered by address. All data concerning environmental barriers are collected and divided into the categories of A, B, and C, which refers to the outdoor environment, the entrance, and the indoor environment, respectively. All items are listed and the user can choose the ratings of "yes," "no," and "not rated." More exact items offer the option to add notes or photos. The dwelling's accessibility score is automatically calculated, and data is automatically saved on the unit and can be exported.

2. Research methods

After having developed the HE app in a semi-controlled manner [11], the next step of development needed to incorporate experiences from its use in the clinical practice. Therefore, we undertook a single case study [17] focused on the HE app as a digitized tool for data collection in occupational therapy. Thus, the purpose of the study was to understand the social and technical issues associated with using the mobile app for data collection. The outcomes were expected to provide an understanding of the realistic use of the HE app and generate input for an evaluation and a final design iteration of the app. For example, there was a need to learn how and to whom the occupational therapist needed to export the data in an actual work situation. Consequently, the export functionality and the design of the final app were not yet fully developed. As such, the HE app was still a prototype during the study.

We contacted municipalities in Denmark to find occupational therapists working with accessibility and home modifications who would be interested in testing the HE app in their daily work. A convenience sample of seven occupational therapists from four municipalities was recruited for data collection. All of those participants worked with accessibility and home modification on a regular basis and had been doing so for at least six months. Furthermore, as familiarity with HE was key, all participants agreed to complete a Housing Enabler course before testing the HE app. The course was necessary to ensure that the participants could use the tool to carry out valid and reliable assessments, especially given the tool's complexity [16]. After completing the HE courses, the seven occupational therapists each completed five HE assessments using the HE app. Data collection took place for four months.

2.1 Online diary

As the HE assessments took place across a wide geographical space and were often were planned with very short notice, observations and interviews could not be carried out on location. Moreover, as the time window for carrying out the investigations covered a period of approximately two months, we could not rely on the therapists to recall investigations carried out in the initial part of the period. Therefore, we developed an online diary that therapists could use to continually document their experiences with the HE app.

The diary was set up as an online reporting tool by means of the survey tool Kalus (www.kalus.dk). A combination of open questions and fixed-choice questions was used. No questions were mandatory, as voluntary responses are known to be more useful. Groups of questions were developed under the themes of background data, today's intervention, HE as a tool for cooperation, next steps in the case, and HE as a digital tool. Prior to its use for data collection, the diary was pretested with colleagues and one of the participants to check for clarity, wording, length, and relevance. The participants were asked to complete the diary within 24 hours of each intervention to ensure detail and accuracy in the reflections. A total of 35 diary reports were sent out to the participants. Of these, 30 were filled out during the focal period.

As the diaries included open-ended and closed questions, we could carry out different analyses. The quantitative elements of the questionnaire were subjected to univariate statistical analyses. Thematic analysis was used for the open questions. In the results section, we refer to open questions from the diaries using quotes followed by (OD).

2.2 Focus group interview

A qualitative descriptive approach in the form of a focus-group interview, as described by Malterud [18], was used to collect data on the participants' thoughts and experiences with the HE application in their daily work. The aim was to gather more detailed information about the occupational therapists' experiences with the HE app, to encourage the participants to discuss and exchange their experiences, and to clarify the information reported in the diaries.

An interview guide containing mainly open-ended questions was prepared ahead of the focus-group interview. Furthermore, a PowerPoint presentation covering the most significant results from the online diaries was put together in order to facilitate the participants' thoughts and reflections during the interview. The points taken from the diary were anonymized to ensure that no one individual felt that he or she was on display during the focus-group interview.

The focus-group interview was conducted by two researchers. The participants were encouraged to speak as frankly as possible and were told that all proposals emerging from the discussions were of interest. Data were collected until saturation was achieved. The focus-group interview lasted 90 minutes and was recorded on video. It was subsequently transcribed verbatim by an external transcriber. As the focus-group was conducted in Danish, the quotes used here have been translated into English. In the following, we refer to the focus group using quotes from the transcript followed by (FG).

2.3 Data analysis

In order to ensure the validity of coding for the analysis, the two researchers were supplemented by another researcher who was not present during the focus-group interview. To systematize the focus-group data and open statements from the diaries, we used a qualitative inductive content analysis inspired by Georgi's Interpretative Phenomenological Approach as described by Malterud [19]. The decision to use this approach was based on our aim of gathering knowledge about the occupational therapists' experiences with the HE app. Georgi describes four iterative stages: stage 1—encounter with the text; stage 2—identify units of analysis; stage 3—code the units of analysis; and stage 4—categorize and summarize themes and points [19]. In line with these stages, the three researchers first read and reread the interview transcript and the statements from the diaries in order to acquire a good grasp of the data. The researchers also took notes on observed points. Then all three researchers individually identified units of analysis and made notes in the text about the various themes. Thereafter, the researchers met to discuss their interim findings and to reach a consensus on several temporary themes. In the next stage, the researchers individually coded the text into the temporary themes. Subsequently, the codes were again discussed, leading to a final agreement on three main themes: 1) the need to collect multiple types of data, 2) the need for structure versus the need for situated data collection, and 3) the application's influence on the interaction between the occupational therapist and the client. In the final stage, the content of the themes was summarized in writing to provide an overview of the essence and points [19].

2.4 Ethical considerations

Participation in the study was voluntary, and the participants along with their employers gave their written consent for the participation and data collection. According to national regulation, no statement from an ethics committee was needed, because the study did not directly focus on patients. Nor was a notification to the Danish Data Protection Agency necessary, because the study does not contain confidential or sensitive personal data. The personal data has been processed in accordance with the Danish Processing of Personal Data Act and subsequent legislation.

3. Results

In this section, we present the results of the empirical study. Thirty-five online diaries were made available to the seven occupational therapists at the beginning of the data-collection process. Of these, 30 were completed by the 7 occupational therapists within the two-month data-collection period. The majority of the diaries related to real cases (80%, 24 cases), while 20% (6 cases) referred to examples the occupational therapists raised themselves. Of the 24 real cases, 8 concerned only a change in the household environment, while others were more complex, with some covering aids for the client (15 cases). In the latter cases, other investigations often had to be undertaken along with the HE assessment. In most cases, the visit was the occupational therapist's first visit in the home (17 cases). In five cases, the occupational therapist had visited once before, while the occupational therapist had paid a visit at least four times before in three cases. In summary, the majority of cases were real cases with complex characters, and many of them were first visits.

As shown in **Table 1**, the duration of each assessment varied. The majority of investigations lasted between 21 and 50 minutes, but a few went beyond this timespan. In assessing time consumption, we must remember that the participants had little experience with HE at the time of data collection, as they had only just finished the introductory course. This point was raised by one of the participants: "The increased time use is more about the HE assessment, which is what causes it. It is not caused by the tablet" (i.e., the use of the online diary) (FG). The time consumption should thus be assessed in this light.

After each investigation, the occupational therapists were asked to rate different aspects of the app in terms of their agreement with various statements. The central tendencies of the ratings appear in **Table 2**. As can be seen in the table, the HE app earned higher ratings in terms of its usability. Thus, learnability, usability, and understandability all have ratings above the average (mean of 4.31, 3.66, and 4.31, respectively). Despite ratings below the average for enhancing the quality of the home visit (mean of 2.78), making the visit go faster (1.86), easing the dissemination of information to colleagues (2.50), and making the home visit better in general (2.38), the technology's usability may be what led to a rating above the average for the technology's flexibility in terms of the therapists' working situation (mean of 3.04). In the following sections, we use the focus-group interview to examine these differences in assessments.

3.1 The need for structure versus the need for situated data collection

The HE application is designed to facilitate a structured workflow. It guides the user through the data-collection process on a step-by-step basis, and the structure ensures that the data is collected in a standardized manner. In some cases, the structure guides the user to focus on aspects of the dwelling that their clinical experience does not. One participant highlighted this point, stating "I think we are asked to focus on some areas that we usually would not have considered" (FG). In this case, the structure of the application is viewed as a positive aspect, as it guides the occupational therapist towards expanded data collection. Consistent data is one of the best-known strengths of structured data collection, and the HE app facilitates this aspect.

The structure also led occupational therapists to collect data at times when they would otherwise not do so. This happened in cases where the focus of the housing adaptation was predetermined, such as when the door or the bathroom needed to be adapted. In this regard, one user wrote: "Problem is limited to one room. The rest [of the HE app data] is not needed in this case of adaptation." In cases like this, the relevant data were so limited that the information collected through the HE app seemed superfluous: "If the question was whether to add a ramp or do something else, I would answer it by heart" (FG). This quote indicates that the occupational therapist felt he or she could save time by avoiding the structure of the HE app and instead relying on his or her clinical knowledge and understanding of the client's

Assessment duration	21–30 mins.	31–40 mins.	41–50 mins.	51–60 mins.	60+ min.	Total
N	8	3	13	2	3	29

Table 1.
Time consumption.

The app:	n	Missing	Mean	Mode
Increases the quality of the investigation	28	2	2.79	3
Made the home visit go faster	28	2	1.86	1
Is flexible in relation to my work	27	3	3.04	3
Eases the dissemination of information to colleagues	22	8	2.50	3
Has made my work more challenging	23	7	2.87	3
Is easy to learn	29	1	4.31	4
Is easy to use	29	1	3.66	4
Is easy to understand	29	1	4.31	4
Made the home visit better	26	4	2.38	1

As the ratings reflect the focal situation, the same OT rated the same statement several times, but each time with a point of departure in the focal investigation. 1 = "highly disagree" and 5 = "highly agree." N = 30.

Table 2.
Ratings from diaries.

needs. This may be viewed as stepping away from the need for data consistency, but each client's particular case seemed to be more in focus: "Often, we have a specific reason for a home visit. (...) Something else may appear during the visit, but we focus on the initial reason for the visit" (FG1).

The app's structure also guides data collection in areas of the dwelling that occupational therapists rarely consider, such as parking spaces and access to outdoor areas. Even though focusing on other areas of the dwelling can be beneficial, collecting data on areas of the dwelling that the clients had not asked to be considered was often viewed as intimidating: "In reality, we would never do anything [in the dwelling] unless people have the need for it" (FG). The HE application's structure was sometimes experienced as conflicting with the client's interests. In this regard, one occupational therapist highlighted a question from a client: "I do not have any problems in the kitchen, so what are you doing in there?" (FG).

The structure of the HE application forces the user to gather data on areas of the dwelling that the occupational therapist may feel are unrelated to the specific case. As one participant pointed out, "there are many useless things to deal with [in the app]." Another stated, "many of the questions (...) are rarely needed." On the other hand, the occupational therapists often have a very specific focus in the dwelling but some areas of the dwelling are missing from the HE app. Notably, the structure of the HE app offered no options to add other information. The occupational therapists, therefore, suggested that an option be added to allow them to elaborate on selected areas that fit the client's case: "What I really need is the ability to enter the size of the bathroom, the sink, and so forth. (...) That would be extremely useful" (FG).

This made it clear that the app's structure had both positive and negative effects. App's are structured by nature, which goes hand in hand with the nature of structured data-collection tools. This is often highlighted as the best way to collect valid and reliable data. At the same time, the structure of the HE app seems to make it difficult to adapt when different situations call for expanding or decreasing certain areas of data. In developing apps for data collection in the field, attention must be paid to the nature of the occupational therapists' data-collection context, which is dynamic and situated. Options for changing the structure when using the HE app could be considered. Such options may include alternative focus areas, and the extension or removal of areas for data collection. Therefore, along with developing the app itself, there is potential for developing the ways in which it is used. Clearly, knowledge of the field is essential for the development of data-collection apps if they are intended to be employed in the field.

3.2 The need to collect multiple types of data

As the HE app is based on the Housing Enabler assessment, it has specific focus areas for data collection. It is meant to be an assessment representing "only a part of the arsenal of methods that should be used in connection with housing adaptations" ([6], p. 22). Therefore, the data collected through the app only covers one aspect of the data the occupational therapist needs (i.e., data on necessary housing adaptions).

This is a challenge, as occupational therapists find it hard to utilize only one method. They often use a variety of methods during the same home visit. Naturally, housing-adaption cases often call for different assessments. Some may require measures aimed at securing the caregiver's work environment, while others may need measures based on the client's occupational needs and functional level. As one occupational therapist explained, "our starting point is the client's activity problems and the work environment" (FG).

When using the HE app the occupational therapists felt restricted, as they generally utilized several methods simultaneously. Despite the fact that the HE app was never intended to replace other necessary assessments, it was found to be too restrictive, as it was bound to one assessment. One participant highlighted this issue, stating that "I simply cannot do without my notes on activity analysis" (FG). The occupational therapists explained that they were accustomed to taking notes on various issues, drawing floor plans, and taking extra measurements in the room using pen and paper. The HE app does not gather multiple types of data. Instead, it only covers data focused on dwelling accessibility. The HE app created a feeling of complexity among the occupational therapists, who usually used several assessments and tacit knowledge in parallel during their home visits. Therefore, the HE app was rejected as a time-consuming "add-on" to the existing arsenal of methods and tacit knowledge. In place of the HE app, the occupational therapists envisioned a tool that would cover several aspects simultaneously: "the activity, the dwelling, and the work environment" (FG). In other words, the occupational therapists called for an app that would cover multiple aspects of their data-collection process. In theory, such a tool may be hard to develop and it may actually increase the complexity of data collection.

In general, the clinical practice calls for an app that embraces several of the assessments or methods used in the field. Although the development of such an app may not be theoretically or technically possible, it is important to learn about the many methods used in the field in order to define the relationship between those methods and the app itself. Consideration of the ways in which the HE app is expected to correspond with and supplement other methods of data collection seems essential for this aspect of clinical practice.

3.3 The HE app's influence on the interaction between the occupational therapist and the client

Occupational therapy is a client-centered field [20]. The use of an app to collect data concerning the client might influence the interaction between the occupational therapist and the client, as well as the approach to and extent of the client-centered practice. The client's situation, personality, and needs differ every time the occupational therapist visits, which also has an impact on the occupational therapists' experiences with using the HE app in the dwelling: "There has been a big difference in how much tranquility the clients have given me to do [the assessment]" (FG). In accordance with the client-centered perspective, the occupational therapists find it necessary to respond to client's current needs and adjust their work processes accordingly: "Then the client comes around and you have to chat a little. And she also wanted to discuss something about the garden" (FG5).

Consequently, most of the occupational therapists felt that measuring the dwelling with the HE app took extra time, as the app requires the user to follow certain steps and to go through a precise number of items. It is not possible to skip items in order to make time for chatting with the client. One occupational therapist said, "I felt as though I used more time because of the Housing Enabler, which was a waste for both the client and I" (OD). Another suggested that "it can be difficult to stay focused on all of the items in the app when you are visiting a very chatty client" (FG). Another issue concerning the occupational therapist's contact with the client was that the app might be perceived as a physical obstacle in the relationship, as it made it difficult for the occupational therapist to maintain eye contact with the client: "I think I use too much time on reading the questions and that I have too little eye contact with the client" (FG).

Importantly, the extra time used on measuring the dwelling was not always regarded as wasted time by the occupational therapists: "The visit took 30–45 minutes longer than it would have without the HE app. However, it is a nice structured tool that ensures that you get all of the details on your first examination of the dwelling" (OD). Another occupational therapist added: "The app gives me peace to work, as the client can understand the necessity of me going around and typing in all of the information into the system. It gives you more peace than going around with a pen, paper, and a tape measure" (OD).

The HE assessment method ensures thorough data collection, and the app makes the assessment appear even more thorough and professional. One participant highlighted this benefit, stating "I think the client felt I was being thorough in terms of the problems he faces with being in a wheelchair. Therefore, from the client's perspective, I think my visit was better than if I had only been concentrating on the accessibility of the dwelling" (OD).

In sum, on one hand, the HE app signals professionalism and can reassure clients that the occupational therapist is doing the job well. Moreover, the app provides the occupational therapist with the peace needed to focus on systematic data collection without interruptions from the client. On the other hand, the tablet can be a physical obstacle in the occupational therapist's contact with the client, as it can hinder eye contact and take time away from social interaction with the client.

4. Discussion

We have presented a study of occupational therapists' use of a digital tool for assessing housing adaptations. Fänge et al. [16] have previously raised the possibility of implementing a tool developed for research in a clinical practice context. The current study suggests that this remains a challenge in relation to occupational therapy. The participants repeatedly indicated that there was a lack of correspondence between the tool and their daily work. Whether this challenge was caused by the technological aspect of the tool or whether it concerns the tool's structure can be discussed. However, the results of this study support Fänge et al. [16] finding that it can be difficult to directly transfer a research tool to clinical practice. Instead, tools can be adjusted to existing practices to ensure wider acceptance by occupational therapists. At the same time, both this study and the study by Fänge et al. [16] investigated users with relatively little experience with the tool. Future research should therefore examine whether these challenges are reduced if the occupational therapists have more knowledge of and experience with the tool.

The current study covers the adoption of a digital tool in clinical practice. We used diaries to capture the immediate impressions about the tool and a follow-up focus-group interview to uncover the bigger picture of the tool's use in clinical practice. The combination of the two data-collection methods was well suited for the research conditions, given that interventions occurred with short notice across a relatively wide geographical area. However, the diary method was challenging to manage from a distance. For example, some participants did not adhere to the recommendation to fill out the diary within 24 hours of the interaction with the client. Screen logging might represent an alternative to this kind of data collection in future studies, as it does not require the participants to remember to fill out a diary during their busy workday.

This study also suffers from several limitations that should be considered before drawing conclusions. First, only seven occupational therapists participated in the study. As the study was not formally implemented in a municipality, it was challenging to recruit a larger number of participants. Second, the participants had not used the tool in paper form before participating in the project. Therefore, the findings reflect their early experiences with a new tool in a new format that challenged their existing work practice related to housing adaptations. Third, the tool used in this study was only a prototype. Therefore, there were instances in which the application shut down in the middle of data collection. Moreover, the report module had not been fully developed at the time of data collection. For this reason, we have not reported on therapists' use of the mobile app after they returned to their offices but solely focused on the use of the tool in the clients' homes.

5. Conclusion

This study has investigated the challenges and possibilities identified by occupational therapists in relation to using a digitized tool on android tablets in clinical practice. We learned that despite the expectation of a common experience in using digital tools in work practices, the occupational therapists still experienced challenges when interacting with the technology. Moreover, they found it challenging when different sources of information were needed, as the technology only covered certain aspects of the problem. At the same time, the technology itself was considered from two different perspectives. On the one hand, technology was viewed as a barrier between the therapist and the client. On the other hand, it symbolized professionalism in interactions with the client and provided a focus for the therapist. After the study's completion, the findings were incorporated into yet another update of the software that reflected the user perspective. More specifically, the export function was completed and the general design was updated.

Some questions were answered by this study, while it gave rise to others. The study was not specifically focused on the role of technology in interactions with clients. However, information on this aspect emerged from the data gathered from both the diaries and the focus-group interview. More focused studies should be carried out to elaborate on this issue. An interesting perspective in this regard might be to investigate how clients experience the role of technology in their interactions with the occupational therapist. Lastly, this study involved a limited number of participants. Therefore, a follow-up study with more participants could provide a more fine-grained picture of the use of the mobile app.

Author details

Tanja Svarre[1*], Marie Bangsgaard Bang[2] and Tine Bieber Lunn[3]

1 Aalborg University, Aalborg, Denmark

2 University College of Northern Denmark, Aalborg, Denmark

3 SOSU Nord, Aalborg, Denmark

*Address all correspondence to: tanjasj@ikp.aau.dk

References

[1] Sonn U, Törnquist K. ADL-taxonomi: en bedömning av aktivitetsförm. Stockholm: Nacka: Förbundet Sveriges Arbetsterapeuter; 2001

[2] Baron K, Kielhofner G, Goldhammer V, et al. A User's Manual for the Occupational Self Assessment (OSA) (Version 1.0). Illinois: Department of Occupational Therapy, University of Illinois; 1999

[3] Law M, Baptiste S, Carswell A, et al. Canadian Occupational Performance Measure. Ottawa: Ottowa COAT Publ. ACE; 2005

[4] Parkinson S, Forsyth K, Kielhofner G. A user's Manual for the Model of Human Occupation Screening Tool (MOHOST). Chicago: Model of Human Occupation Clearinghouse, Department of Occupational Therapy, College of Applied Health Sciences, University of Illinois at Chicago; 2004

[5] Clearinghouse EATS. Dansk IPPA: Et redskab til at afdække aktivitetsproblemer i hverdagen og evaluere indsatser. Odense: Socialstyrelsen; 2013. Available from: http://www.etf.dk/sites/default/files/uploads/public/documents/Evidens_og_kvalitetsudvikling/dansk_ippa_manual_pdfa.pdf

[6] Agarwal R, Gao G, DesRoches C, et al. The digital transformation of healthcare: Current status and the road ahead. Information Systems Research. 2010;**21**:796-809

[7] Free C, Phillips G, Felix L, et al. The effectiveness of M-health technologies for improving health and health services: A systematic review protocol. BMC Research Notes. 2010;**3**:250

[8] Silva BMC, Rodrigues JJPC, de la Torre DI, et al. Mobile-health: A review of current state in 2015. Journal of Biomedical Informatics. 2015;**56**:265-272

[9] Ventola CL. Mobile devices and apps for health care professionals: Uses and benefits. P T. 2014;**39**:356-364

[10] Iwarsson S, Slaug B. Housing Enabler – A Method for Rating/Screening and Analysing Accessibility Problems in Housing: Manual for the Complete Instrument and Screening Tool. 2nd ed. Lund & Staffanstorp: Veten & Skapen HB and Slaug Enabling Development; 2010

[11] Svarre T, Lunn TB, Helle T. Transforming paper-based assessment forms to a digital format: Exemplified by the Housing Enabler prototype app. Scandinavina Journal of Occupational Therapy. 2017;**24**:438-447

[12] Kujala S. User involvement: A review of the benefits and challenges. Behaviour & Information Technology. 2003;**22**:1-16

[13] Liu L, Cruz AM, Rincon AR, et al. What factors determine therapists' acceptance of new technologies for rehabilitation – A study using the Unified Theory of Acceptance and Use of Technology (UTAUT). Disability and Rehabilitation. 2015;**37**:447-455

[14] Walthouwer MJL, Oenema A, Soetens K, et al. Implementation of web-based interventions by Dutch occupational health centers. Health Promotion International. 2017;**32**:818-830

[15] Sezgin E, Yıldırım SÖ. A literature review on attitudes of health professionals towards health information systems: From e-Health to m-Health. Procedia Technology. 2014;**16**:1317-1326

[16] Fänge A, Risser R, Iwarsson S. Challenges in implementation of research methodology in community-based occupational therapy: The

Housing Enabler Example. Scandinavian Journal of Occupational Therapy. 2007;**14**:54-62

[17] Yin RK. Case Study Research: Design and Methods. 5th ed. Thousand Oaks, Calif: Sage; 2014

[18] Malterud K. Fokusgrupper som forskningsmetode for medisin og helsefag. Oslo: Universitetsforlaget; 2012

[19] Malterud K. Kvalitative metoder i medisinsk forskning. Oslo: Universitetsforlaget; 2003

[20] Townsend EA, Polatajko HJ. Menneskelig aktivitet II: En ergoterapeutisk vision om sundhed, trivsel og retfærdighed muliggjort gennem betydningsfulde aktiviteter. Copenhagen: Munksgaard; 2008